MW01069094

The Encyclopedia of

MEDICAL ROBOTICS

Volume 4

Rehabilitation Robotics

The Encyclopedia of MEDICAL ROBOTICS

Volume 4

Rehabilitation Robotics

Editor-in-chief

Jaydev P Desai
Georgia Institute of Technology, USA

Edited by

Sunil Agrawal
Columbia University, USA

World Scientific

NEW JERSEY • LONDON • SINGAPORE • BEIJING • SHANGHAI • HONG KONG • TAIPEI • CHENNAI • TOKYO

Published by

World Scientific Publishing Co. Pte. Ltd.
5 Toh Tuck Link, Singapore 596224
USA office: 27 Warren Street, Suite 401-402, Hackensack, NJ 07601
UK office: 57 Shelton Street, Covent Garden, London WC2H 9HE

Library of Congress Cataloging-in-Publication Data
Names: Desai, Jaydev P., editor. | Patel, R. V. (Rajni V.), editor. | Ferreira, Antoine, editor. | Agrawal, Sunil Kumar, editor.
Title: The encyclopedia of medical robotics / editor in chief, Jaydev P. Desai (Georgia Institute of Technology, USA); edited by, Rajni V. Patel (University of Western Ontario, Canada), Antoine Ferreira (Institut National des Sciences Appliquées Centre Val de Loire, campus Bourges, France), Sunil K. Agrawal (Columbia University, USA).
Description: New Jersey : World Scientific, 2017. | In 4 volumes. | Includes bibliographical references and index. | Contents: volume 1. Minimally invasive surgical robotics -- volume 2. Micro and nano robotics in medicine -- volume 3. Image-guided Surgical Procedures and Interventions -- volume 4. Rehabilitation robotics
Identifiers: LCCN 2017042862| ISBN 9789813232228 (hc: set : alk. paper) | ISBN 9789813232259 (hc: v.1 : alk. paper) | ISBN 9789813232273 (hc: v.2 : alk. paper) | ISBN 9789813232297 (hc: v.3 : alk. paper) | ISBN 9789813232310 (hc: v.4 : alk. paper)
Subjects: | MESH: Robotics | Robotic Surgical Procedures | Minimally Invasive Surgical Procedures | Rehabilitation--instrumentation | Biomedical Technology
Classification: LCC RD29.7 | NLM QT 36.2 | DDC 617.00285--dc23
LC record available at https://lccn.loc.gov/2017042862

British Library Cataloguing-in-Publication Data
A catalogue record for this book is available from the British Library.

For any available supplementary material, please visit
https://www.worldscientific.com/worldscibooks/10.1142/10770#t=suppl

Desk Editors: Dr. Sree Meenakshi Sajani/Amanda Yun

Typeset by Stallion Press
Email: enquiries@stallionpress.com

Printed in Singapore

PREFACE

The Encyclopedia of Medical Robotics combines contributions in four distinct areas of Medical robotics, namely: *Minimally Invasive Surgical Robotics, Micro and Nano Robotics in Medicine, Image-guided Surgical Procedures and Interventions*, and *Rehabilitation Robotics*. The volume on *Minimally Invasive Surgical Robotics* focuses on robotic technologies geared toward challenges and opportunities in minimally invasive surgery and the research, design, implementation and clinical use of minimally invasive robotic systems. The volume on *Micro and Nano Robotics in Medicine* is dedicated to research activities in an emerging interdisciplinary technology area raising new scientific challenges and promising revolutionary advancement in applications such as medicine and biology. The size and range of these systems are at or below the micrometer scale and comprise assemblies of micro- and nanoscale components. The volume on *Image-guided Surgical Procedures and Interventions* focuses primarily on the use of image guidance during surgical procedures and the challenges posed by various imaging environments and how they related to the design and development of robotic systems as well as their clinical applications. This volume also has significant contributions from the clinical viewpoint on some of the challenges in the domain of image-guided interventions. Finally, the volume on *Rehabilitation Robotics* is dedicated to the state of the art of an emerging interdisciplinary field where robotics, sensors, and feedback are used in novel ways to relearn, improve, or restore functional movements in humans.

ABOUT THE EDITOR

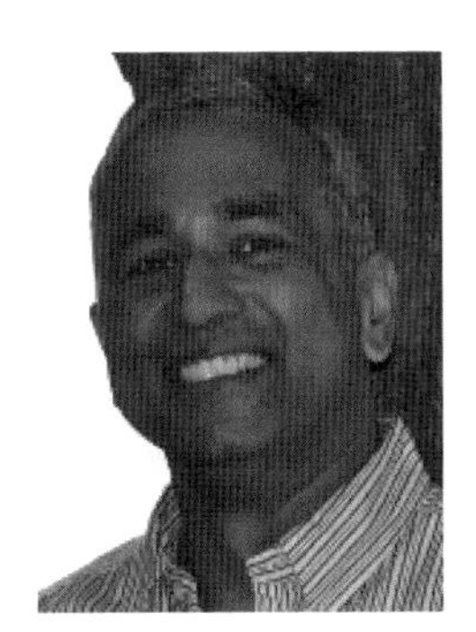

Sunil K. Agrawal received a PhD in Mechanical Engineering from Stanford University in 1990. He is currently a Professor and Director of Robotics and Rehabilitation (ROAR) Laboratory at Columbia University, located both in engineering and medical campuses of Columbia University. He has published close to 500 journal and conference papers. Dr. Agrawal is a Fellow of the ASME and AIMBE. His honors include an NSF Presidential Faculty Fellowship from the White House in 1994, a Bessel Prize from Germany in 2003, and a Humboldt US Senior Scientist Award in 2007. He is a recipient of 2016 Machine Design Award from the ASME for "seminal contributions to design of robotic exoskeletons for gait training of stroke patients" and 2016 Mechanisms and Robotics Award from the ASME for "cumulative contributions and being an international leading figure in mechanical design and robotics". He is a recipient of several Best Paper awards in ASME and IEEE sponsored robotics conferences. He has held positions of a Distinguished Visiting Professor at Hanyang University in Korea, a Professor of Robotics at the University of Ulster in Northern Ireland, and a Visiting Professor at the Biorobotics Institute of SSSA in Pisa. He actively serves on editorial boards of conferences and journals.

CONTENTS

Chapter 1

ROBOT-AIDED GAIT TRAINING

Robert Riener

Sensory-Motor Systems Lab, Department of Health Sciences and Technology, ETH Zurich, Switzerland

Spinal Cord Injury Center, University Hospital Balgrist, Medical Faculty, University of Zurich, Switzerland

Robotic rehabilitation devices have become increasingly important and popular in clinical and rehabilitation environments to facilitate prolonged duration of training, increased number of repetition of movements, improved patient safety, less strenuous operations by therapists, and eventually to improve the therapeutic outcome. After presenting the rationale of robot-aided movement therapy, this article shows several design criteria that are relevant for the development of effective and safe rehabilitation robots. Several examples of gait rehabilitation robots are then presented that are in the developmental status or already commercially available. Novel patient-cooperative strategies are described, such as impedance control, assistance-as-needed control and tunnel (path) control. Such patient-cooperative strategies can increase movement variability, patient activity, and patient motivation; all of this can have a positive effect on the therapeutic outcome. This chapter finishes with a short overview about existing clinical trials that have been performed showing that the application of rehabilitation devices is at least as effective as the application of conventional therapies. It concludes with the finding that further clinical studies are required to find predictors for the success of a robot-aided treatment.

1. Introduction

1.1. *Sociomedical need and motivation*

Loss of the ability to walk and grasp represents a major disability for millions of individuals worldwide, and a major expense for health care and social support systems. More than 700,000 people in the U.S. suffer from a stroke each year; 60–75% of these individuals will live beyond 1 year after the incident, resulting in a stroke survivor population of about 3 million people.[1,2] Almost two-thirds of all stroke survivors have no functional ability and cannot move without assistance in the acute phase following the incident.[3] Similarly, for many of the 10,000 Americans who are affected by a traumatic spinal cord injury (SCI) per year, the most visible lingering disability is the lost or limited ability to walk.[4]

One major goal in the rehabilitation of patients suffering from a movement disorder, such as stroke or SCI, is the retraining of locomotor function. The approach to stroke physiotherapy is diverse, as are the theoretical bases assumed by the physiotherapists who provide the therapy.[5–10] Traditional methodology includes neuro-developmental training (NDT),[11] the motor relearning program,[12] proprioceptive neuromuscular facilitation,[13] and the Rood approach.[14]

1.2. *Rationale for gait therapy*

Task-oriented repetitive movements can improve muscular strength and movement coordination in patients with impairments due to neurological or orthopedic problems. A typical repetitive movement is the human gait. Treadmill training has been shown to improve gait and lower limb motor function in patients with locomotor disorders. Manually assisted treadmill training was first used approximately 20 years ago as a regular therapy for patients with SCI or stroke. Its use is steadily increasing. Numerous clinical studies support the effectiveness of the training, particularly in SCI and stroke patients.[15–17] Recently, a large randomized clinical trial, known as the LEAPS study, has confirmed that walking training on a treadmill using body-weight support and practice overground at clinics was superior to usual care in improving walking, regardless of the severity of initial impairment.[18]

Lower extremity movement therapy also serves to prevent secondary complications such as muscle atrophy, osteoporosis, and spasticity. It was observed that longer training sessions and a longer total training duration have a positive effect on the motor function. In a meta-analysis comprising nine controlled studies with 1,051 stroke patients, Kwakkel *et al.*[19] showed that increased training intensity yields positive effects on neuromuscular function and (ADL). This study did not distinguish between upper and lower extremities. The finding that the rehabilitation progress depends on the training *intensity* motivates the application of robot-aided therapies.

1.3. *Rationale for robot-aided gait training*

Manually assisted gait training has several major limitations. Treatment for stroke, SCI and other neurological diseases is very costly and accounts for a large percentage of health care budgets.[20] The training is labor-intensive, and, therefore, training duration is usually limited by personnel shortage and fatigue of the therapist, not by that of the patient. During treadmill training, therapists often suffer from back pain because the training has to be performed in an ergonomically unfavorable posture. The disadvantageous consequence is that the training sessions are shorter than required to gain an optimal therapeutic outcome. Finally, manually-assisted gait training lacks repeatability and objective measures of patient performance and progress.

In contrast, with automated, i.e. robot-assisted gait training, the duration and number of training sessions can be increased, while reducing the number of therapists required per patient. Long-term automated gait therapy can be an efficient way to make intensive gait training affordable for clinical use. One therapist may be able to train two or more patients at once. Thus, personnel costs can be significantly reduced and more patients can be treated satisfying the need for a higher treatment capacity due to the increasing number of age-related neurological patients.

Furthermore, the robot provides quantitative measures, thus allowing the observation and quantitative assessment of the rehabilitation process. Even more, some of the recorded data can be online-processed and displayed to the patient as "biofeedback" signals so that the patient immediately understands how she or he performs. This can help the patient to try to improve the walking pattern and performance during the robot-aided training sessions. This kind of feedback can be further exploited via the application of virtual reality (VR) technologies. Allowing the patient to perform a gait task within a virtual environment does not only allow instructing the patient in an easy, convenient, and a very intuitive way, but it also increases the patient's engagement during task execution and the general motivation to participate in the rehabilitation program.

These advantages of the use of robots as compared to conventional therapy are based on common wisdom and plausibility. Not many publications exist that prove these arguments yet.

2. Basic Design Criteria

2.1. *Therapeutic versus assistive systems*

Robotic aids can be distinguished with respect to their application on the patient. There are two main application types: *robots for therapy* and *robots for assistance*. Robots for therapy are mainly used in a clinical environment, thus being shared by several patients, with the goal to improve body function as well as activities of daily living (ADL) and participation in society. This article focuses on training systems being used in therapeutic hospital units. In contrast, robots for assistance are used in home and outside environments in order to assist an individual patient in daily life activities enabling her or him to participate in different societal situations and events. The goal is not to get a therapeutic effect, though a positive therapeutic effect can be often observed. Assistive robotic devices range from wheelchairs, actuated prostheses and mobile service robots to assistive manipulators, which can be mounted onto wheelchairs or desks.

2.2. *Robot actuation and patient interaction*

Therapeutic systems can be split into *passive*, *active*, and *interactive systems*. In *passive systems*, no actuation is implemented to move the patient limbs. Instead, limbs are passively stabilized, fixed, or limited in the range of motion. Typical technical components are stiff frames, bearings, elastic springs and pulleys and ropes with counter weights.

Active systems are equipped with electromechanical, pneumatic, hydraulic, and other drives to actively move patient's limbs. The devices are either open-loop controlled or different position and force control strategies are implemented. Most motorized rehabilitation robots are powered by electromagnetic motors.[21] The motor torques can be applied directly at the joints, or transmitted via Bowden cables to the robot–human interaction points. The advantage of fluidic actuators is that they can produce a rather high force-density (force to load ratio) at the robot–human interaction points. Heavy parts, such as the compressor and/or the reservoir can be placed in the static frame or base of the robot, and the forces can be transmitted via tubes to the interaction points, so that the moving parts of the robot can be made rather lightweight. The long tubes can lead to high compliance in pneumatic systems and high inertia in hydraulic systems. Together with the high friction of the piston and cylinder combination, this can make an accurate position and/or force control very challenging. Furthermore, the risk of leakages is another disadvantage, especially of hydraulic systems.

Interactive systems are active systems that are characterized by sophisticated user-interactive control strategies that allow reacting to the patient's voluntary effort. Depending on the underlying control paradigm, the motors can control the interaction forces or torques between the patient and the robot, thus allowing the robotic device to support the human limb against gravity, compensating gravitational forces and making it easier for the patient to move her or his limb. Such interactive systems are often based on impedance control strategies. Impedance controllers are well established in the field of robotics and human–system interaction. Hogan first introduced them in the early eighties of the last century.[22] The basic idea of the impedance control strategy applied to robot-aided therapies is to allow a variable deviation from a predefined trajectory rather than imposing a rigid movement pattern. The deviation depends on the patient's effort and behavior. Also, other control strategies are possible to allow robot–patient interaction, such as model adaptive, assist-as-needed or so-called patient-driven controllers.[23–26] Interactive systems require position and/or force sensors to measure the user–machine interaction and feed the controllers. Several requirements must be fulfilled when designing and applying a robot for therapy, for instance, the robot should be rather "transparent" and "human-friendly",[27] i.e. safe, small, lightweight, quiet, etc.

2.3. *Robot complexity*

The robot complexity in terms of the number and type of joints and adjustability is another criterion of differentiation among robotic devices. It is crucial that the robot is adapted or adaptable to the human limb anthropometry in terms of range of motion, the number of degrees of freedom (DOF), and the segment lengths.

One must be aware that increasing complexity of the robotic structure results in an increased size and number of DOF, which can yield disadvantageous dynamic properties, such as increased mass to be moved, reduced stiffness, higher backlash, joint friction, etc. These disadvantages can affect certain safety aspects of the robot, especially when used in the vicinity or in close interaction with a human subject.

2.4. *Exoskeletal versus end-effector-based approach*

End-effector-based robots are connected to a patient's limb or joint at the end-effector of the robot (Fig. 1). An important advantage of these robots is that they are easy to adjust to different limb lengths. A disadvantage is that, in general, the limb posture and/or the individual joint interaction torques are not fully determined by the robot because the patient and the robot interact just through one point — the robot's end-effector (Fig. 2). From a mechanical point of view, an end-effector-based robot is easier to build and to use because the robot's axes generally do not need to align with the human-joint rotation axes.

In contrast, the mechanical structure of an exoskeletal robot resembles the human arm anatomy, and the robot's joints usually correspond with the human joints. Thus, robotic joint axes of rotation should align with the human axes of rotation to avoid mechanical stress in the attachment points and/or in the human joints and unwanted movements of the exoskeleton with respect to the human limb. This becomes difficult at more complex joints, where the center

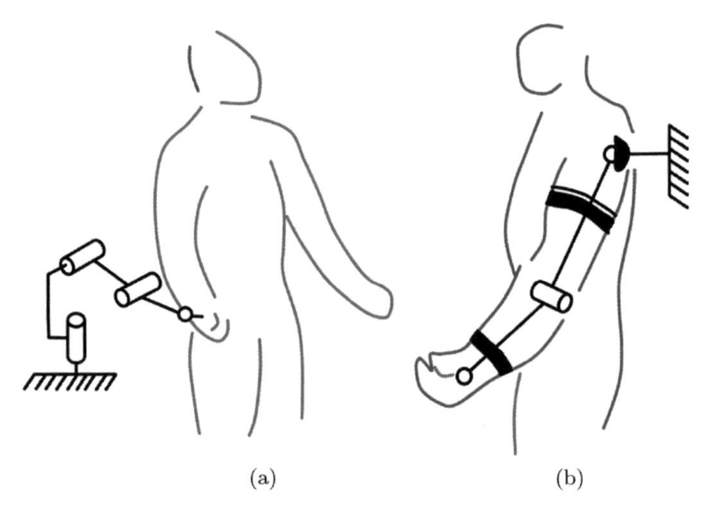

Figure 1. Schematic view of (a) end-effector-based and (b) exoskeleton robots (taken from Ref. 21).

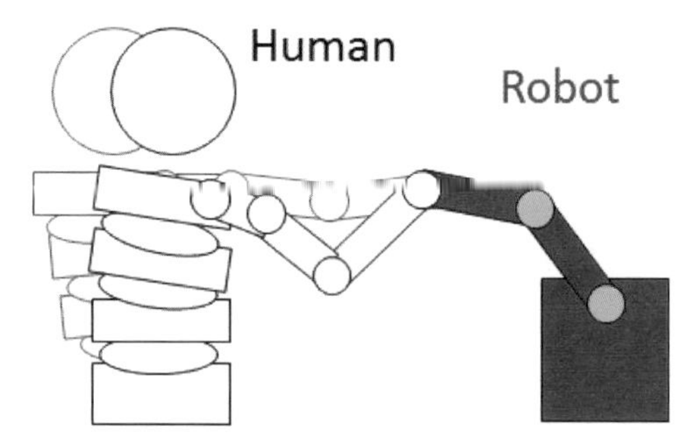

Figure 2. Limb posture and/or the individual joint interaction torques are not fully determined in end-effector-based robotic systems.

of rotation moves over a wide range with varying joint angle (such as at the shoulder joint or along the vertebral column, e.g. the lumbosacral joint). As the human limb has been attached to the exoskeleton at several points, adaptation to different body sizes is, therefore, more difficult than in end-effector-based systems because the length of each robot segment must be adjusted to the respective limb length of the patient. However, exoskeletal devices can better guide the body limb, thus leading to a determined body posture and movement — assuming that anatomical and technical joints can be arranged in good alignment. Thus, mechanical end stops can be used in a convenient way to prevent the joint from hyperextension or hyperflexion, which is another advantage of exoskeletal robots.

3. Examples of Gait Rehabilitation Robots

3.1. *End-effector-based systems*

One of the first commercially available systems for locomotion therapy was the "Gait Trainer" developed by Hesse and Uhlenbrock.[28] The device is being sold by the German company "Reha-Stim" in Berlin. It operates like a conventional elliptical trainer, where the subject's feet are strapped into two footplates moving the feet along a trajectory that is similar to a gait trajectory. The patient wears a harness, which is connected via ropes to the frame of the device to support the body weight of the patient. The patient can be easily mounted onto the device, without time consuming adjustments, as the human thighs and shanks do not need to be attached, but only the feet. As the device does not control knee and hip joint angles, the patient often needs continuous assistance by at least one therapist — unless the patient has sufficient knee extension as is often the case after stroke. Forces or torques can only be measured in the moving plates and not in the leg joints.

As the Gait Trainer moves each leg only in 1-DOF, Hesse and colleagues from the Fraunhofer Institute IPK developed a more complex device, called the "HapticWalker"[29] (Fig. 3). The device comprises two end-effector-based platforms

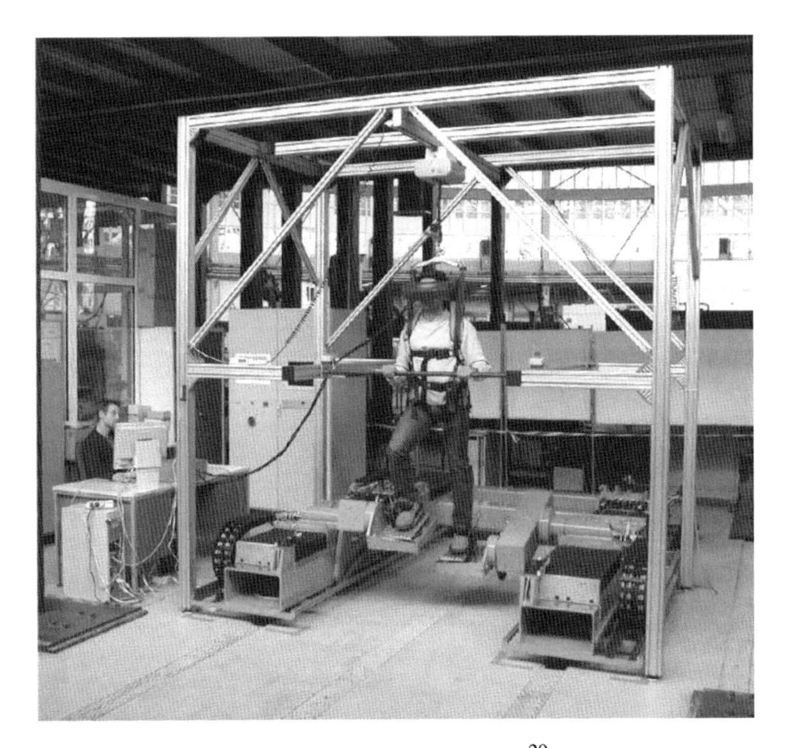

Figure 3. The HapticWalker.[29]

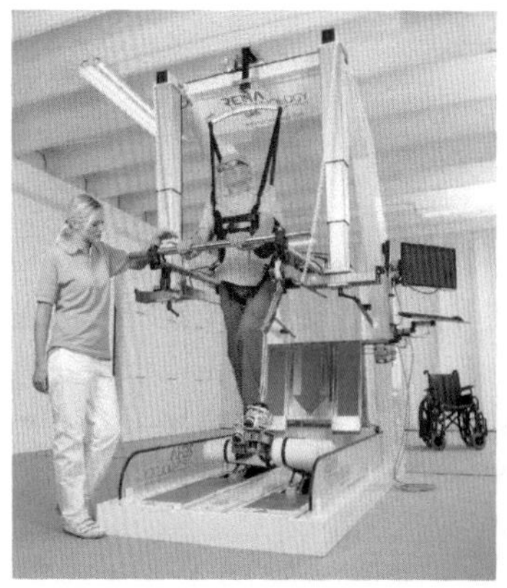
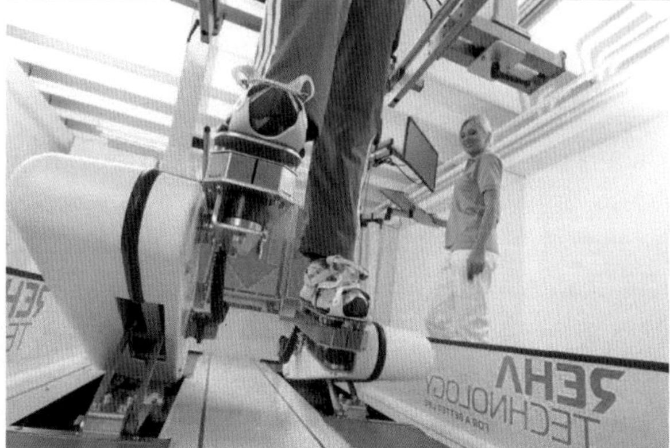

Figure 4. The G-EO system gait training robot (courtesy of Reha Technology AG).

that move each foot in 3-DOF. The body weight is supported by a body weight support system that is also used to lift the patient onto the device. The HapticWalker is able to perform walking trajectories in the sagittal plane with speeds of up to 5 km/h and 120 steps/min. It is possible to apply different gait trajectories in order to train scenarios like walking on elevated terrains or ascending and descending stairs. As the device with its strong drives and stiff construction can display rather high bandwidths, high frequency effects can also be simulated such as they occur when walking on rough ground or when stumbling or sliding.

Based on the knowledge gained with Gait Trainer and HapticWalker, Hesse *et al.*[30] developed G-EO robot (EO is Latin meaning "I walk"), which is commercially made available by the company Reha Technology AG in Switzerland (www.rehatechnology.com) (Fig. 4). As in the HapticWalker, G-EO consists of two footplates, which move each foot with 3-DOF in the sagittal plane and enables the training of freely programmable tasks such as stair climbing. The patient is additionally secured by a harness that is connected to a lifting system. The maximal step length and step height are 55 and 24 cm, respectively. The maximum gait speed is 2–3 km/h.[30]

Another end-effector-based robot developed by the group of D. Reinkensmeyer together with colleagues from UCLA and University of Louisville was ARTHUR, which is a backdrivable 2-DOF planar robot to measure and assist the stepping of the right leg. This robot uses a two-coil linear motor and a pair of lightweight linkages to drive the robot's apex, which is attached to the subject through a revolute joint and running shoe modified to include an embedded footplate.[24,31]

3.2. *Exoskeletal systems*

An alternative to end effector based systems are exoskeletal systems. Already in 1995, the research team of the Spinal Cord Injury Center of the University

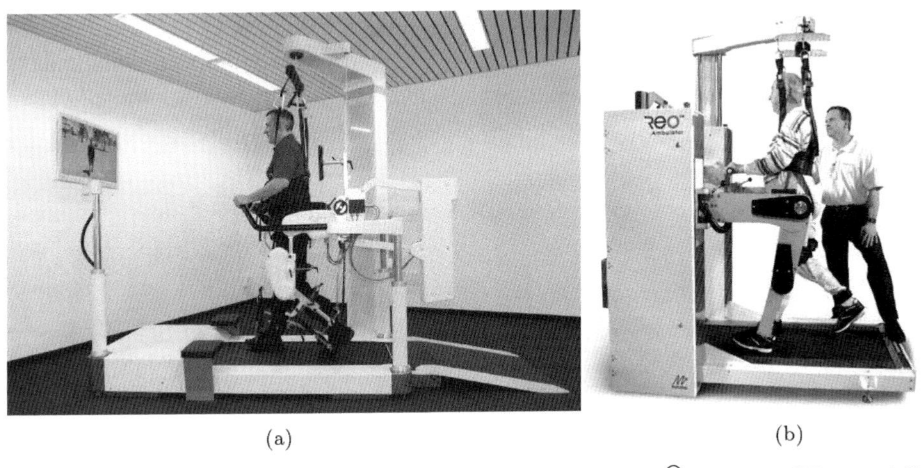

Figure 5. The commercially available gait-driven orthoses (a) Lokomat® (courtesy of Hocoma AG, Switzerland) and (b) AutoAmbulator, also known as ReoAmbulator (courtesy of Motorika Ltd.).

Hospital Balgrist in Zurich, Switzerland, an interdisciplinary group of physicians, therapists, and engineers, began to work on a driven gait orthosis that would essentially replace the arduous physical labor of therapists in the administration of locomotor training.[32,33] Some years later, the device, called "Lokomat", became commercially available from Hocoma AG, Volketswil, Switzerland. The Lokomat® is a bilaterally driven gait orthosis that is used in conjunction with a body weight support system and treadmill (Fig. 5). The Lokomat moves the patient's legs through the gait cycle in the sagittal plane. The Lokomat hip and knee joints are actuated by linear drives integrated into an exoskeletal structure. Passive foot lifters support ankle dorsiflexion during the swing-phase. The leg motion can be controlled with highly repeatable predefined hip and knee joint trajectories on the basis of a conventional position control strategy. The orthosis is fixed to the rigid frame of the bodyweight support system via a parallelogram construction that allows passive vertical translations of the orthosis, while keeping the orientation of the robotic pelvis segment constant. The patient is fixed to the orthosis with straps around the waist, thighs, and shanks. The angular positions of each leg are measured by potentiometers attached to the lateral sides of the hip and knee joints of the orthosis. The hip and knee joint trajectories can be manually adjusted to the individual patient by changing amplitude and offsets. Knee and hip joint torques of the orthosis are measured by force sensors integrated into the orthosis in series with the linear drives. The signals may be used to determine the interaction torques between the patient and the device, which allows estimation of the voluntary muscle effort produced by the patient. This important information may be optimally used for various control strategies as well as for specific biofeedback and assessment functions. The Lokomat geometry can be adjusted to an adult subject's individual anthropometry. A new Lokomat was designed and developed in 2006 to accommodate pediatric patients with body heights between approximately 1.00 and 1.50 m. More than 800 Lokomat robots have been already sold worldwide (till end of 2016).

Another commercially available exoskeletal gait training robot is the AutoAmbulator, which was developed in cooperation with the HealthSouth network of rehabilitation hospitals in the U.S. (Fig. 5). As the Lokomat, the AutoAmbulator is a 4-DOF treadmill-based rehabilitation device, which consists of actuated robotic orthoses that guide the patient's knee and hip joints within the sagittal plane.[34] Multiple sensors perform continuous monitoring and adjustment of power and speed according to the patient's physical requirements. An interactive display with multiple scene modes works to increase patient motivation and add variation to the repetitive training exercises. The patient is fitted with a harness and lifted from his wheelchair on to the treadmill by the overhead body weight support system. The robotic exoskeleton is then strapped to the patient's legs at the thigh and ankle. The therapist controls the device through a touch screen panel or a remote control unit. Gait speed can be up to 3.2 km/h.[34] In Europe, the device is sold as "ReoAmbulator" (www.motorika.com).

Some more actuated orthotic devices that can be applied for gait training in a clinical setting have been developed, however, these are not (yet) commercially available. One of these is the LOPES device (Fig. 6). LOPES is a treadmill-based robotic exoskeleton that combines an actuated pelvis segment with a leg exoskeleton. The pelvis can move in translational directions, whereas the legs have two active rotary DOF at the hip (flexion–extension and abduction/adduction) and one active DOF at the knee (flexion–extension). The leg joints of the robot are actuated with Bowden-cable-driven series elastic actuators. The lateral pelvis translation is also equipped with the same actuation principle, whereas the anterior/posterior

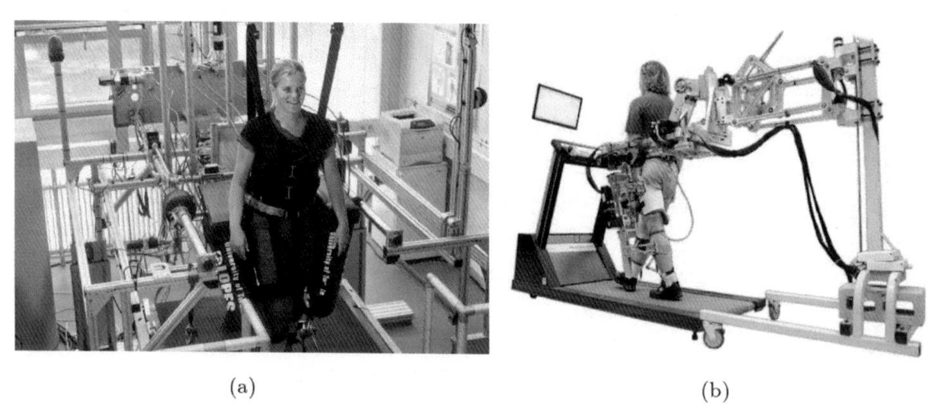

(a) (b)

Figure 6. (a) The research gait exoskeletons: LOPES (courtesy of H. van der Kooij, University of Twente) and (b) ALEX II (courtesy of S. Agrawal, University of Columbia).

motion is driven by a linear actuator. The joints are impedance controlled to allow bi-directional mechanical interaction between the robot and the training subject. The device allows both "patient-in-charge" and "robot-in-charge" modes. In the patient-in-charge mode, the robot follows the movements of the patient, allowing a relatively undisturbed movement of the non-parametric side of a hemiplegic subject. In the robot-in-charge mode, the robot is able to move the legs of a weak or passive subject in a gait-like pattern.[35] In 2014, a new version, LOPES II, has been finalized that actuates a similar number of degrees, but uses another actuation method, compared to the original device.

Another gait rehabilitation robot is the Active Leg Exoskeleton ALEX.[36] ALEX is a motorized orthosis (Fig. 6). A so-called walker supports the weight of the device, and the orthosis has several passive and actuated DOF with respect to the walker. The trunk of the orthosis (connected to the walker) has 3-DOF, namely, vertical and lateral translations and rotation about the vertical axis. The human trunk is secured to the orthosis with a hip brace. All the DOFs in the trunk are passive and held in position by springs. The hip joint of the orthosis has 2-DOF with respect to trunk of the orthosis allowing actuated hip flexion–extension and passive abduction/adduction movements. The flexion–extension DOF is actuated using a linear actuator, the abduction/adduction DOF is passive and held by a spring. The knee joint has one actuated DOF that is also actuated by a linear actuator. The thigh and shank segments contain telescopic units so that they can be adjusted to the human limb lengths. The foot segment is attached to the shank of the leg with one passive DOF ankle joint (plantar-/dorsiflexion). The foot segment also allows limited inversion–eversion motion at the ankle due to its structurally flexible design. The actuators in the hip and knee joint can generate about 50 Nm peak torques at the joints. Joint angles are measured via encoders built into the linear actuators. Interaction torques in the leg can be measured via two force-torque sensors, one mounted between the thigh segment and the leg, the other mounted between shank segment and the foot brace on the human leg.

David Reinkensmeyer from UC Irvine together with colleagues from UCLA developed the exoskeletal device "PAM" (pelvic assist manipulator), which is a device that assists the pelvic motion during human gait training on a treadmill[37] and "POGO" (pneumatically operated gait orthosis), which moves the patient's legs with linear actuators attached to a frame placed around the subject.[38]

3.3. *Body weight support systems*

Body weight support systems applied to gait therapy normally consist of a harness system worn by the patient that is connected via ropes and pulleys to a counterpoise

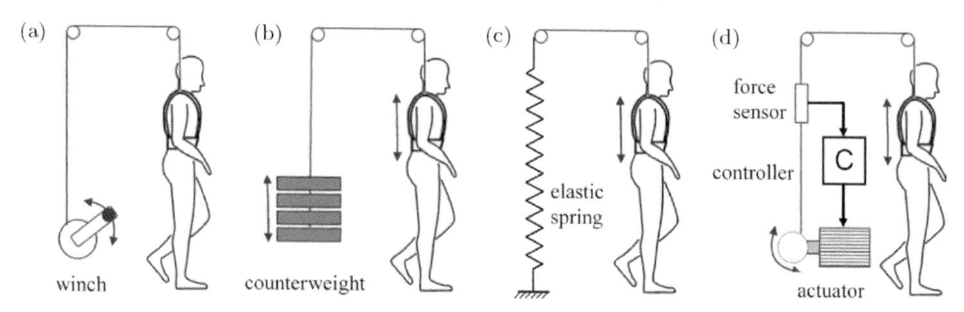

Figure 7. Illustration of the most common body weight support systems: (a) static BWS with rope and winch; (b) passive dynamic BWS with adjustable counterweights; (c) passive dynamic BWS with elastic spring; and (d) active dynamic BWS with force sensor and electric winch, according to Frey *et al.*[39]

to unload the patient. Different counterpoise systems can be distinguished (see also Ref. [39]). They can be characterized by different complexities, actuation principles, compliance and force constancy at the connection point to the patient.

3.3.1. *Static systems*

In static systems, the harness is attached to an overhead suspension, usually a system composed of ropes and pulleys connected to a winch (Fig. 7(a)). The winch actuation can be driven manually[40] or automatically by an electric actuation[41] or a fluidic system.[42] The winch is wound-up until the rope supports the desired unloading. More advanced systems use a force transducer that measures the weight support during hoisting. The drive stops as soon as the desired patient unloading is reached. The main disadvantage of static systems is the limitation of vertical movement of the center of mass. Thus, the constancy of the patient unloading during walking is not guaranteed and the execution of a physiologic gait pattern may be hampered.

3.3.2. *Passive counterweight systems*

A counterweight can be used to dynamically unload part of the patient's body weight. The counterweight is connected to the patient harness by a rope-and-pulley system (Fig. 7(b)).[43] However, the counterforce comprises not only the counterweight's gravitational force but also an inertial component, resulting from accelerations of the counter mass when moving the body up and down during walking. These inertial forces cause deviations of the suspension force from the desired value. Further disadvantages of common counterweight systems are that only discrete force values can be chosen and that the adjustments have to be done manually.

3.3.3. *Passive elastic systems*

Elastic components such as a metal spiral spring or a bungee cord can be used to unload the subject (Fig. 7(c)).[44–46] The amount of unloading is determined by the amount of tension of the elastic element. Compared to counterweights, the advantage of this approach is that inertial effects can be neglected. However, the suspension force is a function of spring length and, therefore, varies due to the vertical movement of the patient. Force variation can be reduced using a spring with low stiffness. This, however, requires a long spring elongation in order to obtain the required working load. Kram *et al.*[46] obtained rather large elongations using a series of springs connected by cables and separated by pulleys. However, in such systems, it is difficult to allow load adjustments over a large range. Passive elastic unloading can also be achieved with a closed pneumatic cylinder filled with compressed gas[47] instead of elastic springs. Gazzani *et al.*[43] proposed a system, where a closed-loop controller is used in order to compensate for small pressure losses due to air leakage.

3.3.4. *Active dynamic systems*

Body weight support can also be realized with active dynamic systems in which a pneumatic, hydraulic, electromagnetic, or any other active force-generating unit produces the desired force during walking (Fig. 7(d)). The vertical position or supporting force to the patient's movement is adjusted by applying a closed-loop approach. Vertical position or force is measured by a position sensor or force sensor, respectively, and fed into a controller that sends commands to the actuator to generate the desired positions or forces. Several groups developed closed-loop systems that are based on pneumatic actuators.[40,48,49] Pneumatic systems can be made to behave rather compliant due to the compressibility of air, thus providing force constancy during small movements. A closed-loop control ensures force constancy over time and during large vertical movements. However, bandwidths are limited to less than 20 Hz, which is insufficient for high performance tasks such as sudden changes of force or movements.[50] In contrast, hydraulic actuators have very high output stiffness, which make the actuator essentially a pure position source. Thus, force control needs to be realized with a position-based force controller, which needs very fast actuators to ensure a high quality force control.[51] In general, this type of closed-loop controller generating a constant force while compensating friction and inertial forces tends to be instable.[52,53] Electromagnetic actuators can either be used as a position source in combination with a position sensor and a closed-loop position control or as a force source in combination with a back-drivable transmission.[54,55] Thus, they comprise the advantages of both fluidic and pneumatic actuators.

3.3.5. *Combined passive elastic and active dynamic system*

A mechatronic body-weight support system called "Lokolift" has been developed to allow a more precise unloading during treadmill walking. The Lokolift combines the key principles of both passive elastic and active dynamic systems.[39,56] In this system, at unloading levels of up to 60 kg and walking speeds of up to 3.2 km/h, the mean unloading error was less than 1 kg and the maximum unloading error was less than 3 kg. This new system can perform changes of up to 20 kg in desired unloading within less than 100 ms. With this innovative feature, not only constant body weight support but also gait-cycle-dependent or time variant changes of the desired force can be realized with a high degree of accuracy. More recently, a spring-based (passive) system has been developed that allows similar results like the Lokolift system.[57]

An extension of the Lokolift system has been presented by Pennycott *et al.*[58] Their device is designed to minimize lateral forces acting on the subject from the body weight support cable. It comprises two pulley systems, referred to as the main and support systems (Fig. 8). The main pulley system allows the pulley connecting the body weight support and the human subject to move laterally in response to movement of the latter. The support pulley system ensures that the cable length of the main pulley system which is directly connected to the main body weight support mechanism is unchanged, irrespective of lateral movements of the pulleys. This constant cable length means that disturbances to the main body

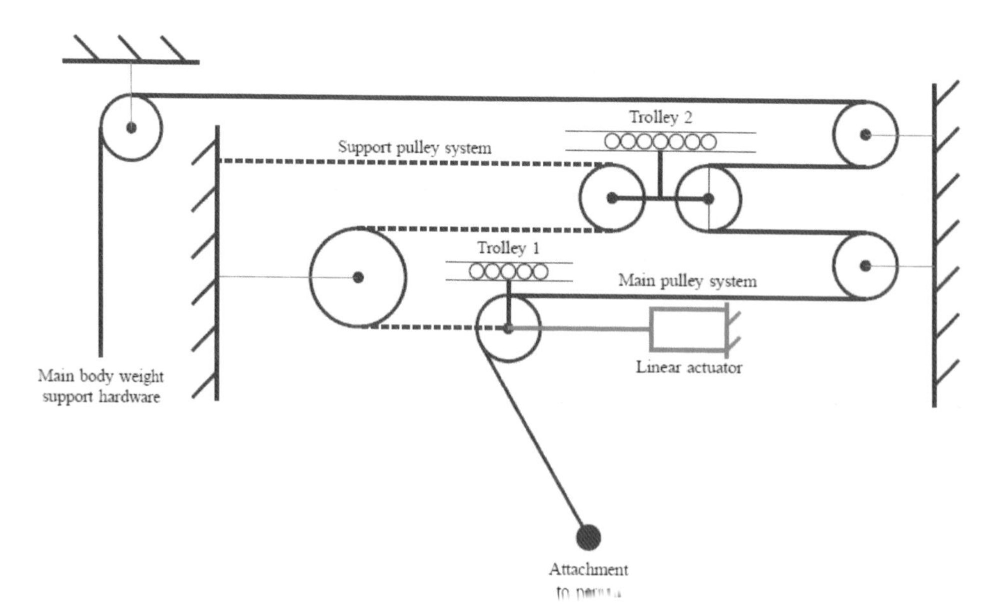

Figure 8. Body weight support system extension to allow also lateral deviations (frontal view).

weight support system, which maintains the magnitude of the body weight support force, are minimized.

3.3.6. *Systems supporting overground walking*

The body weight support systems presented above are designed to unload part of the patient's weight during treadmill training. As the devices are only 1-DOF systems, they have limitations because the subject is always stabilized with respect to the vertical, thus leading to a pendulum-restoring effect. This might simplify balance training tasks and can also cause non-physiological training effects.

Therefore, special body-weight support principles can be applied to overground walking in order to allow the patient to perform unhindered movements and train balance. Systems for overground walking need additional DOF, in order to allow the patient propagating in walking direction, and perhaps also in lateral direction. Therefore, the position of the pulley guiding the cable to the user needs to move in the horizontal direction or plane.

One example is the Zero-G,[59] which provides support by means of a trolley that runs on a rail and contains a pulley mechanism. A more advanced and more complex system is the FLOAT, which allows the connection point towards the user to move in 3 active translational DOF.[60] FLOAT is a cable-based robot supporting the patient with a 3D force vector in a large workspace (Fig. 9). Four cables are spanned by winches and guided over pulleys to the patient, where they are

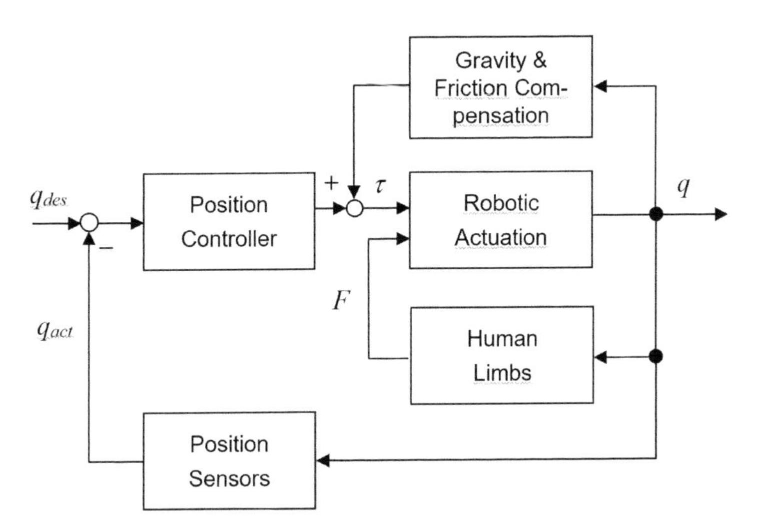

Figure 9. Position controller with friction and gravity compensation. Symbols: q is the vector of generalized positions or joint angles; τ is the vector of generalized joint torques; F is the interaction force between human limbs and the robot; index *des* refers to the desired reference signal; index *act* refers to the actual, measured signal.

connected to a single node on the harness worn by the patient.[60] The pulleys are mounted on carts running on two parallel rails. The carts on the same rail are connected by an additional cable and form one trolley. The position of the trolleys are measured and controlled such that the pulleys form the corners of a rectangle above the subject. The force transmitted by the cables are also measured and controlled by the winches in order to produce the desired force vector to optimally support the patient.[60]

4. Control Strategies

4.1. *Conventional controllers*

4.1.1. *Position controller*

Many rehabilitation robots apply conventional position controllers, where the measured joint angles are fed into a conventional PD controller[33] that determines a reaction to the actual error value (amplified by a factor P) and another reaction to the derivative error (amplified by a factor D) that is based upon the rate at which the error has been changing. Note that in a position controller, the robot does not systematically allow for deviation from the predefined gait pattern.

If the performance of such a simple linear position controller is not sufficient, the controller can be extended by a computed torque approach, in which the equations of motion of the robot's direct dynamic model are inverted to achieve the input into the robotic drives required to achieve the desired motion from the desired joint kinematics.[61,62] Alternatively, simpler sub-models simulating specific characteristics can be incorporated in a feedforward manner to compensate for viscous (friction), gravitational, and other properties (Fig. 9).

4.1.2. *Adaptive position controller*

The main disadvantage of position controllers is that they are based on a fixed reference trajectory, were individual adjustments are difficult to perform. Such adjustments have to be carried out manually based on qualitative observations made by the therapist or the patient. This limitation can be overcome by certain automatic adaptation principles. Jezernik *et al.* developed several control algorithms (Fig. 10) that can automatically adapt the predefined reference trajectory of different reference-based controllers to the individual motion of a patient.[63–65] Hereby, the involvement of human natural control leads to promoted patient activity during the exercise. The basis of the automatic reference trajectory adaptation algorithms is to modify the reference trajectory, and thus the robot motion, in a way

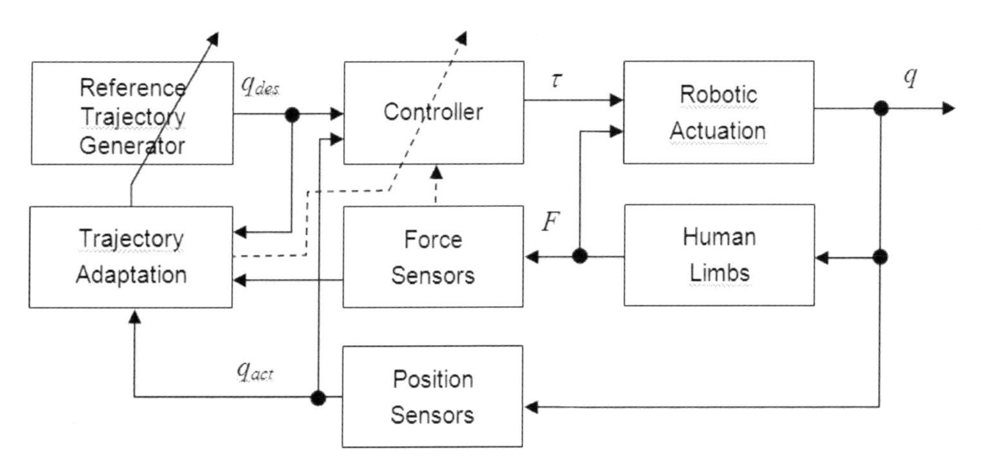

Figure 10. Principle of automatic position reference trajectory adaptation applied to any adaptive reference-based control strategy, such as position or impedance control.[63–65] Controller can be combined with gravity and friction compensation, see Fig. 9. Robotic components moved by the human (cuffs, exoskeletal links, bearings, etc.) have to be considered within the "Human Limbs" or "Robotic Actuation" block, depending on where exactly the force sensors are mounted between robot and human.

that is desired by the patient. Thus, the robot motion is derived from the mechanical interaction between the patient and the robot, which can be measured by the robotic interaction force sensors. The reference trajectories can be adjusted via adaptation of the trajectory parameters by online optimization. To accomplish this, a suitable parameterization of the trajectories is needed. Based upon measurements of "free" joint trajectories (i.e. when a healthy person was moving without any robotic device), it was found that a simple parameterization containing amplitude scaling, amplitude offset, and time-stretching of a nominal reference trajectory could yield a new desired reference trajectory that provides a satisfactory approximation of all variations observed during measurements.

Assuming a symmetric and periodic movement pattern, such as gait, identical parameters can be applied to the left and right joints. In the adaptive controller applied to the Lokomat,[63,64] the total number of independent adaptation parameters for the knee and hip joints was five: two for the amplitude range in hip and knee (amplitude scaling), two for the amplitude offset in hip and knee, and only one for the temporal scaling, which had to be identical for all four joints in order to provide motion synchrony. The allowed parameter changes were limited to 20% of their nominal values (multiplicative parameters) and $\pm 4^\circ$ (bias/offset of additive parameters). In this way, it was guaranteed that the adapted trajectories remained physiological.

Different versions of the reference trajectory adaptation algorithms were developed and successfully tested in computer simulations and evaluated in experiments with healthy and SCI subjects. SCI subjects were all incomplete paraplegic patients with a remaining ability to generate minor lower limb forces. One version of the algorithm provided gait pattern adaptation by estimating the human–robot interaction torques from the force recordings and then attempting to minimize these by adapting the parameters of the reference angle trajectories. Thus, the robot motion got entrained with the desired human motion. The variation in the torque was calculated from a mathematical model describing the dynamics of human leg including the Lokomat.[64] The minimization of the cost functional was performed over the parameter space spanned by the three parameters of amplitude scaling, amplitude offset, and time-stretching (see also Ref. [65]). In another algorithm, the estimated human–robot interaction torques were used to adapt the trajectory parameters in order to obtain the estimated change in the trajectory accelerations desired by the patient. The cost functional could be estimated from the measured interaction force using a dynamic model of Lokomat and human leg.[64] In both algorithms, the parameters that have generated adaptation of reference position trajectories were allowed to change every 2 s. The time-course of parameter changes was additionally low-pass filtered. Therefore, the gait pattern change usually occurred after several steps and took at least 5–10 s.

4.2. *Patient cooperative controllers*

4.2.1. *Rationale for the use of cooperative controllers*

Many rehabilitation devices work with patients in a "master–slave" relationship, thus forcing the patients to follow a predetermined motion without consideration of active voluntary efforts of the patient. In that traditional position control mode, the human subject often remains passive and the robot disregards the active contribution of the subject. Furthermore, the robot does not systematically allow for deviation from the predefined movement pattern.

However, rigid execution and repetition of the same pattern is not optimal for learning. In contrast, the variability and possibility to make errors are considered as essential components of practice for motor learning. Bernstein's demand that training should be "repetition without repetition"[66] is considered to be a crucial requirement and is also supported by recent advances in computational models describing motor learning.[67] More specifically, a recent study by Lewek *et al.*[68] demonstrated that intralimb coordination after stroke was improved by manual training, which enabled kinematic variability, but was not improved by position-controlled Lokomat training, which reduced kinematic variability to a minimum. Furthermore, Cai *et al.* applied a novel technical approach that allowed spinalized mice to deviate from a desired path.[25,69] The mice could move their hind limb freely within a moving window inside a virtual tunnel while walking on a treadmill. Mice trained with that moving window approach improved faster than those trained with a classical position control strategy. Many other groups could make similar conclusions, all indicating that more freedom and more active participation during the movement lead to a better outcome in terms of a faster learning and/or better performance after the learning, as has been shown in studies with different kinds of active/passive/haptic movement guidance and in constraint-induced movement therapy (CIMT).[70–77]

Thus, in future applications, it should be ensured that (i) the robot assists only as needed so that the patient can contribute to the movement with own voluntary effort and (ii) the limb movement deviates from a given and repetitive trajectory. We call this kind of robotic behavior "patient-cooperative". It is expected that patient-cooperative strategies will stimulate active participation by the patient. They also have the potential to increase the motivation of the patient because changes in muscle activation will be reflected in the walking pattern, causing consistently a feeling of success. It is assumed that patient-cooperative strategies will maximize the therapeutic outcome. Intensive clinical studies with large patient populations still have to be carried out to prove these hypotheses.

Patient-cooperative control strategies were developed to "recognize" the patient's movement intention and motor abilities by monitoring muscular efforts and adapt the robotic assistance to the patient's contribution, thus giving the patient more movement freedom and variability than during position control.[26,65,78] It is recommended that the control and feedback strategies should do the same as a qualified human therapist, i.e. they assist the patient's movement only as much as needed and inform the patient how to optimize voluntary muscle efforts and coordination in order to achieve and improve a particular movement.

4.2.2. *Impedance controller*

The first step in incorporating a variable deviation from a predefined leg trajectory into the system, thus giving the patient more freedom, may be achieved using an impedance control strategy. Impedance controllers are well established in the field of robotics and human–system interaction, and were first introduced by Hogan about 30 years ago.[22] They have been applied in robot-aided upper extremity therapy of stroke patients.[79] The basic idea of the impedance control strategy applied to robot-aided training is to allow a variable deviation from a predefined joint or limb trajectory rather than imposing a rigid movement pattern. This amount of deviation depends upon the patient's effort and behavior. An adjustable torque is applied at each joint depending on the deviation of the current joint position from the desired trajectory. This torque is usually defined as a zero order (stiffness)

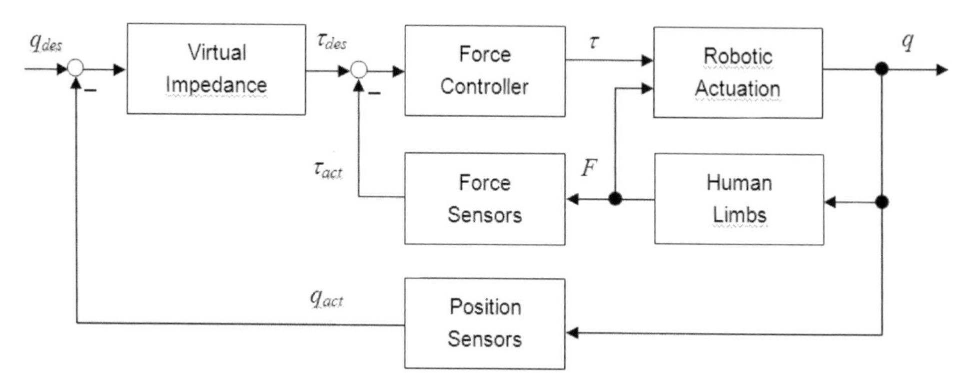

Figure 11. Example of an impedance control architecture for a rehabilitation robot (see also Refs. [33, 65]). Controller can be combined with gravity and friction compensation, see Fig. 9. Robotic components moved by the human (cuffs, exoskeletal links, bearings, etc.) have to be considered within the "Human Limbs" or "Robotic Actuation" block, depending where exactly the force sensors are mounted between the robot and the human.

or higher order (usually first or second order) function of angular position and its derivatives. This torque is more generally called mechanical impedance.[22] Figure 11 depicts a block diagram of an impedance controller.

One version of an impedance controller was initially tested in several healthy subjects with no known neurological deficits and also in several subjects with incomplete paraplegia using the Lokomat.[65] In the impedance control mode, angular deviations increased with increasing robot compliance (decreasing impedance) as the robot applied a smaller force to guide the human legs along a given trajectory. Inappropriate muscle activation, produced by high muscle tone, spasms, or reflexes, can affect the movement and may yield a physiologically incorrect gait pattern, depending on the magnitude of the impedance chosen. In contrast, several subjects who used the system with the impedance controller stated that the gentle behavior of the robot feels good and comfortable (personal experience of subjects told to the authors). The disadvantage of a standard impedance controller is that the patient needs sufficient voluntary effort to move along a physiologically correct trajectory, which limits the range of application to patients with only mild lesions. In addition, the underlying gait trajectory allows no flexibility in time, i.e. leg position can deviate only orthogonally but not tangentially to the given trajectory.

In general, satisfactory impedance control behavior was observed with zero and low virtual impedance values set in the controller. However, it is well known that due to limited sampling times and sensor noise, experimentally verified impedance controllers may become unstable at higher impedances.[52,65,80,81] Therefore, instead of an impedance controller, an admittance controller can be used because it has better stability at high impedances. Compared to the above-mentioned force-based impedance controller, the admittance controller can also be called position-based impedance controller.[52] To avoid performance and stability problems, the user can choose either an impedance or an admittance control architecture. The impedance values can be chosen by the therapist based on their experience. This depends on the amount of voluntary muscle force the patient can produce in order to contribute to the desired movement. Subjects with a high level of voluntary control, e.g. incomplete SCI patients after some weeks of training, can move with lower impedances.

4.2.3. *Assistance-as-needed controller*

A prevailing paradigm for supporting patients is the concept of "assistance-as-needed" (AAN).[24,82] Such robot-aided training strategies have been developed based on the common clinical practice of physical therapists: robotic devices provide just enough assistance to allow participants to practice the task, while reducing the assistance based on real-time measurement of the patient's performance to encourage the individual to learn and execute the movement on their own. Recently developed robotic therapy control algorithms provide assistance-as-needed during movement tasks like reaching,[83] walking,[31] and wheelchair steering[71] based on computational models of human motor adaptation and optimization theory. These algorithms have two key features: they update their parameters based on real-time measurement of recent performance errors ("error-based learning"), and they decrease their assistance when performance errors are small due to a "forgetting" or "slacking" term.

The most commonly employed AAN is of the form:

$$R_{k+1} = f_R R_k - g_k |x_k - x_{d,k}|,$$

where R_k is the control parameter that is adapted (e.g. the gain of robot assistance force, or the robot stiffness), k refers to the kth movement, f_R is the robot forgetting factor, g_R is the robot learning gain, x_k is the performance variable (e.g. measured position) and $x_{d,k}$ is the desired performance variable (e.g. desired position). If f_R is chosen such that $0 < f_R < 1$, then the error-based learning algorithm reduces the control parameter when the performance error $|x_k(t) - x_{d,k}(t)|$ is small, with the effect of always challenging the patient.

An algorithm of this form was employed to adjust the workspace-dependent impedance gains of a gait-assisting robot during walking training of spinal cord injured subjects.[31] The success of this algorithm was based on the mechanical nature of the robot, i.e. the robot was highly backdrivable. However, pneumatically or hydraulically driven robots are intrinsically not backdrivable, and thus when the robot stiffness is reduced to zero, the amount of force to influence the robot is excessive for many patients.

More sophisticated AAN approaches have been defined as adaptive controllers able to provide mechanically compliant assistance during the movement, while still allowing patients to be challenged. A compliant robot must calculate an appropriate amount of force to compensate for undesired robot-dynamics and cancel for patient-dependent disabilities. In one study, a sliding-type adaptive controller[83] was used to develop a radial-basis function model of the participant's impairment during a reaching task. In order to avoid patients to rely on the assistance, a "forgetting" factor reduced the robot assistance when tracking error was small. A similar adaptive algorithm that reduces the assisting force based on real-time measures of tracking error was developed for the investigation of gait-like movements using an MR-compatible stepping device (MARCOS).[84]

There is recent evidence that training with AAN improves rehabilitation outcomes. One study in spine-injured mice compared a position-dependent, velocity force field with a fixed training trajectory, and an AAN strategy.[25] It was found that training with AAN increased significantly the number of steps and periodicity. In a more recent study, training with an AAN robotic arm/hand device (Pneu-WREX)[85] after chronic stroke resulted in an almost significant greater reduction of the Fugl-Meyer score than training with conventional tabletop therapy.[86] Finally, a recent pilot study with 12 spine injured patients reported that training with the robotic gait trainer LOPES using an AAN algorithm for hip flexion improved the ability and quality of walking.[87]

4.2.4. *Tunnel controller* (*path controller*)

All approaches using classical impedance control share the disadvantage of imposing a defined timing of movements on the patient. As spatial and temporal corrections are coupled in these control strategies, it is not possible to achieve freedom in timing without losing guidance in space. If the impedance setting is too stiff, patients feel passively moved; if it is too soft, patients are not corrected in space and might move in undesired patterns. A solution to this problem was first proposed for the upper extremity robot MIT-MANUS.[88] The controller of the robot simulated a virtual tunnel in space. Patients could autonomously move their hands through this tunnel. If they did not move forward as desired, the moving "back wall" of this tunnel carried their hand along after a certain amount of time. Cai *et al.*[25] applied two similar concepts to spinalized mice using a miniature rehabilitation robot. Firstly, they created a virtual tunnel similar to the approach for the MIT-MANUS, but without a moving "backwall". The mice could move their hind limb freely within this tunnel while walking on a treadmill. Secondly, they trained the mice with a "moving window" that allowed some freedom, but kept them synchronized to the treadmill. Mice trained with the "moving window" approach improved faster than those trained with a classical position control strategy. Banala *et al.*[36] implemented the virtual tunnel approach of Cai *et al.*[25] for their ALEX and tested the approach with healthy and stroke subjects.

Likewise motivated by the work of Cai *et al.*,[25] Duschau-Wicke *et al.* developed a similar approach for the Lokomat.[78] However, to focus more on leg postures than on end-effector position, they designed a torque field tunnel in joint space rather than a force field in Cartesian space. Pilot studies indicated that training of incomplete SCI subjects requires more control over the amount of freedom provided by the controller than training of healthy subjects. The incomplete SCI subjects could not cope with the freedom of timing that was possible in a plain virtual tunnel. Consequently, Duschau-Wicke *et al.*[78] superposed the "moving window" approach and the virtual tunnel from Cai *et al.*[25] to one control strategy. The moving window restricts the domain of possible leg postures to a region within the virtual tunnel. The window size determines how much freedom in timing the subjects experience within the tunnel. As this algorithm allows subjects to move actively along the spatial *path* of a defined walking pattern, it is referred to as "path control". The additional freedom provided by this patient-cooperative control strategy is combined with a training task, in which patients have to autonomously control their legs within the given freedom. A visual display shows both the patients' movements and the reference movements which the patients are supposed to track (Fig. 12).

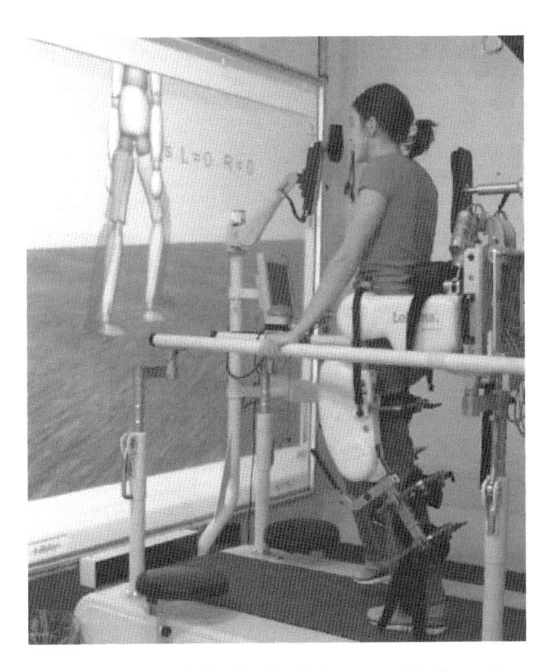

Figure 12. Healthy subject training in the Lokomat with the path control strategy.

In the path controller, the controller enables the impedance along the path to vary in order to obtain satisfactory movement particularly at critical phases of the movement (e.g. before heel contact). This is comparable to fixing the patient's feet to soft rails, thus limiting the accessible domain of foot positions calculated as functions of hip and knee angles. The patients are free to move along these "virtual rails". In order to supplement these *corrective* actions of the Lokomat, a *supportive* force field of adjustable magnitude can be added. Depending on the actual position of the patient's legs, the supportive forces act in the direction of the desired path. The support is derived from the desired angular velocities of the predefined trajectory at the current path location. Supportive forces make it possible to move along the path with reduced effort. Compared to the impedance controller, the path controller gives the patient more freedom in timing, while he/she can still be guided through critical phases of the gait, providing a safe and variable repetitive gait therapy. The reference trajectory has been recorded from healthy subjects[32] and is used as set point for the underlying impedance controller. The treadmill speed is selected by the therapist. A dynamic set point generation algorithm is used to minimize the Euclidean distance between the reference trajectory and the actual trajectory.

An adjustable zero band of a predefined width creates a virtual tunnel around the reference trajectory. The width of the zero band has been designed heuristically based upon the evidence and experience from pre-trials. The width was computed to permit larger spatial variation during late swing and early stance-phase to account for the large variability of knee flexion at heel strike. Additionally, the reference trajectory has been adapted to a less pronounced loading response and more knee flexion during swing-phase so that the desired zero band spreads symmetrically around the reference. In this way, a genealizable tunnel was obtained that could accommodate all subjects and enable additional variability and support. Within the tunnel, the controller is in the so-called "free run" mode, i.e. the output of the impedance is zero, and gravity and friction torques of the robot are compensated. Therefore, subjects can move freely and with their own timing as long as they stay within the tunnel. Leg postures outside the tunnel are corrected by the impedance controller. The spring constant of the virtual impedance is chosen as a function of the distance to the tunnel wall. These measurements were experimentally determined such that the wall of the tunnel felt comfortably soft to the subjects. A nonlinear stiffness function has been implemented to allow for a compromise between soft contact with the wall and strong corrections for larger deviations. An additional damping constant was determined as a function of the stiffness such that the system is critically damped. Adjustable supportive torques can be superimposed to the controller output. To determine the direction of support, a torque vector is calculated by differentiating the reference trajectory with respect to the relative position in the gait cycle. Thus, the direction of the torque vector is tangential to the movement path in joint space. The supportive torques are not only important in helping a patient to overcome weaknesses but also reduce the effect of the uncompensated inertia of the robot. More details and data regarding the path controller may be found in Ref. 78.

Several experimental studies have been performed on healthy subjects, incomplete SCI, and hemiplegic persons after stroke. Duschau-Wicke *et al.*[89] could show that the path controller increases active participation of individuals with incomplete SCI during robot-aided gait training, when compared to non-cooperative robot-aided gait training. In their study, 11 patients with incomplete SCI participated in a single training session with the gait rehabilitation robot, Lokomat. The patients were exposed to different training modes in random order. Joint angles and torques of the robot as well as muscle activity and heart rate of the patients were recorded. Kinematic variability, interaction torques, heart rate and muscle activity were compared between the different conditions. Patients showed more spatial and temporal kinematic variability, reduced interaction torques, a higher increase of heart rate and more muscle activity in the patient-cooperative path control mode with individually adjusted support than in the non-cooperative position control mode.

In another study performed by the same group,[90] two individuals with chronic incomplete SCI and two with chronic stroke did an intensive training with the Lokomat gait rehabilitation robot which was operated in the patient-cooperative path-control mode for a period of 4 weeks with 4 training sessions of 45 min per week (i.e. 16 sessions in total). At baseline, after 2 and 4 weeks, walking function was assessed with the 10-meter walking test. Additionally, muscle activity of the major leg muscles, heart rate and the Borg scale were measured under different walking conditions including a non-cooperative position control mode to investigate the short-term effects of patient-cooperative versus non-cooperative robot-aided gait training. It was observed that patient-cooperative robot-aided gait training was tolerated well by all subjects and performed without difficulties. The subjects trained more actively and with more physiological muscle activity than in a non-cooperative position-control mode. One subject showed a significant and relevant increase of gait speed after the therapy, the three remaining subjects did not show significant changes.

Another intensive training study was performed at the Rehabilitation Institute of Chicago (RIC).[91] They tested the feasibility of the path controller developed by Duschau-Wicke *et al.*[78] also using the Lokomat in mitigating post-stroke gait impairments of a 52-year-old male stroke survivor. Their gait training paradigm combined the patient-cooperative robot-aided walking with a target-tracking task for the ankle movement. The training lasted for 4 weeks with three training sessions per week (i.e. 12 sessions in total). The subject's neuromotor performance and recovery were evaluated using biomechanical, neuromuscular and clinical measures recorded at various time-points (pre-training, post-training, and 6-weeks after training). Krishnan *et al.* could show that this kind of interactive robotic training resulted in considerable increase in target-tracking accuracy and reduction in the kinematic variability of the ankle trajectory during robot-aided treadmill walking. These improvements also transferred to overground walking as characterized by larger propulsive forces and more symmetric ground reaction forces. Training also resulted in improvements in muscle coordination, which resembled patterns observed in healthy controls. These changes were accompanied by a reduction in motor cortical excitability of the vastus medialis, medial hamstrings, and gluteus medius muscles during treadmill walking. Importantly, active robotic training resulted in substantial improvements in several standard clinical and functional parameters, such as Timed-Up-and-Go (TUG) test, 6-min walk test, single leg balance, maximum gait velocity, lower extremity Fugl-Meyer test, etc. These improvements persisted during the follow-up evaluation at 6 weeks.

The same group could repeat this positive outcome in a second single case study,[92] which was performed with a 62-year-old male with right temporal lobe ischemic stroke. The baseline lower extremity Fugl-Meyer score of the subject was 10 on a scale of 34, which represented severe impairment in the paretic leg. The subject underwent 4 weeks of training with three sessions per week (i.e. 12 sessions in total) of conventional robotic training with the Lokomat, where the robot provided full assistance to leg movements while walking, followed by 12 sessions of patient-cooperative robotic control training, where the robot provided minimal guidance based on the path control strategy.[78] Clinical outcomes were evaluated before and immediately after the 4-week training phases. These were self-selected and fast walking speed, 6-min walk test, timed up and go test, and the lower extremity Fugl-Meyer score. Results showed that clinical outcomes changed minimally after full guidance robotic training, but improved considerably after 4 weeks of reduced guidance robotic training.

The path controller has been extended and transferred to further application areas, such as the patient-cooperative training of the upper extremities using the arm therapy robot ARMin[93–96] and the pediatric arm therapy robot PASCAL[97] or the learning of complex movement tasks in sports using the parallel cable robot R3[98] which have been applied to rowing[99–101] and tennis.[102,103]

4.2.5. *Robot transparency*

When controlling the robot such that it assists only when needed, there will be certain instants or even longer phases in time, where the robot should not be felt by the patient, i.e. where robot should provide virtual support. There are several approaches to achieve transparency of a robot (see Refs. [104, 105]). One of the best means is to minimize the robot's mass. Then, its dynamics cause only small interaction forces between the human subject and the robot. However, mass reduction is limited when higher forces and powers are needed requiring a more robust mechanical design. Inertial forces generated by the actuators can be reduced by suitable actuation concepts, e.g. using Series Elastic Actuators.[106] However, it is difficult to avoid the insertion of additional inertia between the actuators and the connection to the human, especially when using an end-effector or exoskeleton attached to the human.

Furthermore, closed-loop force control, for example, using impedance or admittance control concepts, is another efficient means to improve transparency because it can reduce the reflected inertia of the robot and its actuators.[22,107,108] However, this reduction is limited, i.e. there will always be inertial forces remaining,[107] and the control scheme requires force or acceleration sensors. As reduction of inertia is limited, a common attempt is to compensate at least robot gravity, and possibly also Coriolis, centrifugal, and friction forces.

A control scheme that explicitly optimizes passive dynamics of haptic devices with regard to interaction forces is the concept of *Generalized Elasticities*.[104,105] Given that the user's preferred movements are approximately known in advance, optimal conservative force fields are derived. The algorithm does not need a model of the human, and the robot's kinematics does not need to resemble that of the human limbs. With conservative force fields, the robot is stable when coupled to any passive system,[109] which is important for safe human–robot interaction. Generalized elasticities have been implemented not only on the gait rehabilitation robot Lokomat but also on other robotic systems.[101] The approach reduced interaction torques compared to closed-loop force control and to gravity compensation, and the gait pattern was more natural regarding gait cadence (i.e. stepping frequency).[105]

The conservative force fields used in the generalized elasticity approach can act jointly with other controllers, like the previously developed Nearest-Neighbor Path Control with Gravity Cancellation.[110] Due to the passive nature of the Generalized elasticities, no stability problems should occur when interacting with other passive concepts. However, the potential of the conservative force fields might be higher, which means that they can take over additional guiding functions as well. By finding a conservative force field that optimally approximates an arbitrary assistive strategy complex controllers can be realized without tedious stability analysis. The fitted force field is intrinsically passive, and it preserves the originally desired assistance in an optimal way.

5. Biofeedback and Augmented Feedback Methods

5.1. *Biofeedback*

5.1.1. *Definition*

Natural as well as artificial optimization processes require detectable performance quantities, which are optimized in a certain way. In the human body, these performance quantities are obtained by proprioceptive feedback of movements, forces, visual impressions, sounds, etc. However, perception may be disturbed or missing either because the user lacks appropriate afferent input from receptors (e.g. after peripheral nervous system injuries) or has not learned to perform the optimization procedure (e.g. after congenital lesions of the central or vegetative nervous system).

In such cases, artificial sensors can be used for recording the performance quantities (or related values that can be used for determining performance) and feeding them back to the user.[111] Because biological quantities are transferred to a biological system (human) via artificial feedback, the term "biofeedback" has been introduced and become widely accepted.

To make the artificial feedback signals perceptible and allow the patient to react to the signal, technical display devices are required, such as graphic monitors, loudspeakers, vibrators, or haptic displays. The kind of display device depends not only on the application and ergonomic issues but also on the pathology (when biofeedback is applied to a patient). For patients with minor lesions, the display can enhance the affected sensory input. In severe cases, another non-affected perceptible modality can be chosen as a substitute for the affected sensory function and allows the patient to perceive even "invisible" information.

5.1.2. *State of the art*

Several research groups suggest novel application of biofeedback principles for gait rehabilitation of patients with stroke,[112–127] cerebral palsy (CP),[128–131] incomplete paraplegia,[132] spina bifida,[133] or arthritis.[134] Many studies detect motor functions or performance by electromyographic (EMG) recordings.[119–122,128,132] As an alternative or extension to EMG recordings, kinematic quantities have also been used, such as joint angles of the ankle and the knee, step length, stance duration and other quantities.[121–126,132–137] Kinetic measures have been used as well, such as ground reaction forces and plantar pressure values.[136,137]

The recorded signals are processed and fed back to the patients via visual displays, acoustic displays, or both. Some research groups also use vibrotactile displays to generate tactile impressions on the skin.[133,135,136]

The clinical evidence for a beneficial effect of biofeedback is controversial. Van Peppen *et al.* did not find a significant difference in gait speed when they pooled seven appropriate studies out of 16 identified in a systematic literature review.[127] The summary effect size of biofeedback on the active range of motion was also not significant (based on four pooled studies). In comparison, Teasell *et al.* did not pool results from different studies but rather counted the studies with positive versus negative outcome effects; from this systematic review, eight of nine studies showed a positive biofeedback effect.[112]

Wolf and Binder-MacLeod investigated the effects of EMG-biofeedback during arm rehabilitation of 22 patients with hemiplegia.[138] In comparison with a control group ($n = 9$), improved neuromuscular parameters were observed, whereas functional changes were absent. In contrast, Inglis *et al.* showed that, compared to conventional therapy, biofeedback improved functional properties, such as muscle force, active range of movement, and motor recovery of patients with hemiplegia.[139] Several further studies reported positive functional effects of EMG biofeedback applied to stroke patients.[140,141]

In conclusion, we interpret the available evidence as demonstrating a positive effect of biofeedback on motor recovery and see the potential for wider benefits in neurological rehabilitation.

5.1.3. *Biofeedback with the Lokomat*

An early implementation of a force-biofeedback strategy for the Lokomat has been described.[142,143] In order to obtain relevant biofeedback values, the gait cycle is divided into stance-phase and swing-phase. For each phase, weighted averages of the forces are calculated at each joint independently, thus yielding two values per stride per joint. Eight biofeedback values are available for each gait cycle from all four joints of the two lower limbs. Because of the bilateral symmetry, four weighting functions are required for the averaging procedure (hip stance, hip swing, knee stance, knee swing). The weighting functions were selected heuristically to provide positive biofeedback values when the patient performs therapeutically reasonable activities (e.g. active weight bearing during stance, sufficient foot clearance during swing, active hip flexion during swing, active knee flexion during early swing, knee extension during late swing). The graphical display of these values has been positively rated by the patients and leads to an increased instantaneous activity by the patients.[144,145] However, there is no direct clinical evidence showing that this training with computerized feedback leads to better rehabilitation outcomes or faster recovery compared with Lokomat training without feedback.

To further increase patient's engagement and motivation, virtual reality, computer game techniques may be used as "augmented feedback" applications to provide virtual environments that encourage active participation during training. A first feasibility study showed that the majority of subjects could navigate through a virtual environment by appropriately controlling and increasing their activity of left and right legs while walking through a virtual underground scenario.[146]

5.2. *Augmented feedback*

In a simple manner, the information can be presented to the patient only by graphical elements, such as numbers, bars, or graphs. A more advanced method is the application of virtual reality (VR) technologies. When used as an additional feedback quantity in rehabilitation, it is also often called "augmented feedback". Here, the measured patient activity, such as gait speed, muscle activity, and leg and foot motion patterns, is displayed by graphical or audiovisual animations and provide a realistic impression to the patient. The goal is for the patient to feel present in a virtual environment while continuously confronted with information about his or her motor performance during the training in an easy, intuitive way. VR can make training therapies more exciting for the patient, thus motivating him or her to train longer and more often. There are plenty of research groups who have applied VR to physical therapy of lower limbs.[147–152] Whole conferences on this topic have been organized in the last years. Several VR applications also exist with the Lokomat.[153–155]

6. Clinical Outcomes

Robotic technology is still very much in development and there are a lot of new devices and technical features that might further enhance the potential of therapeutic training. Nevertheless, there have already been more than 200 clinical investigations applying the Lokomat technology to different patient groups. It was applied for the therapy of patients with SCI, hemiplegia after stroke, traumatic brain injuries, multiple sclerosis, Parkinson's disease, cerebral palsy and other pathologies (see Ref. [156]). Most of these studies show positive outcomes with the Lokomat compared to conventional therapies or usual care.

A majority of clinical studies were carried out with stroke subjects. Often cited are the ones from Hidler *et al.*[157] and Hornby *et al.*[158] who applied the Lokomat on sub-acute and chronic stroke patients, respectively, and compared it with conventional gait therapy. Both studies showed that participants who received conventional training experienced greater gains in gait parameters such as walking speed, walking distance or single limb stance than those trained on the Lokomat.

Hidler *et al.* and Hornby *et al.* concluded that for stroke participants, conventional gait training interventions appear to be more effective than robotic-assisted gait training. However, both studies included only ambulatory patients, although the Lokomat is recommended to be used primarily for non-ambulatory patients. Furthermore, the Lokomat was used in most simple control modes (position controller, or impedance controller with reduced guidance force) without any other feature such as augmented feedback or biofeedback functions. Of course, this kind of mode cannot compete with the quality and gentleness of a trained therapist or more advanced robotic features, such as cooperative and self-adaptive control strategies.

A recent Cochrane report[159] analyzing 17 trials with 837 stroke patients revealed that people who receive electromechanical-assisted gait training, such as that provided by the Lokomat or the Gait Trainer, in combination with physiotherapy after stroke, that are more likely to achieve independent walking than people who receive gait training without these devices. Specifically, people in the first 3 months after stroke and those who are not able to walk seem to benefit most from this type of intervention. The role of the type of devices is not clear. Further research should consist of a large definitive, pragmatic, phase III trial, undertaken to address specific questions such as "what frequency or duration of electromechanical-assisted gait training might be most effective?" and "how long does the benefit last?". One of the latest studies was the one by Dundar *et al.*[160] who compared conventional physiotherapy and robotic training combinded with conventional therapy, on 107 sub-acute and chronic stroke patients. They found that robotic training combined with conventional therapy produced better improvement in a large number of different stroke scales.

7. Conclusion and Outlook

Robotic rehabilitation devices have become increasingly important and popular in clinical and rehabilitation environments to facilitate prolonged duration of gait training, increased number of repetition of movements, improved patient safety, and less strenuous operation by therapists. Novel sensor, display, and control technologies made possible the improvement of the function, usability and accessibility of the robots by increasing patient participation and improving performance assessment. Improved and standardized assessment tools provided by robots will be an important prerequisite for the intra- and intersubject comparison that the researcher and the therapist require to evaluate the rehabilitation process of individual patients and entire patient groups. Furthermore, gait rehabilitation robots offer an open platform for the implementation of advanced technologies, which will provide new forms of training for patients with gait disorders.

One of the most important features of any training is that the patients should be as active as possible. This can affect not only the possible gains in motor learning but could also potentially help reduce the severity of the secondary complications of neurological patients such as cardiovascular disease, decubitus, and osteoporosis. A robot designed for a high level of transparency would enhance active patient participation and achieve low robotic interference for the more able patients, while retaining the option of more support when it is really needed. A compact, low weight design incorporating passive elements and a sufficient number of DOF to allow different aspects of the movement to be trained will help achieve a high level of voluntary effort, enhance training variation and, thus promote more effective motor learning. Furthermore, with the use of cooperative control strategies and particular augmented feedback (i.e. virtual reality) technologies, patients can be encouraged not only to increase engagement during movement training but also to improve their motivation to participate in the therapy sessions.

Some clinical trials have been performed showing that the application of gait rehabilitation devices is at least as effective as the application of conventional therapies. However, further clinical studies are required to find predictors for the success of a therapeutical treatment. From such investigations, one can expect to figure out choices of technical features (technical complexity, actuation, kind of feedback, etc.) have to be applied to which kinds of patient characteristics (kind of pathology, severity, time since lesion, anthropometry, etc.) in order to obtain the best therapeutic outcome.

Acknowledgments

Special thanks go to Volker Bartenbach, Urs Keller, Laura Marchal-Crespo, Domen Novak, Verena Klamroth, and Dario Wyss for their contributions to this chapter. Parts of this chapter have been published earlier (see Ref. [161]).

References

1. WHO (2003). The World health report, Shaping the future: World Health Organization.
2. M. Kelly-Hayes, J. T. Robertson, J. P. Broderick, P. W. Duncan, L. A. Hershey, E. J. Roth, *et al.* (1998). The American Heart Association stroke outcome classification: executive summary, *Circulation* 97(24):2474–2478.
3. H. S. Jørgensen, H. Nakayama, H. O. Raaschou and T. S. Olsen. (1995). Recovery of walking function in stroke patients: the Copenhagen Stroke Study, *Archives of Physical Medicine and Rehabilitation* 76(1):27–32.
4. R. Waters, R. Adkins, J. Yakura and I. Sie. (1998). Donal Munro Lecture: functional and neurologic recovery following acute SCI, *The Journal of Spinal Cord Medicine* 21(3):195–199.
5. A. Pennycott, D. Wyss, H. Vallery and R. Riener. (2012). Towards more effective robotic gait training for stroke rehabilitation, *Journal of NeuroEngineering and Rehabilitation* 9(65).

6. K. H. Mauritz. (2002). Gait training in hemiplegia, *European Journal of Neurology* 9(s1): 23–29.
7. I. Davidson and K. Waters. (2000). Physiotherapists working with stroke patients: a national survey, *Physiotherapy* 86(2):69–80.
8. R. Dickstein, S. Hocherman, T. Pillar and R. Shaham. (1986). Stroke rehabilitation three exercise therapy approaches, *Physical Therapy* 66(8):1233–1238.
9. S. Lennon. (2003). Physiotherapy practice in stroke rehabilitation: a survey, *Disability and Rehabilitation* 25(9):455–461.
10. C. Partridge and S. Edwards. (1996). The bases of practice — neurological physiotherapy, *Physiotherapy Research International* 1(3):205–208.
11. B. Bobath. (1990). *Adult Hemiplegia: Evaluation and Treatment*, Heinemann Medical Books, Oxford.
12. J. H. Carr and R. B. Shepherd. (2003). *Stroke rehabilitation: guidelines for exercise and training to optimize motor skill.* https://www.amazon.com/Stroke-Rehabilitation-Guidelines-Exercise-Training/dp/0750647124.
13. M. Knott, D. E. Voss, H. D. Hipshman and J. B. Buckley. (1968). *Proprioceptive Neuromuscular Facilitation: Patterns and Techniques*, Hoeber Medical Division, Harper & Row.
14. S. A. Stockmeyer. (1967). An interpretation of the approach of Rood to the treatment of neuromuscular dysfunction, *American Journal of Physical Medicine and Rehabilitation* 46(1):900–956.
15. V. Dietz, G. Colombo, L. Jensen and L. Baumgartner. (1995). Locomotor capacity of spinal cord in paraplegic patients, *Annals of Neurology* 37(5):574–582.
16. S. Hesse, C. Bertelt, M. Jahnke, A. Schaffrin, P. Baake, M. Malezic, *et al.* (1995). Treadmill training with partial body weight support compared with physiotherapy in nonambulatory hemiparetic patients, *Stroke* 26(6):976–981.
17. H. Barbeau and S. Rossignol. (1994). Enhancement of locomotor recovery following spinal cord injury, *Current Opinion in Neurology* 7(6):517–524.
18. S. E. Nadeau, S. S. Wu, B. H. Dobkin, S. P. Azen, D. K. Rose, J. K. Tilson, S. Y. Cen and P. W. Duncan. (2013). Effects of task-specific and impairment-based training compared with usual care on functional walking ability after inpatient stroke rehabilitation: LEAPS trial, *Neurorehabilitation and Neural Repair* 27(4):370–380.
19. G. Kwakkel, R. C. Wagenaar, T. W. Koelman, G. J. Lankhorst and J. C. Koetsier. (1997). Effects of intensity of rehabilitation after stroke a research synthesis, *Stroke* 28(8):1550–1556.
20. M. J. Riddoch, G. W. Humphreys and A. Bateman. (1995). Stroke: stroke issues in recovery and rehabilitation, *Physiotherapy* 81(11):689–694.
21. T. Nef and R. Riener. (2012). Three-Dimensional Multi-Degree-of-Freedom Arm Therapy Robot (ARMin). In: V. Dietz, Z. Rymer and T. Nef (Eds.). *Neurorehabilitation Technology.* London: Springer, pp. 141–157.
22. N. Hogan. (1985). Impedance control: An approach to manipulation: Parts I, II and III, *Journal of Dynamic Systems, Measurement, and Control* 107:1–23.
23. S. Jezernik, R. Schärer, G. Colombo and M. Morari. (2003). Adaptive robotic rehabilitation of locomotion: a clinical study in spinally injured individuals, *Spinal Cord* 41(12):657–666.
24. J. L. Emken, J. E. Bobrow and D. J. Reinkensmeyer. (Eds.) (2005). Robotic movement training as an optimization problem: designing a controller that assists only as needed. *Proceedings of the 2005 IEEE 9th International Conference on Rehabilitation Robotics June 28–July 1*, Chicago, IL, USA. (see also http://ieeexplore.ieee.org/abstract/document/1501108/).
25. L. L. Cai, A. J. Fong, C. K. Otoshi, Y. Liang, J. W. Burdick, R. R. Roy, *et al.* (2006). Implications of assist-as-needed robotic step training after a complete spinal cord injury on intrinsic strategies of motor learning, *Journal of Neuroscience* 26(41):10564–10568.
26. R. Riener and T. Fuhr. (1998). Patient-driven control of FES-supported standing up: a simulation study. *IEEE Transactions on Rehabilitation Engineering* 6(2):113–124.

27. M. Zinn, B. Roth, O. Khatib and J. K. Salisbury. (2004). A new actuation approach for human friendly robot design, *The International Journal of Robotics Research* 23(4–5):379–398.
28. S. Hesse and D. Uhlenbrock. (2000). A mechanized gait trainer for restoration of gait, *Journal of Rehabilitation Research and Development* 37(6):701–708.
29. H. Schmidt, S. Hesse, R. Bernhardt and J. Krüger. (2005). HapticWalker — a novel haptic foot device, *ACM Transactions on Applied Perception* (*TAP*) 2(2):166–180.
30. S. Hesse, A. Waldner and C. Tomelleri. (2010). Research innovative gait robot for the repetitive practice of floor walking and stair climbing up and down in stroke patients, *Journal of NeuroEngineering and Rehabilitation* 7(30).
31. J. L. Emken, S. J. Harkema, J. A. Beres-Jones, C. K. Ferreira and D. J. Reinkensmeyer. (2008). Feasibility of manual teach-and-replay and continuous impedance shaping for robotic locomotor training following spinal cord injury. *IEEE Transactions on Biomedical Engineering* 55(1):322–334.
32. G. Colombo, M. Joerg, R. Schreier and V. Dietz. (2000). Treadmill training of paraplegic patients using a robotic orthosis, *Journal of Rehabilitation Research and Development* 37(6):693–700.
33. R. Riener, L. Lünenburger, I. C. Maier, G. Colombo and V. Dietz. (2010). Locomotor training in subjects with sensori-motor deficits: an overview of the robotic gait orthosis Lokomat, *Journal of Healthcare Engineering* 1(2):197–216.
34. R. G. West. (2004). Powered gait orthosis and method of utilizing same. U.S Patent No. 6,689,075.
35. J. F. Veneman, R. Kruidhof, E. E. Hekman, R. Ekkelenkamp, E. H. Van Asseldonk and H. van der Kooij. (2007). Design and evaluation of the LOPES exoskeleton robot for interactive gait rehabilitation. *IEEE Transactions on Neural Systems and Rehabilitation Engineering: a Publication of the IEEE Engineering in Medicine and Biology Society* 15(3):379–386.
36. S. K. Banala, S. K. Agrawal and J. P. Scholz. (Eds.) (2007). Active Leg Exoskeleton (ALEX) for gait rehabilitation of motor-impaired patients. *Proceedings of the 2007 IEEE 10th International Conference on Rehabilitation Robotics*, June 12–15, Noordwijk, The Netherlands.
37. D. Aoyagi, W. E. Ichinose, S. J. Harkema, D. J. Reinkensmeyer and J. E. Bobrow. (2007). A robot and control algorithm that can synchronously assist in naturalistic motion during body-weight-supported gait training following neurologic injury. *IEEE Transactions on Neural Systems and Rehabilitation Engineering* 15(3):387–400.
38. D. J. Reinkensmeyer, D. Aoyagi, J. L. Emken, J. Galvez, W. Ichinose, G. Kerdanyan, S. Maneekobkunwong, K. Minakata, J. A. Nessler, R. Weber, R. R. Roy, R. deLeon, J. E. Bobrow, J. E. Harkema and V. R. Edgerton. (2006). Tools for understanding and optimizing robotic gait training, *Journal of Rehabilitation Research and Development* 43(5), 657–670.
39. M. Frey, G. Colombo, M. Vaglio, R. Bucher, M. Jorg and R. Riener. (2006). A novel mechatronic body weight support system. *IEEE Transactions on Neural Systems and Rehabilitation Engineering* 14(3):311–321.
40. K. Gordon, D. Ferris, M. Roberton, J. Beres and S. Harkema. (Eds.) (2000). The importance of using an appropriate body weight support system in locomotor training. Society for Neuroscience Proceedings.
41. H. Barbeau, M. Wainberg and L. Finch. (1987). Description and application of a system for locomotor rehabilitation, *Medical and Biological Engineering and Computing* 25(3):341–344.
42. K. E. Norman, A. Pepin, M. Ladouceur and H. Barbeau. (1995). A treadmill apparatus and harness support for evaluation and rehabilitation of gait, *Archives of Physical Medicine and Rehabilitation* 76(8):772–778.
43. F. Gazzani, A. Fadda, M. Torre and V. Macellari. (2000). WARD: a pneumatic system for body weight relief in gait rehabilitation. *IEEE Transactions on Rehabilitation Engineering* 8(4):506–513.

44. G. Chen, D. Schwandt, H. Van der Loos, J. Anderson, D. Ferris, F. Zajac, *et al.* (Eds.) (2001). Compliance-adjustable, force-sensing harness support for studying treadmill training in neurologically impaired subjects, *Proceedings of the 6th Annual Gait and Clinical Movement Analysis Meeting*, Sacramento, CA, USA.
45. J. He, R. Kram and T. A. McMahon. (1991). Mechanics of running under simulated low gravity, *Journal of Applied Physiology* 71(3):863–870.
46. R. Kram, A. Domingo and D. P. Ferris. (1997). Effect of reduced gravity on the preferred walk-run transition speed, *Journal of Experimental Biology* 200(4):821–826.
47. G. Cook. (2002). Exercise hoist. US Patent No. US 2002/0065173 A1.
48. C.-Y. Lee, K.-H. Seo, C. Oh and J.-J. Lee. (2003). Newly designed rehabilitation robot system for walking-aid with pneumatic actuator, *International Journal of Human-Friendly Welfare Robotic Systems* 4:42–46.
49. S. Kim, H. Shin, S.-H. Jung, J.-J. Lee and B.-O. Kim. (2002). Supporting force control of walking training robots, *International Journal of Human-Friendly Welfare Robotic Systems* 3:2–7.
50. J. M. Hollerbach, I. W. Hunter and J. Ballantyne. (Eds.) (1992). A comparative analysis of actuator technologies for robotics, *The Robotics Review* 2; MIT Press.
51. M. Frey, J. Hoogen, R. Burgkart and R. Riener (2006). 9 DOF Haptic Display of the Munich Knee Joint Simulator. *Presence-Teleoperators and Virtual Environments* 15:570–587.
52. D. A. Lawrence, editor. (1988). Impedance control stability properties in common implementations. *Proceedings of the 1988 IEEE International Conference on Robotics and Automation*; Philadelphia: IEEE.
53. K. Gordon, B. Svendesen, S. J. Harkema and S. El-alami. (2003). Closed-loop force controlled body weight support system. US Patent 2003/0153438 A1.
54. D. Kelsey and A. Walls. (1993). Therapeutic unloading apparatus and method. US Patent 5,273,502.
55. D. Surdilovic and R. Bernhardt. (Eds.) (2004). STRING-MAN: a new wire robot for gait rehabilitation. Robotics and Automation, *IEEE International Conference on ICRA'04*; New-Orleans.
56. G. Colombo, R. Bucher and R. Riener. (2008). Device for adjusting the height of and the relief force acting on a weight. EP Patent 1,586,291 B1.
57. G. Colombo and R. Bucher. (2010). Device for Adjusting the Prestress of an Elastic Means Around a Predetermined Tension or Position. US Patent 8,192,331 B2.
58. A. Pennycott, H. Vallery, D. Wyss, M. Spindler, A. Dewarrat and R. Riener. (2013). A Novel Body Weight Support System Extension for Balance Training, *IEEE International Conference on Rehabilitation Robotics (ICORR)*; Seattle, USA.
59. J. Hidler, D. Brennan, I. Black, D. Nichols, K. Brady and T. Nef. (2011). ZeroG: overground gait and balance training system, *Journal of Rehabilitation Research and Development* 48(4):287.
60. H. Vallery, O. Lutz, J. Von Zitzewitz, G. Rauter, M. Fritschi, C. Everarts, *et al.* (2013). Multidirectional Transparent Support for Overground Gait Training, *IEEE International Conference on Rehabilitation Robotics (ICORR)*; Seattle, USA.
61. C. H. An, C. G. Atkeson, J. D. Griffiths and J. M. Hollerbach. (1989). Experimental evaluation of feedforward and computed torque control. Robotics and Automation, *IEEE Transactions on* 5(3):368–373.
62. R. Kelly and R. Salgado. (1994). PD control with computed feedforward of robot manipulators: A design procedure. *IEEE Transactions on Robotics and Automation* 10(4):566–571.
63. S. Jezernik, K. Jezernik and M. Morari. (Eds.) (2002). Impedance control based gait-pattern adaptation for a robotic rehabilitation device, *Proceedings of the 2nd IFAC Conference on Mechatronic Systems*; Berkeley.

64. S. Jezernik, G. Colombo and M. Morari. (2004). Automatic gait-pattern adaptation algorithms for rehabilitation with a 4-DOF robotic orthosis. *IEEE Transactions on Robotics and Automation* 20(3):574–582.
65. R. Riener, L. Lunenburger, S. Jezernik, M. Anderschitz, G. Colombo and V. Dietz. (2005). Patient-cooperative strategies for robot-aided treadmill training: first experimental results. *IEEE Transactions on Neural Systems and Rehabilitation Engineering* 13(3):380–394.
66. N. A. Bernstein. (1967). *The Co-ordination and Regulation of Movements*. Pergamon Press Ltd, first English edition.
67. V. S. Huang and J. W. Krakauer. (2009). Robotic neurorehabilitation: a computational motor learning perspective, *Journal of NeuroEngineering and Rehabilitation* 6(1):5.
68. M. D. Lewek, T. H. Cruz, J. L. Moore, H. R. Roth, Y. Y. Dhaher and T. G. Hornby. (2009). Allowing intralimb kinematic variability during locomotor training poststroke improves kinematic consistency: a subgroup analysis from a randomized clinical trial, *Physical Therapy* 89(8):829–839.
69. L. L. Cai, A. J. Fong, C. K. Otoshi, Y. Q. Liang, J. G. Cham, H. Zhong, *et al.* (Eds.) (2005). Effects of consistency vs. variability in robotically controlled training of stepping in adult spinal mice. Rehabilitation Robotics, *9th International Conference on ICORR*, Chicago: IEEE.
70. A. W. Dromerick, D. F. Edwards and M. Hahn. (2000). Does the application of constraint-induced movement therapy during acute rehabilitation reduce arm impairment after ischemic stroke? *Stroke* 31(12):2984–2988.
71. L. Marchal-Crespo and D. J. Reinkensmeyer. (2008). Haptic guidance can enhance motor learning of a steering task, *Journal of Motor Behavior* 40(6):545–557.
72. C. J. Winstein, P. S. Pohl and R. Lewthwaite. (1994). Effects of physical guidance and knowledge of results on motor learning: support for the guidance hypothesis, *Research Quarterly for Exercise and Sport* 65(4):316–323.
73. J. E. Harris and J. J. Eng. (2010). Strength training improves upper-limb function in individuals with stroke a meta-analysis, *Stroke* 41(1):136–140.
74. A. Domingo and D. P. Ferris. (2009). Effects of physical guidance on short-term learning of walking on a narrow beam, *Gait and Posture* 30(4):464–468.
75. A. A. A. Timmermans, H. A. M. Seelen, R. D. Willmann and H. Kingma. (2009). Technology-assisted training of arm-hand skills in stroke: concepts on reacquisition of motor control and therapist guidelines for rehabilitation technology design, *Journal of NeuroEngineering and Rehabilitation* 6(1).
76. M. A. Perez, B. K. Lungholt, K. Nyborg and J. B. Nielsen. (2004). Motor skill training induces changes in the excitability of the leg cortical area in healthy humans, *Experimental Brain Research* 159(2):197–205.
77. R. Shadmehr and F. A. Mussa-Ivaldi. (1994). Adaptive representation of dynamics during learning of a motor task, *Journal of Neuroscience* 14(5):3208–3224.
78. A. Duschau-Wicke, J. von Zitzewitz, A. Caprez, L. Lunenburger and R. Riener. (2010). Path control: a method for patient-cooperative robot-aided gait rehabilitation, *IEEE Transactions on Neural Systems and Rehabilitation Engineering* 18(1):38–48.
79. H. I. Krebs, N. Hogan, M. L. Aisen and B. T. Volpe. (1998). Robot-aided neurorehabilitation, *IEEE Transactions on Rehabilitation Engineering* 6(1):75–87.
80. J. Hoogen, R. Riener, G. Schmidt. (2002). Control aspects of a robotic haptic interface for kinesthetic knee joint simulation, *Control Engineering Practice* 10(11):1301–1308.
81. R. J. Adams, M. R. Moreyra and B. Hannaford. (Eds.) (1998). Stability and performance of haptic displays: Theory and experiments, Proceedings ASME International Mechanical Engineering Congress and Exposition, Anaheim, CA, USA.
82. D. J. Reinkensmeyer, D. Aoyagi, J. L. Emken, J. A. Galvez, W. Ichinose, G. Kerdanyan, *et al.* (2006). Tools for understanding and optimizing robotic gait training, *Journal of Rehabilitation Research and Development* 43(5):657–670.

83. E. T. Wolbrecht, V. Chan, D. J. Reinkensmeyer and J. E. Bobrow. (2008). Optimizing compliant, model-based robotic assistance to promote neurorehabilitation. *IEEE Transactions on Neural Systems and Rehabilitation Engineering* 16(3):286–297.
84. C. Hollnagel, H. Vallery, R. Schädler, I. G.-L. López, L. Jaeger, P. Wolf, *et al.* (2013). Nonlinear adaptive controllers for an over-actuated pneumatic MR-compatible stepper, *Medical and Biological Engineering and Computing* 51(7):799–809.
85. E. T. Wolbrecht, D. J. Reinkensmeyer and J. E. Bobrow. (2010). Pneumatic control of robots for rehabilitation, *The International Journal of Robotics Research* 29(1):23–38.
86. D. J. Reinkensmeyer, E. T. Wolbrecht, V. Chan, C. Chou, S. C. Cramer and J. E. Bobrow. (2012). Comparison of Three-Dimensional, Assist-as-Needed Robotic Arm/Hand Movement Training Provided with Pneu-WREX to Conventional Tabletop Therapy After Chronic Stroke, *American Journal of Physical Medicine and Rehabilitation* 91(11):232–241.
87. B. M. Fleerkotte, J. H. Buurke, B. Koopman, L. Schaake, H. van der Kooij, E. H. F. van Asseldonk, *et al.* (2013). Effectiveness of the Lower Extremity Powered ExoSkeleton (LOPES) Robotic Gait Trainer on Ability and Quality of Walking in SCI Patients, *Converging Clinical and Engineering Research on Neurorehabilitation*: Springer, 161–165. See here: https://link.springer.com/chapter/10.1007/978-3-642-34546-3_26.
88. H. I. Krebs, J. J. Palazzolo, L. Dipietro, M. Ferraro, J. Krol, K. Rannekleiv *et al.* (2003). Rehabilitation robotics: Performance-based progressive robot-assisted therapy, *Autonomous Robots* 15(1):7–20.
89. A. Duschau-Wicke, A. Caprez and R. Riener. (2010). Patient-cooperative control increases active participation of individuals with SCI during robot-aided gait training, *Journal of Neuroengineering and Rehabilitation* 7(43):1–13.
90. A. Schück, R. Labruyère, H. Vallery, R. Riener and A. Duschau-Wicke. (2012). Feasibility and effects of patient-cooperative robot-aided gait training applied in a 4-week pilot trial, *Journal of Neuroengineering and Rehabilitation* 9(1):31.
91. C. Krishnan, R. Ranganathan, S. S. Kantak, Y. Y. Dhaher and W. Z. Rymer. (2012). Active robotic training improves locomotor function in a stroke survivor, *Journal of Neuroengineering and Rehabilitation* 9(1):1–13.
92. C. Krishnan, D. Kotsapouikis, Y. Y. Dhaher and W. Z. Rymer. (2013). Reducing Robotic Guidance During Robot-Assisted Gait Training Improves Gait Function: A Case Report on a Stroke Survivor, *Archives of Physical Medicine and Rehabilitation* 94(6): 1202–1206.
93. M. Guidali, P. Schlink, A. Duschau-Wicke, R. Riener. (Eds.) (2011). Online learning and adaptation of patient support during ADL training. *IEEE International Conference on Rehabilitation Robotics (ICORR)*; IEEE.
94. M. Guidali, A. Duschau-Wicke, S. Broggi, V. Klamroth-Marganska, T. Nef and R. Riener. (2011). A robotic system to train activities of daily living in a virtual environment, *Medical and Biological Engineering and Computing* 49(10): 1213–1223.
95. M. Guidali, A. Duschau-Wicke, M. Büchel, A. Brunschweiler, T. Nef and R. Riener. (2009). Path control — a strategy for patient-cooperative arm rehabilitation. AUTOMED; Berlin: Fortschritt-Berichte VDI, Reihe 17, Nr. 274.
96. M. Guidali, M. Büchel, V. Klamroth, T. Nef and R. Riener. (Eds.) (2009). Trajectory planning in ADL tasks for an exoskeletal arm rehabilitation robot, Proceedings of the European Conference on Technically Assisted Rehabilitation, Berlin.
97. U. Keller, G. Rauter and R. Riener. (2013). Assist-as-needed path control for the PASCAL rehabilitation robot. *IEEE International Conference on Rehabilitation Robotics (ICORR)*; Seattle.
98. J. Von Zitzewitz, A. Morger, G. Rauter, L. Marchal-Crespo, F. Crivelli, D. Wyss, *et al.* (2013). A reconfigurable, tendon-based haptic interface for research into human-environment interactions, *Robotica* 31:441–453.

99. G. Rauter, R. Sigrist, L. Marchal-Crespo, H. Vallery, R. Riener and P. Wolf. (Eds.) (2011). Assistance or challenge? Filling a gap in user-cooperative control, in *IEEE/RSJ International Conference on Intelligent Robots and Systems (IROS)* 3068–3073.
100. G. Rauter, J. von Zitzewitz, A. Duschau-Wicke, H. Vallery and R. Riener. (Eds.) (2010). A tendon-based parallel robot applied to motor learning in sports. Biomedical Robotics and Biomechatronics (BioRob), *International Conference on 3rd IEEE RAS and EMBS* 82–87.
101. G. Rauter, N. Gerig, H. Vallery, R. Sigrist, R. Riener and P. Wolf. (2013). Hybrid Path Control Enables Haptic Guidance Along Self-Crossing Paths, *IEEE Transactions on Robotics.* submitted.
102. L. Marchal-Crespo, G. Rauter, D. Wyss, J. von Zitzewitz, R. Riener. (Eds.) (2012). Synthesis and control of an assistive robotic tennis trainer. *4th IEEE RAS & EMBS International Conference on Biomedical Robotics and Biomechatronics (BioRob)* 355–360.
103. L. Marchal-Crespo, M. Bannwart, R. Riener and H. Vallery. (2014) The effect of haptic guidance on learning a hybrid rhythmic-discrete motor task. *IEEE Transactions on Haptics* 8:222–234.
104. H. Vallery, A. Duschau-Wicke and R. Riener. (Eds.) (2009). Generalized elasticities improve patient-cooperative control of rehabilitation robots. *2009 IEEE 11th International Conference on Rehabilitation Robotics Kyoto International Conference Center*; Japan, June 23–26.
105. H. Vallery, A. Duschau-Wicke and R. Riener. (Eds.) (2009). Optimized passive dynamics improve transparency of haptic devices. *2009 IEEE International Conference on Robotics and Automation, 2009. ICRA '09*; Kobe, Japan. pp. 01-306, Publication date: 09/5/12.
106. G. A. Pratt, M. M. Williamson, P. Dillworth, J. E. Pratt and A. Wright. (Eds.) (1995). Stiffness Isn't Everything, *The 4th International Symposium on Experimental Robotics (ISER)*; Springer-Verlag.
107. E. Colgate and N. Hogan. (Eds.) (1989). An analysis of contact instability in terms of passive physical equivalents. *Proceedings of the IEEE International Conference on Robotics and Automation (ICRA)*; Scottsdale, AZ, USA, pp. 404–409.
108. B. Siciliano and O. Khatib. (2008). *Springer Handbook of Robotics*. Springer.
109. J. E. Colgate. (1988). *The Control of Dynamically Interacting Systems*. Massachusetts Institute of Technology.
110. A. Duschau-Wicke, J. von Zitzewitz, M. Wellner, A. König, L. Lunenburger and R. Riener. (Eds.) (2007). Path control a strategy for patient-cooperative training of gait timing, *Proceedings of the 7th Automed Workshop*; Munich.
111. R. Riener, L. Lünenburger and G. Colombo. (2006). Human-centered robotics applied to gait training and assessment, *Journal of Rehabilitation Research and Development* 43(5): 679–694.
112. R. W. Teasell, S. K. Bhogal, N. C. Foley and M. R. Speechley. (2003). Gait retraining post stroke, *Topics in Stroke Rehabilitation* 10(2):34–65.
113. D. Novak, J. Ziherl, A. Olensek, M. Milavec, J. Podobnik, M. Mihelj, *et al.* (2010). Psychophysiological responses to robotic rehabilitation tasks in stroke. *IEEE Transactions on Neural Systems and Rehabilitation Engineering* 18(4):351–361.
114. D. Novak, M. Mihelj, J. Ziherl, A. Olensek and M. Munih. (2011). Psychophysiological measurements in a biocooperative feedback loop for upper extremity rehabilitation. *IEEE Transactions on Neural Systems and Rehabilitation Engineering* 19(4):400–410.
115. D. Novak, M. Mihelj and M. Munih. (2011). Psychophysiological responses to different levels of cognitive and physical workload in haptic interaction, *Robotica* 29(03):367–374.
116. A. Koenig, D. Novak, X. Omlin, M. Pulfer, E. Perreault, L. Zimmerli, *et al.* (2011). Real-time closed-loop control of cognitive load in neurological patients during robot-assisted gait training. *IEEE Transactions on Neural Systems and Rehabilitation Engineering* 19(4): 453–464.

117. A. Koenig, X. Omlin, L. Zimmerli, M. Sapa, C. Krewer, M. Bolliger, *et al.* (2011). Psychological state estimation from physiological recordings during robot assisted gait rehabilitation, *Journal of Rehabilitation Research and Development* 48(4):367–386.
118. A. Koenig, X. Omlin, J. Bergmann, L. Zimmerli, M. Bolliger, F. Müller, *et al.* (2011). Controlling patient participation during robot-assisted gait training, *Journal of Neuroengineering and Rehabilitation* 8(1):14.
119. C. Cozean, W. Pease and S. Hubbell. (1988). Biofeedback and functional electric stimulation in stroke rehabilitation, *Archives of Physical Medicine and Rehabilitation* 69(6):401–405.
120. J. D. Moreland, M. A. Thomson and A. R. Fuoco. (1998). Electromyographic biofeedback to improve lower extremity function after stroke: a meta-analysis, *Archives of Physical Medicine and Rehabilitation* 79(2):134–140.
121. A. Mandel, J. Nymark, S. Balmer, D. Grinnell and M. O'Riain. (1990). Electromyographic versus rhythmic positional biofeedback in computerized gait retraining with stroke patients, *Archives of Physical Medicine and Rehabilitation* 71(9):649–654.
122. G. R. Colborne, S. J. Olney and M. P. Grifin. (1993). Feedback of ankle joint angle and soleus the rehabilitation of hemiplegic gait, *Archives of Physical Medicine and Rehabilitation* 74(10):1100–1106.
123. M. E. Morris, T. M. Bach and P. A. Goldie. (1992). Electrogoniometric feedback: its effect on genu recurvatum in stroke, *Archives of Physical Medicine and Rehabilitation* 73(12):1.
124. A. S. Aruin, S. Rob Larkins, Gouri Chaudhuri, Alexander. (2000). Knee position feedback: its effect on management of pelvic instability in a stroke patient, *Disability and Rehabilitation* 22(15):690–692.
125. R. Montoya, P. Dupui, B. Pages and P. Bessou. (1994). Step-length biofeedback device for walk rehabilitation, *Medical and Biological Engineering and Computing* 32(4):416–420.
126. M. Batavia, J. G. Gianutsos and M. Kambouris. (1997). An augmented auditory feedback device, *Archives of Physical Medicine and Rehabilitation* 78(12): 1389–1392.
127. R. P. Van Peppen, G. Kwakkel, S. Wood-Dauphinee, H. J. Hendriks, P. J. Van der Wees and J. Dekker. (2004). The impact of physical therapy on functional outcomes after stroke: what's the evidence? *Clinical Rehabilitation* 18(8):833–862.
128. J. E. Bolek. (2003). A preliminary study of modification of gait in real-time using surface electromyography, *Applied Psychophysiology and Biofeedback* 28(2):129–138.
129. A. Koenig, K. Brutsch, L. Zimmerli, M. Guidali, A. Duschau-Wicke, M. Wellner, *et al.* (Eds.) (2008). Virtual environments increase participation of children with cerebral palsy in robot-aided treadmill training. Virtual Rehabilitation, *Virtual Rehabilitation*, IEEE.
130. K. Brütsch, T. Schuler, A. Koenig, L. Zimmerli, S. Mérillat, L. Lünenburger, *et al.* (2010). Influence of virtual reality soccer game on walking performance in robotic assisted gait training for children, *Journal of Neuroengineering and Rehabilitation* 7(1):15.
131. K. Brutsch, A. Koenig, L. Zimmerli, S. Merillat-Koeneke, R. Riener, L. Jancke, *et al.* (2011). Virtual reality for enhancement of robot-assisted gait training in children with neurological gait disorders, *Journal of Rehabilitation Medicine* 43(6):493–499.
132. J. Petrofsky. (2001). The use of electromyogram biofeedback to reduce Trendelenburg gait, *European Journal of Applied Physiology* 85(5):491–495.
133. C. Phillips, R. Koubek and D. Hendershot. (1991). Walking while using a sensory tactile feedback system: potential use with a functional electrical stimulation orthosis, *Journal of Biomedical Engineering* 13(2):91–96.
134. S. Hirokawa and K. Matsumura. (1989). Biofeedback gait training system for temporal and distance factors, *Medical and Biological Engineering and Computing* 27(1):8–13.
135. M. C. F. De Castro and Jr. A. Cliquet. (2000). Artificial sensorimotor integration in spinal cord injured subjects through neuromuscular and electrotactile stimulation, *Artificial Organs* 24(9):710–717.

136. M. Batavia, J. G. Gianutsos, A. Vaccaro and J. T. Gold. (2001). A do-it-yourself membrane-activated auditory feedback device for weight bearing and gait training: A case report, *Archives of Physical Medicine and Rehabilitation* 82(4):541–545.
137. V. G. Femery, P. G. Moretto, J.-M. G. Hespel, A. Thévenon and G. Lensel. (2004). A real-time plantar pressure feedback device for foot unloading, *Archives of Physical Medicine and Rehabilitation* 85(10):1724–1728.
138. S. L. Wolf and S. A. Binder-Macleod. (1983). Electromyographic biofeedback applications to the hemiplegic patient changes in upper extremity neuromuscular and functional status, *Physical Therapy* 63(9):1393–1403.
139. J. Inglis, M. Donald, T. Monga, M. Sproule and M. Young. (1984). Electromyographic biofeedback and physical therapy of the hemiplegic upper limb, *Archives of Physical Medicine and Rehabilitation* 65(12):755–759.
140. J. Crow, N. Lincoln, F. Nouri and Wd. Weerdt. (1989). The effectiveness of EMG biofeedback in the treatment of arm function after stroke, *Disability and Rehabilitation* 11(4):155–160.
141. R. E. Schleenbaker and A. G. Mainous. (1993). Electromyographic biofeedback for neuromuscular reeducation in the hemiplegic stroke patient: a meta-analysis, *Archives of Physical Medicine and Rehabilitation* 74(12):1301–1304.
142. L. Lünenburger, G. Colombo, R. Riener and V. Dietz. (Eds.) (2004). Biofeedback in gait training with the robotic orthosis Lokomat. Engineering in Medicine and Biology Society, *26th Annual International Conference of the IEEE on IEMBS'04*; IEEE.
143. L. Lünenburger, G. Colombo and R. Riener. (2007). Biofeedback for robotic gait rehabilitation, *Journal of Neuroengineering and Rehabilitation* 4(1):1.
144. R. Banz, M. Bolliger, G. Colombo, V. Dietz and L. Lünenburger. (2008). Computerized visual feedback: an adjunct to robotic-assisted gait training, *Physical Therapy* 88(10):1135–1145.
145. R. Banz, M. Bolliger, S. Muller, C. Santelli and R. Riener. (2009). A method of estimating the degree of active participation during stepping in a driven gait orthosis based on actuator force profile matching, *IEEE Transactions on Neural Systems and Rehabilitation Engineering* 17(1):15–22.
146. L. Lünenburger, M. Wellner, R. Banz, G. Colombo and R. Riener. (Eds.) (2007). Combining immersive virtual environments with robot-aided gait training, *IEEE 10th International Conference on ICORR* 421–424.
147. M. Girone, G. Burdea, M. Bouzit, V. Popescu and J. Deutsch. (2000). Orthopedic rehabilitation using the "Rutgers ankle" interface, *Studies in Health Technology and Informatics* 89–95.
148. M. Ohsuga, Y. Tatsuno, F. Shimono, K. Hirasawa, H. Oyama and H. Okamura. (1998). Development of a bedside wellness system, *Cyberpsychology and Behavior* 1(2):105–112.
149. G. Riva. (1998). Virtual reality in paraplegia: A VR-enhanced orthopaedic appliance for walking and rehabilitation, *Stud Health Technol Inform.* 58:209–218.
150. J. Fung, F. Malouin, B. McFadyen, F. Comeau, A. Lamontagne, S. Chapdelaine, *et al.* (Eds.) (2004). Locomotor rehabilitation in a complex virtual environment. Engineering in Medicine and Biology Society, *26th Annual International Conference on IEMBS'04*; IEEE.
151. J. Patton, G. Dawe, C. Scharver, F. Mussa-Ivaldi and R. Kenyon. (Eds.) (2004). Robotics and virtual reality: the development of a life-sized 3-D system for the rehabilitation of motor function. Engineering in Medicine and Biology Society, *26th Annual International Conference on IEMBS'04*; IEEE.
152. E. Keshner, R. Kenyon and Y. Dhaher. (Eds.) (2004). Postural research and rehabilitation in an immersive virtual environment. Engineering in Medicine and Biology Society, *26th Annual International Conference on IEMBS'04*; IEEE.
153. A. Koenig, X. Omlin, J. Bergmann, L. Zimmerli, M. Bolliger, F. Müller, *et al.* (2011). Controlling patient participation during robot assisted gait training, *Journal of Neuroengineering and Rehabilitation* 8(1):14.

154. A. Koenig, K. Brutsch, L. Zimmerli, M. Guidali, A. Duschau-Wicke, M. Wellner, *et al.* (Eds.) (2008). Virtual environments increase participation of children with cerebral palsy in robot-aided treadmill training. *Virtual Rehabilitation*; IEEE.
155. K. Brütsch, T. Schuler, A. Koenig, L. Zimmerli, S. Mérillat, L. Lünenburger, *et al.* (2010). Influence of virtual reality soccer game on walking performance in robotic assisted gait training for children, *Journal of Neuroengineering and Rehabilitation* 7(1):15.
156. R. Riener, L. Lünenburger, I. C. Maier, G. Colombo and V. Dietz. (2010). Locomotor training in subjects with sensorimotor deficits: an overview of the robotic gait orthosis Lokomat, *Journal of Health Engineering* 1(2):197–216.
157. J. Hidler, D. Nichols, M. Pelliccio, K. Brady, D. D. Campbell, J. H. Kahn and T. G. Hornby. (2009). Multicenter randomized clinical trial evaluating the effectiveness of the Lokomat in subacute stroke, *Neurorehabilitation and Neural Repair* 23(1):5–13.
158. T. G. Hornby, D. D. Campbell, J. H. Kahn, T. Demott, J. L. Moore and H. R. Roth. (2008). Enhanced gait-related improvements after therapist- versus robotic-assisted locomotor training in subjects with chronic stroke. A randomized controlled study, *Stroke* 39:1786–1792.
159. J. Mehrholz, C. Werner, J. Kugler and M. Pohl. (2013). Electromechanical-assisted training for walking after stroke, *Cochrane Database of Systematic Reviews* 7.
160. U. Dundar, *et al.* (2014). A Comparative Study of Conventional Physiotherapy Versus Robotic Training Combined with Physiotherapy in Patients with Stroke, *Topics in Stroke Rehabilitation* 21.6:453–461.
161. R. Riener. (2012). Rehabilitation Robotics. *Foundations and Trends in Robotics* 3(1–2): 1–137.

Chapter 2

RESEARCH AND DEVELOPMENT TRENDS IN ROBOT-ASSISTED WALKING REHABILITATION INCORPORATING POSTURAL BALANCING

K. H. Low and Lei Li

School of Mechanical and Aerospace Engineering
Nanyang Technological University, 50 Nanyang Avenue, Singapore 639798

In recent years, robotic technology has been suggested in walking rehabilitation to replace traditional manual-assisted training. However, the effectiveness of the robot-assisted walking training does not show clear superiority to manually-assisted training. One of the possible reasons may be due to the limited balance training activities provided in the current walking rehabilitation robots. On the other hand, high falling rate is observed in both stroke patients and elderly persons, which demonstrates the importance of walking postural balance training. In this chapter, a review of walking postural balance training is therefore devoted to investigate the current advancements, limitations and discuss about possible solutions. Firstly, the mechanism of walking postural balance control is studied through three aspects: proactive (or anticipatory) walking postural balance control, reactive walking postural balance control, and balance state feedback. Next, a review of the existing robotic technology for the walking rehabilitation is presented by focusing on the aspect of postural balance training. Finally, the chapter discusses possible ways to improve balance training activities during robot-assisted walking training through robotic hardware and control algorithm. In conclusion, balance-training activities are essential in a rehabilitation program. More and more rehabilitation systems are shifting their attention toward postural balance-training capabilities. Nevertheless, it is still unclear which are the optimal approaches to enhance the balance-training properties. Rigorous clinical evidences are needed to support these new approaches. We are optimistic that with careful research and consideration on the principle of human postural balance and its application to robot design and control, the efficiency of robot-assisted rehabilitation walking training can be improved.

1. Introduction

It is commonly known that the human locomotion control system has a heuristic structure and consists of the supra-spinal system (cerebrum and cerebellum), spinal cord, and the musculoskeletal system that interact with each other through sensory feedback to achieve stable locomotion.[1] Because of the complex interactions between different systems, various diseases (stroke, Parkinson disease, spinal cord injury (SCI), myopathies, and sensory deficits), traumatic accidents or aging can cause the dysfunction of the sub-systems as shown in Fig. 1.

Among the various diseases, stroke is the primary cause of long-term disability[2,3] and patients often experience poor walking capabilities. Due to the lack of effective medical drug treatment, most stroke patients mainly rely on physical rehabilitation.[4] in order to regain the ability to walk. Among various rehabilitation strategies,[5,6] task-specific training is currently the most promising rehabilitation strategy,[7] which suggests that "the best way to improve walking is to walk".[8]

Therapist-assisted body weight support (BWS) gait rehabilitation was the first and is the most widely used method to realize task-specific training principle. It is carried out by suspending the subject to be trained over a treadmill using a cable-harness apparatus with therapists guiding the movements of the patient's pelvis and lower limbs. The cable-harness system can provide partial body support, which facilitates walking training. However, for the therapist-assisted BWS gait rehabilitation approach, labor costs are high since three therapists have to be engaged to train a single subject. Therefore, robot-assisted walking rehabilitation was recently proposed as a solution to this limitation. In robot-assisted walking rehabilitation which is becoming increasingly popular,[9] the training subject is aided by a robotic device instead of therapists. Besides the ability of reducing the physical demand on therapists, a robot can not only provide quantifiable assistance but also track the performance of the training subject by measuring the biofeedback from the subject.[10–12]

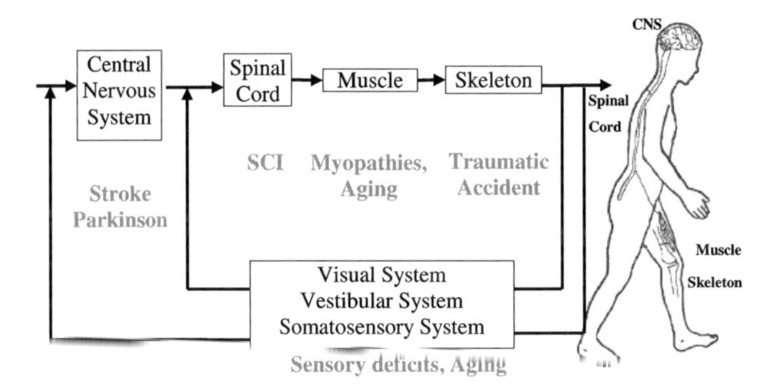

Figure 1. Human locomotion control system.

A number of researches have shown the effectiveness of robot-assisted gait training for stroke patients. Improvements of the quality of walking are shown in different aspects as summarized in Ref. [9]. However, robot-assisted rehabilitation has not shown a clear superiority compared with therapist-assisted rehabilitation. Some research results showed that therapist-assisted training[13,14] is better, while some proved the superiority of robot-assisted rehabilitation.[15,16] There are also some studies that showed limited differences between the two training methods on functional gait improvements.[17,18]

It can be seen that, despite the rapid development of the robot-assisted walking rehabilitation, the technology and training method have not fulfilled the expectations of the rehabilitation field. One of the possible reasons may be due to the lack of balance training in current walking rehabilitation robots.[19] As pointed out in Ref. [9], numerous mechanical constraints can result in poor balance training in current rehabilitation robots. At the same time, falls are observed to be common in all stages of stroke (acute, rehabilitative, and chronic).[20] These incidents cause serious injury which reduces independence and the quality of life of patients.[21] In addition, the deterioration of balance function in aged people increases their risk of falling which results in more than 11,000 deaths each year.[22] All these evidences emphasize the importance of balance training during walking rehabilitation.

Thus, this chapter contributes to the review of current methods in walking balance rehabilitation research and includes suggestions on possible future directions to improve balance training in robot-assisted walking rehabilitation. This review includes a biomechanical study of postural balance control and rehabilitation robots with the function of postural balance training. First, the mechanism of walking postural balance control is explained in Sec. 2. The essential elements of walking postural balance control are identified and grouped into proactive walking postural balance control (Sec. 2.1) and reactive walking postural balance control (Sec. 2.2). In addition, different biofeedbacks related to balance are reviewed (Sec. 2.3). Then, the existing robotic technology for walking rehabilitation is reviewed in Secs. 3 and 4. Section 3 focuses on robotic systems with proactive walking postural balance control training abilities, while Sec. 4 focuses on robotic systems with reactive walking postural balance control training abilities. Finally, better walking rehabilitation robot designs, control algorithms and more appropriate rehabilitation strategies, which are needed to cover the current gaps in walking rehabilitation, are discussed in Sec. 5.

2. Mechanism of Postural Balance Control During Walking

Postural balance control is defined as the act of maintaining, achieving or restoring a state of balance during any posture or activity.[23,24] Postural balance control consists of two parts: postural orientation control and postural equilibrium control.[25] Postural orientation control is defined as the task-specific coordination of different body segments with respect to the environment.[25] On the other hand, postural equilibrium control (maintaining balance) is defined as the coordination of different body segments to regulate the movement of Center of Mass (CoM) during both self-initiated and externally triggered disturbances.[25] Usually, postural balance control requirements are both task- and environment-dependent.

In the case of the walking function, the postural orientation control and equilibrium control are equivalent to gait pattern control and walking equilibrium control:

- Gait pattern control
  — It refers to the control of the walking gait pattern, which is the limb movement pattern of a person during walking that aims to maintain posture and facilitate movement.
- Walking equilibrium control
  — Walking equilibrium control involves the use of different body segment movement strategies such as ankle, hip, and stepping strategies to stabilize the body's CoM when facing perturbation during walking.

The walking postural balance control is affected by both the gait pattern control and the walking equilibrium control. As summarized in Ref. [20], gait deficits include reduced propulsion at push-off (PO), decreased hip and knee flexion during the swing-phase, reduced stability during the stance-phase, while balance deficits can comprise postural stability during quiet standing, and cause delays and less coordinated responses to both self-induced and external balance perturbations.

The first step in finding the optimal balance training approaches is to understand the underlying mechanism of postural balance control. The mechanisms used in gait pattern control and walking equilibrium control are different. The mechanism that is used in gait pattern control is defined as a proactive balance control mechanism while the mechanism that is used in walking equilibrium control is defined as a reactive balance control mechanism. Both the mechanisms are investigated in the following sections.

2.1. *Proactive (anticipatory) walking postural balance control mechanism*

Proactive (anticipatory) postural balance control is defined as the action of modifying postural balance prior to a potentially destabilizing movement in order to avoid instability. The proactive walking postural balance control during walking can be divided into four sub-tasks. Walking is considered to be stable if the four sub-tasks have been achieved:

- Task 1: Weight bearing of stance knee
- Task 2: Up-trunk posture
- Task 3: Bodyweight transfer
- Task 4: Sufficient foot clearance and pre-position for weight acceptance.

Reduced muscular strength, which is usually caused by stroke-induced Central Nervous System damage, often results in reduced weight bearing on the paretic knee and stabilizing the trunk on the paretic hip. The key element in completing Tasks 1 and 2 is the muscle strength and appropriate triggering of the muscle movements. Enough muscle strength is needed to produce the joint torques to keep the desired posture. However, the effect of direct muscle strength training on improving functional walking is not clear.[26] For example, walking speed and distance are not increased when additional resistance during leg cycling is included in bodyweight-supported gait training.[27] The hypothesis is that the balance of the patient is improved because of the compensation movement strategies[28,29] rather than the improvement in the strength of the paretic leg.[30,31] Thus, it is highlighted that training the appropriate muscle triggering mechanism is necessary when designing the rehabilitation programs in enhancing Tasks 1 and 2.

For Task 3, the transfer of support requires the coordination of two legs in a closed loop structure to move the CoM from the trailing leg to the leading leg. The poor quality of bodyweight shift will cause an unbalanced state when the walking enters the single stance-phase. Traditional training methods such as shifting of bodyweight using a force platform,[32,33] compelled bodyweight shift by means of a shoe insert,[34] raising a foot on a step,[35] walking with wall support,[36] etc. are used and have proven to be effective. In contrast, in the current robotic-assisted walking rehabilitation programs, the training of Task 3 is limited due to mechanical constraints at the pelvis. Thus, an improved mechanical pelvic mechanism design is needed.

Lastly, the subject has to produce enough foot clearance to prevent stumbling during the swing-phase of gait. This can be trained by performing a stepping action repeatedly. This feature has already been highlighted in most of the robot-assisted walking training systems. Future attention is needed to focus on how to reduce the inertia added on the leg to increase the transparency of the system. A detailed review on robotic systems covering the proactive walking postural balance training is presented in Sec. 3.

2.2. *Reactive walking postural balance control mechanism*

Reactive postural balance control is defined as the ability to regain balance after an unexpected perturbation. Appropriate control of ground reaction force (GRF) is needed to counter the disturbances. Controlling GRF is a difficult task as subjects cannot control the GRF directly. Subjects can only modulate the GRF through dynamic interactions with the Base of Support (BoS).

Different strategies are employed to create dynamic interactions depending on the different levels of instability:

- Minimal Instability
  - The "Ankle Strategy" is a simple response that involves rotation at the ankle. It is used in the case of small perturbations and the torque provided by the ankle joint limits its effect.
- Medium Instability
  - The "Hip Strategy" is a more complex response that involves rotation at the hip. When the perturbation is larger and the CoM is required to adjust quickly, the hip strategy is usually employed.
- Maximum Instability
  - "Stepping Strategy" and "Grasping Strategy" involve multiple segments of the body. They are employed when the ankle and hip strategies are not enough to recover to equilibrium state. For example, the stepping strategy is employed to change the position and the areas of the BoS in order to make the CoM inside BoS.

A three-segment model (shank, thigh, and trunk) without a swing-leg is used here to illustrate the principle of different strategies in regulating the movements of CoM. The dynamics discussed here are restricted to the sagittal plane but can be easily extended to study lateral dynamics. The dynamics of the three segments model shown in Fig. 2(a) are equivalent to the inverted pendulum model with a point mass and rotation inertia I shown in Fig. 2(b).[37] The dynamic equation of the pendulum model can be expressed as[37]

$$\begin{aligned} ml^2\ddot{\theta}_1 &= mgl\sin\theta_1 - 2ml\dot{l}\dot{\theta}_1 - \tau \\ m\ddot{l} &= F - mg\cos\theta_1 + ml\dot{\theta}_1{}^2 \end{aligned} \quad \text{with} \quad \begin{aligned} F &= f(\tau_a, \tau_k, \tau_h, \theta_a, \theta_k, \theta_h) \\ I\ddot{\theta}_b &= \tau, \end{aligned} \tag{1}$$

where θ_1 is the angle of the line which connects the Center of Pressure (CoP) and CoM, θ_b is the rotational angle of the inertia I with respect to the centerline of the pendulum, l is the distance from the CoP to the CoM, τ is the net torque about CoP created by the rotational inertia, F is the nonlinear mapping from joint torques to effective force on the point mass along the direction from the ground pivot to the mass, and P is the CoP point where the resultant ground reaction force F_{GRF} is applied.

It can be seen from Eq. (1) that there are three ways to relate CoM motion to its corresponding CoP. The first method is to change the location of the CoP, P, which

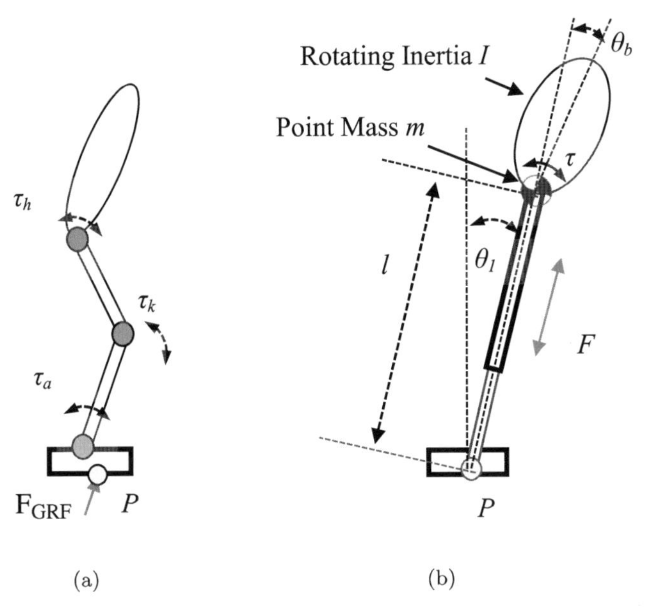

Figure 2. Simplified dynamic models of a human: (a) three-segment model in sagittal plane and (b) inverted pendulum model with rotational inertia.

changes the direction of the ground reaction force. This changes the motion of the CoM in such a way that if the CoP is to the left of the point mass, the mass will accelerate to the right and *vice versa*. By moving the CoP, the CoM motion can be controlled, but only to the extent that the CoP remains inside the BoS. Since the most effective way to change the location of the CoP is by the motion of the ankle joint, this method is named as the ankle strategy.

The second method is to rotate the inertia of the trunk (pitch the trunk forward or backward), and this is named as the hip strategy. A rotational acceleration $\ddot{\theta}_b$ of trunk inertia will create an acceleration of the CoM. The hip strategy is employed if the perturbation is medium and the rotation of the upper body forward can prevent the subject from falling backward and *vice versa*.

The third and least effective method is to change l, which is the distance from the CoP to the CoM. This method can be achieved by using the knee joint. However, compared to the previous two methods, this is the least effective method as l is restricted by biomechanics and must always be greater than zero.

In the situation when large perturbation occurs, a step has to be made to regain balance. Theoretical work on the stepping strategy can be found in Ref. [38] where the correct foot stepping point is defined and named as the Capture Point. In the theorem of Capture Point, the biped model would reach the upright balanced state if it were to instantaneously place the swing-foot on the Capture Point as shown in Fig. 3. The Capture Point in sagittal plane can be derived by using the orbital

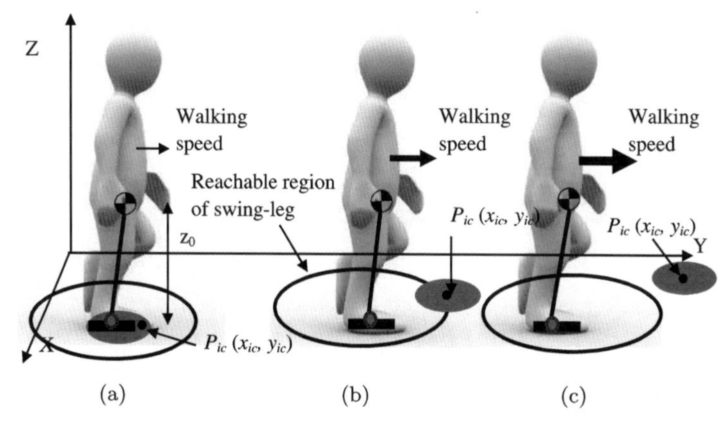

Figure 3. Illustration of human balance state by Capture Point (black dot) and Capture Region (represented by red circle) using a biped model.

energy principle and the conserved quantity named as the Linear Inverted Pendulum Orbital Energy.[39] The same principle can be applied to study the lateral dynamics. The Linear Inverted Pendulum Orbital Energy in sagittal plane can be expressed as

$$E_{\text{LIPM},x} = \frac{1}{2}\dot{x}^2 - \left(\frac{g}{2z_0}\right)(x - x_{\text{ankle}})^2, \tag{2}$$

when $E_{\text{LIPM},x} = 0$, x eventually comes to rest above x_{ic}. Substituting $E_{LIPM,x} = 0$ into (2) and solving for x_{ic} yield

$$x_{ic} = x + \dot{x}\sqrt{\frac{z_0}{g}}. \tag{3}$$

If the biped steps over the capture point x_{ic}, then the velocity $\dot{x}$ will be less than zero when the balanced state is reached. Then, the biped will fall backwards due to gravity. If the biped steps before the capture point x_{ic}, then the velocity $\dot{x}$ will be greater than zero when the balanced state is reached and the biped will continue to fall forward. When the rotational inertia is considered, the Capture Point can be extended into a Capture Region (CR).[38] When the CR intersects the BoS, the human can modulate its CoP to balance without taking a step (Fig. 3(a)). When the CR and the BoS are apart, a step must be taken to let the biped to come to a stop (Fig. 3(b)). If the CR is not covered by the reachable region of the swing-foot, more than one step is required to let the biped to come to a stop (Fig. 3(c)).

Numerous balance-training methods that are non-robotic and task-specific have been developed to target reactive postural balance control. These include balancing on various support surfaces, walking over obstacles, walking with various challenges and responses to perturbations including both self-induced (e.g. weight-shifting) and externally applied.[40] Decreases in the number of falling occurrences and increase in the activity levels in the participants[40,41] have been observed using these approaches. Various robotic systems have recently been developed to reproduce these effects by using electric motors to create similar perturbations. A brief review on robotic systems covering the reactive walking postural balance training is presented in Sec. 4.

2.3. *Balance evaluation index*

In general, walking postural stability is achieved by controlling the interactions between the CoM and BoS in order to regulate the motion of CoM. Some metrics developed to measure the postural stability in both the biomechanical field and the bipedal robotic field have been discussed in the following sections.

2.3.1. *Center of pressure (CoP)*

A biped is considered to be statically stable if the Projection of Center of Mass (PCoM), which is the project point of the CoM on the ground, lies within the BoS. Compared to PCoM, a more suitable index that considers dynamics is the CoP. The CoP is a point where the resultant vertical forces are applied to the foot. The CoP can also be described as a point where the sum of forces could be applied without generating a moment about it and is hence called the Zero Moment Point (ZMP). The biped that is considered to be dynamically stable is the CoP/ZMP which lies within the BoS. Figure 4 shows the relationship between the CoP and the PCoM in different phases of walking. In the initial swing, the CoP and PCoM coincide since there is no acceleration of CoM as shown in Fig. 4(a). The CoP remains within the BoS and is thus considered to be balanced. During the middle-stance-phase, the CoP moves behind the PCoM since the CoM accelerates forward. The biped is still considered stable as the CoP is within the BoS as shown in Fig. 4(b). In the pre-landing phase, the CoP moves in front of the PCoM as shown in Fig. 4(c) as the biped starts to decelerate. Then, the CoP will keep on moving forward until it reaches the edge of the foot as shown in Fig. 4(d). Meanwhile, the CoM that is out of the BoS will create a moment causing the subject to fall around the edge of the BoS. The swing-leg needs to land in time to prevent the fall.

2.3.2. *Extrapolated center of mass (XcoM)*

The extrapolated center of mass (XcoM) is suggested as a complementary measurement to the position of CoM and CoP. It has been discussed in Ref. [42] that the velocity of CoM is an important factor in balance control since even if the CoP

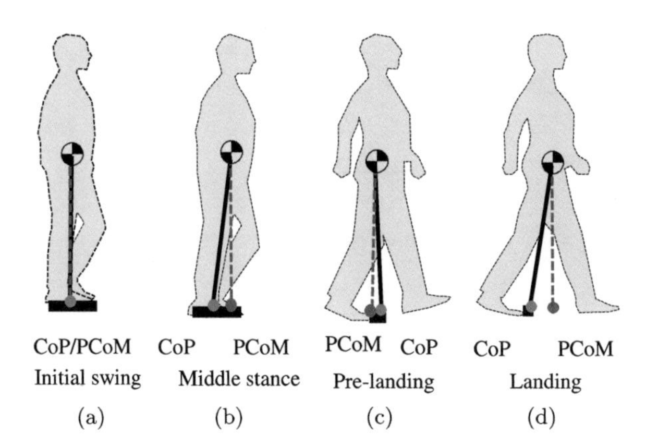

Figure 4. The use of CoP (indicated by dot in blue) as a measure of balance.

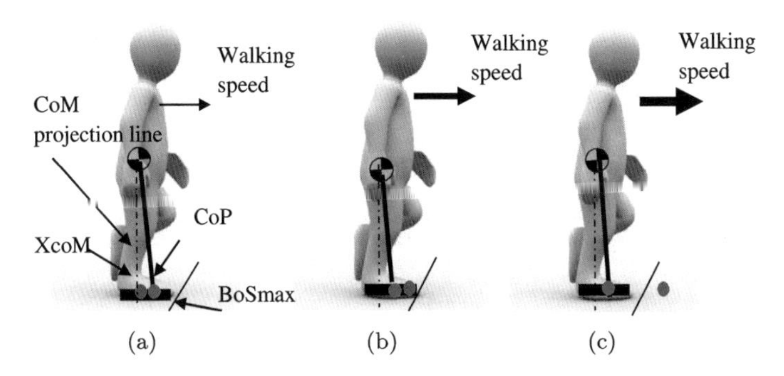

Figure 5. Illustration of human balance state by using XcoM.

is inside the BoS, loss of balance may still happen if CoM velocity points outward. By the same principle, balance can still be recovered even if the CoP is at the edge of the BoS but with the CoM velocity pointing towards BoS. The following three situations describe the balance state in terms of XcoM:

(i) Situation (a): CoM < XcoM < CoP < BoSmax: In the situation shown in Fig. 5(a), the CoM will never pass the CoP point and the velocity will eventually change direction causing the human to fall backwards or sideways. This happens when there is not enough propulsion force provided during walking.
(ii) Situation (b): CoM < CoP < XcoM < BoSmax: In this situation shown in Fig. 5(b), the CoM will pass the CoP point and accelerate forward. However, the subject can modulate their CoP position to balance and does not need to take a step.
(iii) Situation (c): CoM < CoP < BoSmax < XcoM.

If the CoM moves too far ahead of the foot, the only way of stabilizing the body is by taking a step as shown in Fig. 5(c).

The above analysis is demonstrated in the sagittal plane and can also be directly used in the lateral balance analysis.

In the following sections, walking rehabilitation robots classified into proactive postural balance and reactive balance training are reviewed. The review includes both the mechanical designs and control strategies employed to target proactive and reactive balance training.

3. Review on Proactive Postural Balance Training Robots

3.1. *Classification of robots with proactive waking postural balance training ability*

The robots with proactive walking postural balance training ability are classified into different types based on similarities in their mechanical design:

(a) Treadmill-based gait trainer: This system refers to treadmill walking training with BWS by hanging the subject with a fixed harness. The exoskeleton and pelvis support mechanism are used to assist legs and pelvis motion.
(b) Harness-based mobile BWS system: In this system, overground walking training is given with BWS by hanging the subject with a fixed harness attached at the pelvis. A mobile platform with either passive or motorized wheels is used to follow the movements of the training subject and provide the support to the harness.
(c) Arm-based mobile BWS system: This is similar to the harness-based mobile BWS system, except that a rigid arm is used in this case to support the body weight at the pelvis.
(d) Mobile overground gait trainer: This system is similar to the harness-based/arm-based mobile BWS system, except that this kind of system has additional lower limb exoskeleton to provide leg assistance and a more complicated rigid arm to provide natural pelvic motion.
(e) Ceiling-guide-based overground BWS system: In this system, overground walking training is given with BWS where the subject is supported using a movable harness attached to a moving guide installed at the ceiling.
(f) Cable-driven, pelvis-assisted system: This system refers to treadmill walking training with force assistance by attaching subject's pelvis to several cables.

The schematic diagrams of different rehabilitation robots with proactive balance abilities are shown in Fig. 6.

The treadmill-based gait trainer is the most popular method so far. Some of the representative devices include ALEX,[43] Lokomat,[44] LOPES[45] and POGO,[46] as shown in Fig. 7. These kinds of systems usually consist of three parts: a BWS

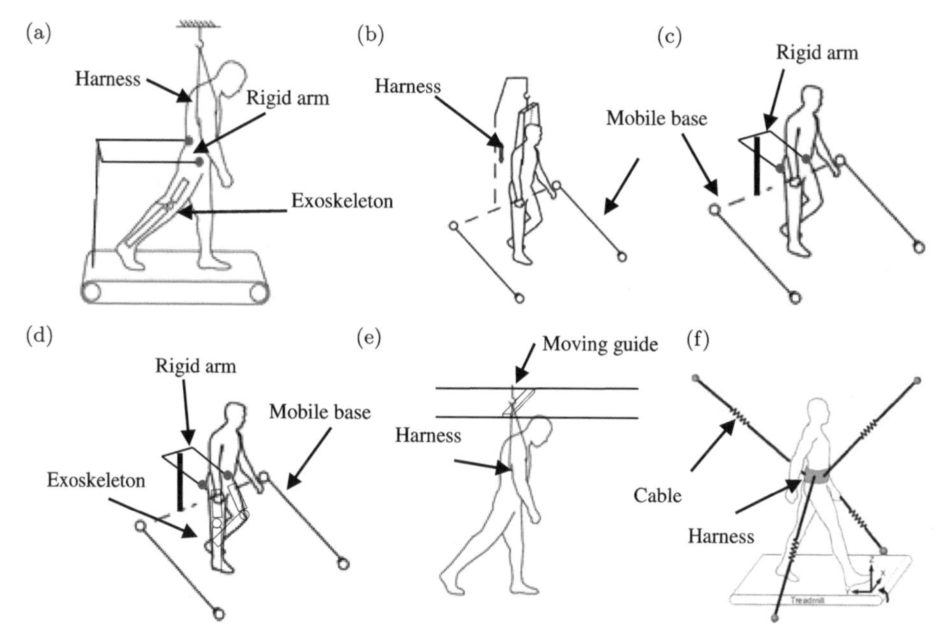

Figure 6. Rehabilitation robot types currently in use: (a) treadmill-based gait trainer; (b) harness-based mobile BWS system; (c) arm-based mobile BWS system; (d) mobile over-ground gait trainer; (e) ceiling-guide-based over-ground BWS system; and (f) cable-driven pelvis-assisted system (figures are modified from [44]).

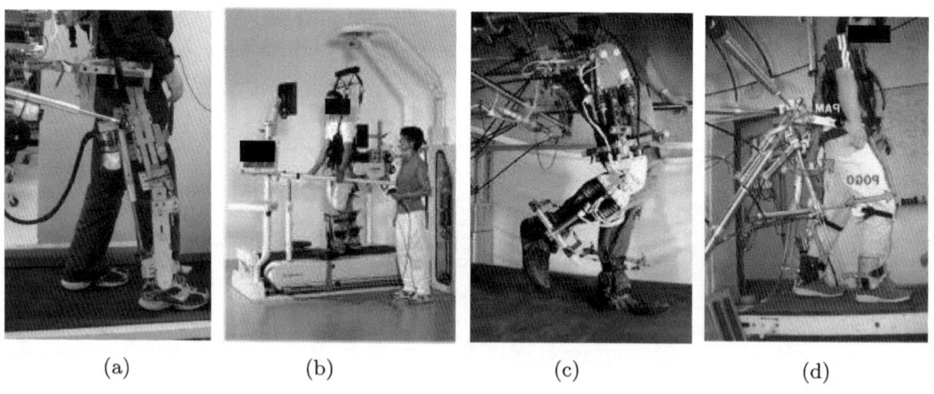

Figure 7. Treadmill-based gait trainer: (a) ALEX,[43] (b) Lokomat,[44] (c) LOPES,[45] and (d) POGO.[46,47]

system to support human bodyweight, a pelvis support mechanism to assist pelvis motion, and an exoskeleton leg to help in leg movements.

Both the harness-based mobile BWS system and the arm-based mobile BWS system use a mobile base to increase the mobility and achieve overground walking. The balance of the system is secured by the mobile base, while the bodyweight of the training subject is supported either by a harness (harness-based) or a

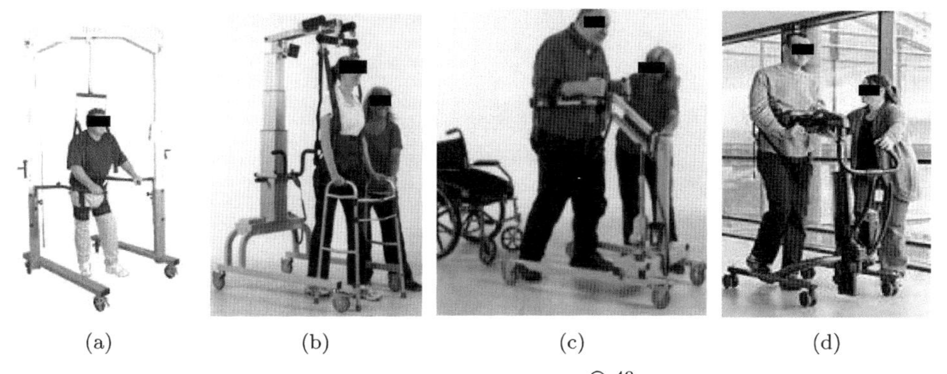

(a) (b) (c) (d)

Figure 8. Harness-based mobile BWS systems: (a) LiteGait®,[48] (b) Biodex unweighing system. Arm-based mobile BWS systems, (c) Mobility Device™ lift walker,[49] and (d) Rifton TRAM.[50]

rigid arm (arm-based). However, the hanging mechanism of harness-based mobile BWS systems (Fig. 8) is usually cumbersome and thus limits the mobility and acceptance of the system. In addition, the harness usually restricts pelvis motion due to the compliance of the strings of harness. Compared to the harness-based system, the use of a rigid arm makes the arm-based system more compact. The rigid structure eliminates the compliance problem in the harness, which allows the mobile platform to follow the subject smoothly.

Training with the harness-based mobile BWS system and the arm-based mobile BWS system with passive wheels often requires multiple therapists both to move the mobile support and to assist the movement of the subject's leg. Motorized arm-based mobile body-weight support systems, such as the KineAssist[51] and GaitTronics[52,53] shown in Fig. 9, attempt to address the issue of passive moving platform. While the mobile overground gait trainer attempts to solve both the unassisted leg movement and passive moving support by adding the exoskeleton and a motorized mobile base together. Usually, these systems are coupled with a complicated pelvic mechanism design to achieve a more natural pelvic motion. However, due to the complexity of the pelvic mechanism, the cost of these systems is high. Some of the representative devices are shown in Fig. 9.

Ceiling-guide-based overground BWS system uses a moveable BWS to allow the training subject to move on different terrains. However, they also require the installation of a large guide to the ceilings. Examples of such devices are Zero-G[47] and FLOAT,[56] which are shown in Fig. 10. However, the BWS with a fixed pulley system imposes lateral forces on the subject and may cause additional disturbance during training.

Cable-driven pelvis-assisted system uses cables to assist pelvis motion, which in turn can influence balance training. Examples of such a system are STRING MAN[57] and A-TPAD[58] which are shown in Fig. 10. However, there is no continuation on the development of STRING MAN,[57] while the A-TPAD[58,59] is still

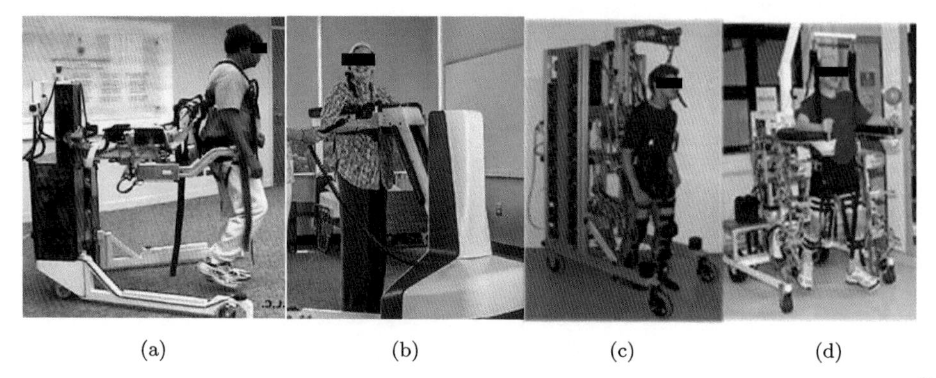

(a) (b) (c) (d)

Figure 9. Motorized arm-based mobile body-weight support systems: (a) KineAssist,[51] (b) GaitTronics.[52] Mobile overground gait trainer, (c) WalkTrainer,[54] and (d) NaTUre-gaits.[55]

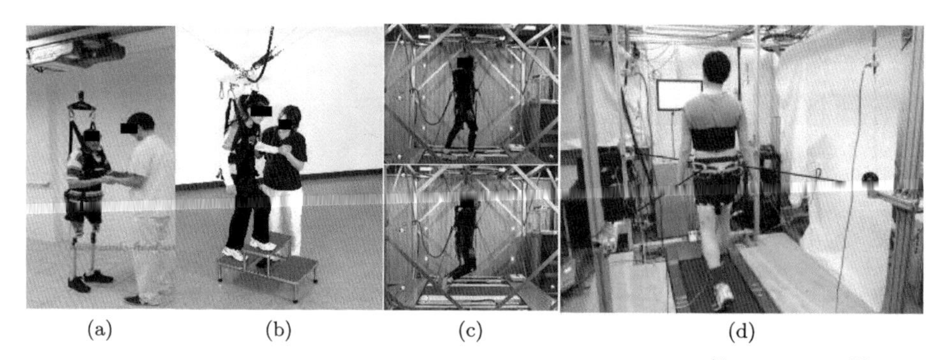

(a) (b) (c) (d)

Figure 10. Ceiling-guide-based over-ground BWS systems: (a) Zero-G,[47] (b) FLOAT.[56] Cable-driven pelvis-assisted system, (c) STRING MAN,[57] and (d) A-TPAD.[58]

under development. Therefore, little clinical results can be found for this method of rehabilitation.

There are also end-effector-based walking rehabilitation robots such as GaitTrainer,[60] HapticWalker,[61] and LokoHelp,[62] which are not included in this review but worth noticing. At the same time, robotic exoskeletons are another option, which can help assist the movement of the people with limited walking ability. This area focuses mainly on postural balance control and emphasizes on the method of coordinating the balance of two coupled dynamic systems.[63–65]

3.2. *Control strategies on proactive walking postural balance training*

All those systems reviewed in the previous sections provide at least one of the three functions in proactive postural balance control:

- Bodyweight support (Task 1)
- Pelvis movements' assistance (Tasks 2 and 3)
- Swing-leg movements' assistance (Task 4).

Different active control strategies have been developed to realize the three functions as described in the following sections.

3.2.1. *Bodyweight support control*

Varying the bodyweight support will alter the joints' torque demand and thus the muscle forces for the lower limbs.[66–68] As a result, it allows the progressive way of training the muscle to regain the ability of bodyweight support in the single support phase. The level of the bodyweight supported can either be kept at a constant level specified by the therapist[69] or can be adaptively changed after each gait cycle through an iterative learning algorithm.[70,71]

3.2.2. *Trajectory-based assistance-as-needed control for pelvis and leg movements*

Based on clinical advice, the robot should not interfere or hinder the subject if the subject moves along the desired trajectory. On the other hand, if the subject's movements deviate from the desired trajectory, an assistive force should be provided to restore the desired movements. Controllers which employ this principle are considered to be "assistance-as-needed" (AAN) since the assistive force will only be applied when the deviation occurs. Impedance-based control is usually used to achieve this kind of AAN effects. Appropriately designed virtual mechanical impedances such as spring and dampers are used to define the interaction mode between the subject and the system. These impedance-based AAN control algorithms have been implemented for both leg movements[72–74] and pelvic motions[46,75] during walking. Compared with passive assistance, where the training subject just "rides" on the robot, this strategy encourages the subject to participate by including his or her efforts during the rehabilitation process.

3.2.3. *Threshold-based assistance-as-needed control for pelvis movements*

Compared to the trajectory-based AAN controller, the threshold-based AAN controller does not need a reference trajectory. This kind of controller is usually an admittance-type controller, which allows the participant to complete a movement without any reference trajectory. The robot will only initiate some forms of assistance after certain performance variables reach a threshold level. This form of threshold-based AAN controller encourages self-initiated movements from the subject, which are essential for motor learning.[76,77] In Ref. [78], the authors use a strategy where the robotic device delivers only the necessary force to restore the balance when loss of balance is detected using XcoM as the balance index.

The assistive force is computed based on the LIPM to bring the subject to a zero velocity stage and is provided to the subject when a fall is detected. In Ref. [52], the user defined an admittance mass-spring-damper interface between the robot and the subject. Unlike the previous method where no force is applied when no falling condition is detected, the subject can feel the resistance force from the robot due to the admittance interface. This is beneficial to patients with severe conditions. The resistance can slow down the motion and allow the subject to be trained in a safer manner. The resistance level can be changed by defining the parameters of the mass-spring-damper model to suit different subjects' conditions. The robot will stop its movements when the falling occurs and thus helps the subject to regain balance.

4. Review on Reactive Postural Balance Training Robots

Other than proactive postural balance training, which is usually done in an assistive manner where external force is used to help stabilize the balance of the training subject, the reactive postural balance training is done in a challenged manner where perturbation is used to destabilize the balance of the training subject. Tables 1 and 2 provide a detailed summary of some of the representative studies for reactive postural balance training robots in walking and standing modes, respectively.

Most of the devices described in Tables 1 and 2 are still in the prototype stage and some of the devices' mechanical structures are shown in Fig. 11. Some of them are tested in healthy human to investigate the normal human response during perturbation while some are aimed at the elderly or Parkinson disease sufferers to study which specific balance training can reduce the chance of falling. There are other methods for inducing perturbation such as using a treadmill to create slipping effects,[88] which are considered dangerous for rehabilitation purposes and are not discussed here.

5. Conclusion and Discussion

This chapter has presented the mechanism of walking postural balance control and a review of the development of walking training robots associated to postural balance control. Additional balance training has proved to be beneficial,[89] but the optimal way to enhance the balance training abilities is still largely unanswered. For further enhancement of postural balance, three directions are suggested for future research.

Among the various types of proactive postural balance training robots, mobile overground gait trainer and cable-driven pelvis-assisted system are more suitable

Table 1. Summary of reactive postural balance training robot during walking.

Device	Target group and rehabilitation focus	Rehabilitation method	System description
CAREN[79]	Walking balance movements strategies (Ankle, Hip Stepping)	Commercial product; replicate the experience of standing on a bus or train	Six hydraulic actuators; manipulating the end-effector surface in each of the six degrees of freedom independently or simultaneously
BaMPer[80]	Walking balance movements strategies (Ankle, Hip Stepping)	Linear perturbation in standing	Translational perturbations up to a maximal acceleration of 9.81 m/s^2, maximal velocity of 0.8 m/s and maximal displacement of 10 cm to any direction in the horizontal plane
Robotic Platform for Gait Study[81]	Standing balance movements strategies (Ankle, Hip Stepping)	Velocity-controlled translational perturbations over the floor surface, rotational perturbations about the ankle joint, and acceleration-controlled vertical translational perturbations; research platform with healthy people trial	With 4-DOF and was designed to provide: Fast (>= 400 mm/s) translation along x axis to allow experimentation on slipping; rotational perturbations up to 100°/s to repeat on stretch reflex studies; +/ − 100 mm translation along both z and x axis; +/ − 10° pitch and roll; linear velocity up to 1 m/linear acceleration up to 1 g

to enhance balance training. The mobile overground gait trainer incorporates two essential features: an overground walking experience and a mobile pelvis support. The mobile pelvis support would allow the subject to practice more real and challenged balance training compared to treadmill walking. If a subject falls while performing rehabilitation on the treadmill, the residual velocity due to inertia will still be present on the treadmill surface even if a hard-brake is applied. This will impose an additional slipping effect on the subject and hinder progress in

Table 2. Summary of reactive postural balance training robot during standing.

Device	Target group and rehabilitation focus	Rehabilitation method	System description
Kung[82]	Standing balance movements strategies (Ankle, Hip)	Rotational perturbation in standing	Pitch and Roll rotations (7.5°/s and 60°/s)
Pneumatic instrumented moving platform[83]	Standing balance movements strategies (Ankle, Hip)	Linear perturbation in standing	The platform can translate from 0 to 0.15 m forward and from 0 to 0.25 m backward over 360 m/s. A force platform that is integrated with the moving platform can be used to quantify balance
Avril Mansfield[84]	Standing balance movement strategies (Stepping, Grasping)	Linear perturbation in standing	For the support-surface translations, displacement, velocity and acceleration of 0.18 m, 0.6 m/s and 2.0 m/s^2 are used, respectively, for forward translations (which evoke backward falling motion), and of 0.27 m, 1.0 m/s and 3.0 m/s^2 are used for the other translation directions (backward, left, right)
J. Hasson[85]	Investigate the possibility of using time-to-contact as a measure to predict when to take a step reaction	Upper body perturbation in standing	A pendulum is used to hit the human's upper body
RotoBit3D[86]	Standing balance training movements strategies (Ankle, Hip)	Three-directional rotational perturbation in standing	Three rotational DOFs, synchronized roll, pitch and yaw, maximum ranges of −10° to +10°; maximum rate of about 50°/s
PROPRIO 5000[87]	Standing balance movements strategies (Ankle, Hip)	Two-directional rotational perturbation in standing	25° both in lateral direction and anterior/posterior direction with a rate range of 12.6°/s to 126°/s

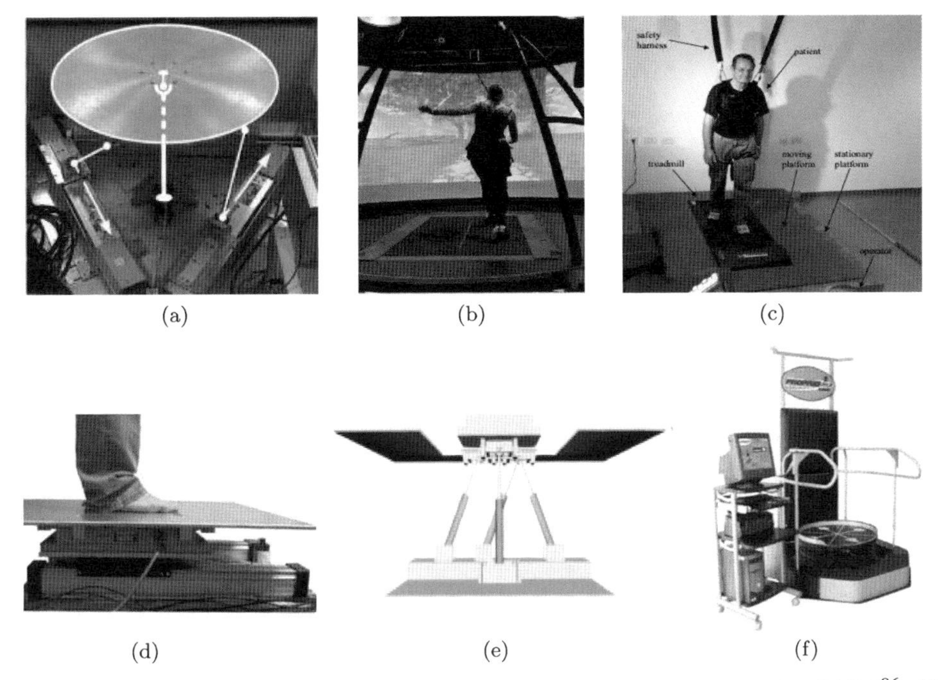

Figure 11. Perturbation-based reactive postural balance training robots. (a) RotoBit3D,[86] (b) CAREN,[79] (c) BaMPer System,[80] (d) Pneumatic instrumented moving platform,[83] (e) Robotic platform for gait study,[81] and (f) PROPRIO 5000.[87]

learning the correct stepping method. On the other hand, the cable-driven pelvis-assisted system has the advantage of an extreme low inertia system and a multi-directional force assistance capability. These features will improve the transparency of the pelvis support mechanism. It is an important feature as an alteration of gait kinematics[13,90,91] and muscle activation patterns[92,93] are observed when the pelvis is constrained by the robot. It is also worth noticing that the cable-driven pelvis-assisted system can also be used in perturbation-based training which makes the system become multifunctional. Currently, both types of systems need more clinical evidence to prove the balance training efficiency. Thus, the first direction is suggested on the clinical studies of the two kinds of systems.

The second direction involves the incorporation of more challenging balance training algorithms. One of the algorithms is to use the admittance control approach to allow the subject to freely move his/her pelvis and the robot would only catch the subject when the intention of falling is detected. This is one of the threshold-based AAN controllers reviewed in Sec. 3. Nevertheless, the methods to detect loss of balance and help the subject to recover from a falling posture still need to be explored. Feedback such as CoP and XcoM provide useful information related to balance control. The time of triggering the assistance and the level of assistance can be based on these indexes to allow the subject to train in achieving balance more effectively.

Perturbation-based rehabilitation has proven to be effective for balance training in aged people, both in simulation and in experiments.[83] However, these training programs focus more on fall prevention and are limited to the elderly. The third direction will be to investigate the ways to incorporate the perturbation-based balance training into the walking rehabilitation for stroke subjects.

In conclusion, even though the field of robot-assisted walking rehabilitation is evolving rapidly, there is still substantial amount of work to be done. We are optimistic that, with careful research and consideration on the principle of human postural balance and its application to the robot design and control, the efficiency of robot-assisted rehabilitation walking training can be improved.

References

1. M. R. Tucker, J. Olivier, A. Pagel, H. Bleuler, M. Bouri, O. Lambercy, *et al.* (2015). Control strategies for active lower extremity prosthetics and orthotics: a review, *Journal of NeuroEngineering and Rehabilitation* 12:1–30.
2. R. Bonita, S. Mendis, T. Truelsen, J. Bogousslavsky, J. Toole and F. Yatsu. (2004). The global stroke initiative, *Lancet Neurol* 3:391–393.
3. C. Warlow, J. Van Gijn, M. S. Dennis, J. M. Wardlaw, J. M. Bamford, G. J. Hankey, *et al.* (2008). Stroke: Practical Management.
4. P. Langhorne, P. Sandercock and K. Prasad. (2009). Evidence-based practice for stroke, *The Lancet Neurology* 8:308–309.
5. B. H. Dobkin. (2004). Strategies for stroke rehabilitation, *The Lancet Neurology* 3: 528–536.
6. A. Pollock, G. Baer, P. Campbell, P. L. Choo, A. Forster, J. Morris, *et al.* (2014). Physical rehabilitation approaches for the recovery of function and mobility following stroke, *Cochrane Database of Systematic Reviews* 4.
7. P. Langhorne, J. Bernhardt and G. Kwakkel. (2011). Stroke rehabilitation, *The Lancet Neurology* 377:1693–1702.
8. S. Hesse. (2008). Treadmill training with partial body weight support after stroke: a review, *NeuroRehabilitation* 23:55–65.
9. A. Pennycott, D. Wyss, H. Vallery, V. Klamroth-Marganska and R. Riener. (2012). Towards more effective robotic gait training for stroke rehabilitation: a review, *Journal of NeuroEngineering and Rehabilitation* 9:65.
10. J. Hidler, D. Nichols, M. Pelliccio and K. Brady. (2005). Advances in the understanding and treatment of stroke impairment using robotic devices, *Topics in Stroke Rehabilitation* 12:22–35.
11. B. T. Volpe, H. I. Krebs and N. Hogan. (2001). Is robot-aided sensorimotor training in stroke rehabilitation a realistic option? *Current Opinion in Neurology* 14:745–752.
12. P. Wang, K. H. Low, A. H. McGregor and A. Tow. (2013). Detection of abnormal muscle activations during walking following spinal cord injury (SCI), *Research in Developmental Disabilities* 34:1226–1235.
13. J. Hidler, D. Nichols, M. Pelliccio, K. Brady, D. D. Campbell, J. H. Kuhn, *et al.* (2009). Multicenter randomized clinical trial evaluating the effectiveness of the Lokomat in subacute stroke, *Neurorehabilitation and Neural Repair* 23:5–13.

14. T. G. Hornby, D. D. Campbell, J. H. Kahn, T. Demott, J. L. Moore and H. R. Roth. (2008). Enhanced gait-related improvements after therapist-versus robotic-assisted locomotor training in subjects with chronic stroke a randomized controlled study, *Stroke* 39:1786–1792.
15. C. Werner, S. Von Frankenberg, T. Treig, M. Konrad and S. Hesse. (2002). Treadmill training with partial body weight support and an electromechanical gait trainer for restoration of gait in subacute stroke patients: a randomized crossover study, *Stroke* 33:2895–2901.
16. A. Mayr, M. Kofler, E. Quirbach, H. Matzak, K. Frohlich and L. Saltuari. (2007). Prospective, blinded, randomized crossover study of gait rehabilitation in stroke patients using the Lokomat gait orthosis, *Neurorehabil Neural Repair* 21:307–314.
17. B. Husemann, F. M*ü*ller, C. Krewer, S. Heller and E. Koenig. (2007). Effects of locomotion training with assistance of a robot-driven gait orthosis in hemiparetic patients after stroke a randomized controlled pilot study, *Stroke* 38:349–354.
18. S. H. Peurala, I. M. Tarkka, K. Pitkänen and J. Sivenius. (2005). The effectiveness of body weight-supported gait training and floor walking in patients with chronic stroke, *Archives of Physical Medicine and Rehabilitation* 86:1557–1564.
19. B. Koopman, J. H. Meuleman, E. H. F. van Asseldonk and H. van der Kooij. (2013). Lateral balance control for robotic gait training. In *IEEE International Conference on Rehabilitation Robotics* 1–6.
20. V. Weerdesteyn, M. de Niet, H. J. van Duijnhoven and A. C. Geurts. (2008). Falls in individuals with stroke, *Journal of Rehabilitation Research and Development* 45:1195–1213.
21. F. A. Batchelor, S. F. Mackintosh, C. M. Said and K. D. Hill. (2012). Falls after stroke, *International Journal of Stroke* 7:482–490.
22. S. RW. (1992). Falls among older persons: a public helth perspective, *Annu Rev Public Health.*
23. A. S. Pollock, B. R. Durward, P. J. Rowe and J. P. Paul. (2000). What is balance? *Clinical Rehabilitation* 14:402–406.
24. M. Mancini and F. B. Horak. (2010). The relevance of clinical balance assessment tools to differentiate balance deficits, *European Journal of Physical and Rehabilitation Medicine* 46:239–248.
25. F. B. Horak. (2006). Postural orientation and equilibrium: what do we need to know about neural control of balance to prevent falls? *Age Ageing* 35 Suppl 2, ii7–ii11.
26. R. W. Bohannon. (2007). Muscle strength and muscle training after stroke, *Journal of Rehabilitation Medicine* 39:14–20.
27. K. J. Sullivan, D. A. Brown, T. Klassen, S. Mulroy, T. Ge, S. P. Azen, *et al.* (2007). Effects of task-specific locomotor and strength training in adults who were ambulatory after stroke: Results of the STEPS randomized clinical trial, *Physical Therapy* 87:1580–1602.
28. G. Kwakkel, B. Kollen and E. Lindeman. (2004). Understanding the pattern of functional recovery after stroke: facts and theories, *Restorative Neurology and Neuroscience* 22: 281–299.
29. A. R. Den Otter, A. C. Geurts, T. Mulder and J. Duysens. (2007). Abnormalities in the temporal patterning of lower extremity muscle activity in hemiparetic gait, *Gait and Posture* 25: 342–352.
30. S. A. Kautz, P. W. Duncan, S. Perera, R. R. Neptune and S. A. Studenski. (2005). Coordination of hemiparetic locomotion after stroke rehabilitation, *Neurorehabilitation and Neural Repair* 19:250–258.
31. J. H. Buurke, A. V. Nene, G. Kwakkel, V. Erren-Wolters, M. J. Ijzerman and H. J. Hermens. (2008). Recovery of gait after stroke: what changes? *Neurorehabilitation and Neural Repair* 22:676–83.
32. M. de Haart, A. C. Geurts, M. C. Dault, B. Nienhuis and J. Duysens. (2005). Restoration of weight-shifting capacity in patients with postacute stroke: a rehabilitation cohort study, *Archives of Physical Medicine and Rehabilitation* 86:755–762.

33. G. Yavuzer, F. Eser, D. Karakus, B. Karaoglan and H. J. Stam. (2006). The effects of balance training on gait late after stroke: a randomized controlled trial, *Clinical Rehabilitation* 20:960–969.
34. A. S. Aruin, N. Rao, A. Sharma and G. Chaudhuri. (2012). Compelled body-weight shift approach in rehabilitation of individuals with chronic stroke, *Topics in Stroke Rehabilitation* 19:556–563.
35. Y. Laufer, R. Dickstein, S. Resnik and E. Marcovitz. (2000). Weight-bearing shifts of hemi-paretic and healthy adults upon stepping on stairs of various heights, *Clinical Rehabilitation* 14:125–129.
36. P. V. Tsaklis, W. J. A. Grooten and E. Franzén. (2012). Effects of weight-shift training on balance control and weight distribution in chronic stroke: a pilot study, *Topics in Stroke Rehabilitation* 19:23–31.
37. J. E. Pratt. (2000). Exploiting inherent robustness and natural dynamics in the control of bipedal walking robots, MIT.
38. J. Pratt, J. Carff, S. Drakunov and A. Goswami. (2006). Capture point: a step toward humanoid push recovery, in *IEEE-RAS International Conference on Humanoid Robots* 200–207.
39. S. Kajita, Y. Tomio and A. Kobayashi. (1992). Dynamic walking control of a biped robot along a potential energy conserving orbit, *IEEE Transactions on Robotics and Automation* 8:431–438.
40. D. Marigold, A. Dawson, J. Inglis, J. Harris and S. Gylfadottir. (2005). Exercise leads to faster postural reflexes, improved balance and mobility, and fewer falls in older persons with chronic stroke, *Journal of American Geriatric Society* 53:416–423.
41. L. A. Vearrier, J. Langan, A. Shumway-Cook and M. Woollacott. (2005). An intensive massed practice approach to retraining balance post-stroke, *Gait and Posture* 22:154–163.
42. A. L. Hof, M. G. J. Gazendam and W. E. Sinke. (2005). The condition for dynamic stability, *Journal of Biomechanics* 38:1–8.
43. S. K. Banala, A. Kulpe and S. K. Agrawal. (2007). A powered leg orthosis for gait rehabilitation of motor-impaired patients. In *Proceedings International Conference on Robotics and Automation*, IEEE, Rome, 4140–4145.
44. D. Novak, P. Reberšek, S. M. M. D. Rossi, M. Donati, J. Podobnik and T. Beravs. (2013). Automated detection of gait initiation and termination using wearable sensors, *Medical Engineering and Physics* 35.
45. E. H. F. Van Asseldonk, J. F. Veneman, R. Ekkelenkamp, J. H. Buurke, F. C. T. Van Der Helm and H. Van Der Kooij. (2008). The effects on kinematics and muscle activity of walking in a robotic gait trainer during zero-force control, *IEEE Transactions on Neural Systems and Rehabilitation Engineering* 16:360–370.
46. D. Aoyagi, W. E. Ichinose, S. J. Harkema, D. J. Reinkensmeyer and J. E. Bobrow. (2007). A robot and control algorithm that can synchronously assist in naturalistic motion during body-weight-supported gait training following neurologic injury, *IEEE Transactions on Neural Systems and Rehabilitation Engineering* 15:387–400.
47. J. Hidler, D. Brennan, I. Black, D. Nichols, K. Brady and T. Nef. (2011). ZeroG: overground gait and balance training system, *Journal of Rehabilitation Research and Development* 48: 287–298.
48. S. Stančin. (2011). MC sensor — a novel method for measurement of muscle tension, *Sensors* 11.
49. P. Lukowicz, F. Hanser, C. Szubski and W. Schobersberger. (2006). Detecting and interpreting muscle activity with wearable force sensors. In K. P. Fishkin, B. Schiele, P. Nixon and A. Quigley, (eds.), *Pervasive Computing, Lecture Notes in Computer Science*, Vol. 3968 PERVASIVE: Springer.

50. P. B. Shull, W. Jirattigalachote, M. A. Hunt, M. R. Cutkosky and S. L. Delp. (2014). Quantified self and human movement: a review on the clinical impact of wearable sensing and feedback for gait analysis and intervention, *Gait and Posture* 40.
51. J. Patton, D. A. Brown, M. Peshkin, J. J. Santos-Munne, A. Makhlin, E. Lewis, *et al.* (2008). KineAssist: design and development of a robotic overground gait and balance therapy device, *Topics in Stroke Rehabilitation* 15:131–139.
52. *GaitTronics*. Available: http://gaittronics.com/.
53. A. Morbi, M. Ahmadi and A. Nativ. (2012). GaitEnable: An omnidirectional robotic system for gait rehabilitation, in *International Conference on Mechatronics and Automation* 936–941.
54. M. Bouri, Y. Stauffer, C. Schmitt, Y. Allemand, S. Gnemmi, R. Clavel, *et al.* (2006). The WalkTrainer: a robotic system for walking rehabilitation, in *IEEE International Conference on Robotics and Biomimetics*, Piscataway, NJ, USA, 1616–1621.
55. W. Ping, K. H. Low and A. H. McGregor. (2011). A subject-based motion generation model with adjustable walking pattern for a gait robotic trainer: NaTUre-gaits, in *IEEE/RSJ International Conference on Intelligent Robots and Systems* Piscataway, NJ, USA, 1743–178.
56. H. Vallery, P. Lutz, J. von Zitzewitz, G. Rauter, M. Fritschi, C. Everarts, *et al.* (2013). Multidirectional transparent support for overground gait training, in *IEEE International Conference on Rehabilitation Robotics* 1–7.
57. D. Surdilovic, Z. Jinyu and R. Bernhardt. (2007). STRING-MAN: Wire-robot technology for safe, flexible and human-friendly gait rehabilitation, in *IEEE International Conference on Rehabilitation Robotics* 446–453.
58. V. Vashista, J. Xin and S. K. Agrawal. (2014). Active Tethered Pelvic Assist Device (A-TPAD) to study force adaptation in human walking, in *IEEE International Conference on Robotics and Automation* 718–723.
59. K. Jiyeon, V. Vashista and S. K. Agrawal. (2015). A novel assist-as-needed control method to guide pelvic trajectory for gait rehabilitation, in *IEEE International Conference on Rehabilitation Robotics* 630–635.
60. S. Hesse and D. Uhlenbrock. (2000). A mechanized gait trainer for restoration of gait, *Journal of Rehabilitation Research and Development* 37:701–708.
61. H. Schmidt, C. Werner, R. Bernhardt, S. Hesse and J. Krüger. (2007). Gait rehabilitation machines based on programmable footplates, *Journal of NeuroEngineering and Rehabilitation* 4:2–2.
62. S. Freivogel, J. Mehrholz, T. Husak-Sotomayor and D. Schmalohr. (2008). Gait training with the newly developed 'LokoHelp'-system is feasible for non-ambulatory patients after stroke, spinal cord and brain injury. A feasibility study, *Brain Injury* 22:625–632.
63. L. Li, K. H. Hoon, A. Tow, P. H. Lim and K. H. Low. (2015). Design and control of robotic exoskeleton with balance stabilizer mechanism in *IEEE/RSJ International Conference on Intelligent Robots and Systems* Hamburg, Germany.
64. W. Shiqian, W. Letian, C. Meijneke, E. van Asseldonk, T. Hoellinger, G. Cheron, *et al.* (2015). Design and control of the MINDWALKER exoskeleton, *IEEE Transactions on Neural Systems and Rehabilitation Engineering* 23:277–286.
65. J. Veneman. (2014). Exoskeletons supporting postural balance — The BALANCE project. In W. Jensen, O. K. Andersen and M. Akay. (eds.), *Replace, Repair, Restore, Relieve — Bridging Clinical and Engineering Solutions in Neurorehabilitation*, vol. 7, Springer International Publishing, pp. 203–208.
66. L. Finch, H. Barbeau and B. Arsenault. (1991). Influence of body weight support on normal human gait: development of a gait retraining strategy, *Physical Therapy* 71:842–855; discussion 855–856.

67. S. M. Colby, D. T. Kirkendall and R. F. Bruzga. (1999). Electromyographic analysis and energy expenditure of harness supported treadmill walking: implications for knee rehabilitation, *Gait and Posture* 10:200–205.
68. A. Danielsson and K. S. Sunnerhagen. (2000). Oxygen consumption during treadmill walking with and without body weight support in patients with hemiparesis after stroke and in healthy subjects, *Archives of Physical Medicine and Rehabilitation* 81:953–957.
69. M. Frey, G. Colombo, M. Vaglio, R. Bucher, M. Jorg and R. Riener. (2006). A novel mechatronic body weight support system, *IEEE Transactions on Neural Systems and Rehabilitation Engineering* 14:311–321.
70. A. Duschau-Wicke, S. Felsenstein, R. Riener, S. C. I. Center, T. Brunsch and A. Hocoma. (2007). Iterative learning support for robot-aided gait rehabilitation, in *International Conference on Rehabilitation Robotics*.
71. L. Trieu Phat, H. B. Lim, Q. Xingda and K. H. Low. (2011). Pelvic motion assistance of NaTUregaits with adaptive body weight support, in *8th Asian Control Conference* 950–955.
72. S. K. Banala, S. K. Agrawal and J. P. Scholz. (2007). Active Leg Exoskeleton (ALEX) for gait rehabilitation of motor-impaired patients, in *IEEE International Conference on Rehabilitation Robotics* 401–407.
73. J. F. Veneman, R. Kruidhof, E. E. Hekman, R. Ekkelenkamp, E. H. Van Asseldonk and H. Van Der Kooij. (2007). Design and evaluation of the LOPES exoskeleton robot for interactive gait rehabilitation, *IEEE Transactions on Neural Systems and Rehabilitation Engineering* 15:379–386.
74. A. Duschau-Wicke, J. von Zitzewitz, A. Caprez, L. Lunenburger and R. Riener. (2010). Path control: a method for patient cooperative robot-aided gait rehabilitation, *IEEE Transactions on Neural Systems and Rehabilitation Engineering* 18:38–48.
75. M. Pietrusinski, I. Cajigas, Y. Mizikacioglu, M. Goldsmith, P. Bonato and C. Mavroidis. (2010). Gait rehabilitation therapy using robot generated force fields applied at the pelvis, in *IEEE Haptics Symposium* 401–407.
76. M. Lotze, C. Braun, N. Birbaumer, S. Anders and L. G. Cohen. (2003). Motor learning elicited by voluntary drive, *Brain* 126:866–872.
77. M. A. Perez, B. K. Lungholt, K. Nyborg and J. B. Nielsen. (2004). Motor skill training induces changes in the excitability of the leg cortical area in healthy humans, *Experimental Brain Research* 159:197–205.
78. H. Vallery, A. Bögel, C. O′Brien and R. Riener. (2012). Cooperative control design for robot-assisted balance during gait, *Automatisierungstechnik Methoden und Anwendungen der Steuerungs-, Regelungs- und Informationstechnik* 60:715.
79. A. Lees, J. Vanrenterghem, G. Barton and M. Lake. (2007). Kinematic response characteristics of the CAREN moving platform system for use in posture and balance research, *Medical Engineering and Physics* 29:629–635.
80. A. Shapiro and I. Melzer. (2010). Balance perturbation system to improve balance compensatory responses during walking in old persons, *Journal of NeuroEngineering and Rehabilitation* 7:1–6, 2010/07/15.
81. J. van Doornik and T. Sinkjaer. (2007). Robotic platform for human gait analysis, *IEEE Transactions on Biomedical Engineering* 54:1696–702.
82. U. M. Küng. (2009). The role of body segment movements on the control of centre of mass during balance corrections, PhD, Faculty of Medicine, University of Basel.
83. K. A. Bieryla. (2009). An investigation of perturbation-based balance training as a fall prevention intervention for older adults, PhD, Mechanical Engineering, Virginia Polytechnic Institute and State University.
84. A. Mansfield, A. Peters, B. Liu and B. Maki. (2007). A perturbation-based balance training program for older adults: study protocol for a randomised controlled trial, *BMC Geriatrics* 7:12.

85. C. J. Hasson, R. E. A. Van Emmerik and G. E. Caldwell. (2008). Predicting dynamic postural instability using center of mass time-to-contact information, *Journal of Biomechanics* 41:2121–2129.
86. X. F. Patane and P. Cappa. (2011). A 3-DOF parallel robot with spherical motion for the rehabilitation and evaluation of balance performance, *IEEE Transactions on Neural Systems and Rehabilitation Engineering* 19:157–166.
87. *PROPRIO® 5000 Reactive Balance Systems*. Available: http://www.perrydynamics.com/products/PROPRIO-5000.aspx.
88. P. Patel and T. Bhatt. (2015). Adaptation to large — magnitude treadmill — based perturbations: improvements in reactive balance response, *Physiological Reports*.
89. N. Alptekin, H. Gok, D. Geler-Kulcu and G. Dincer. (2008). Efficacy of treatment with a kinaesthetic ability training device on balance and mobility after stroke: a randomized controlled study, *Clinical Rehabilitation* 22:922–930.
90. J. Hidler, W. Wisman and N. Neckel. (2008). Kinematic trajectories while walking within the Lokomat robotic gait-orthosis, *Clinical Biomechanics* 23:1251–1259.
91. J. F. Veneman, J. Menger, E. H. van Asseldonk, F. C. van der Helm and H. van der Kooij. (2008). Fixating the pelvis in the horizontal plane affects gait characteristics, *Gait and Posture* 28:157–163.
92. J. F. Israel, D. D. Campbell, J. H. Kahn and T. G. Hornby. (2006). Metabolic costs and muscle activity patterns during robotic- and therapist-assisted treadmill walking in individuals with incomplete spinal cord injury, *Physical Therapy* 86:1466–1478.
93. J. M. Hidler and A. E. Wall. (2005). Alterations in muscle activation patterns during robotic-assisted walking, *Clinical Biomechanics* 20:184–193.

Chapter 3

A COOPERATIVE ROBOTIC ORTHOSIS FOR GAIT ASSISTANCE

Andrea Parri*, Tingfang Yan*, Francesco Giovacchini*, Mario Cortese*, Marco Muscolo*, Matteo Fantozzi*, Guido Pasquini†, Federica Vannetti†, Raffaele Molino Lova†, and Nicola Vitiello*,†

**The BioRobotics Institute, Scuola Superiore Sant'Anna, 34 viale Rinaldo Piaggio, Pontedera (Pisa), 56025, Italy*

†Don Carlo Gnocchi Foundation 256, Via di Scandicci, Firenze, 50143, Italy

In an era where the aging of population and the increased incidence of gait impairments are dominant trends, the need for devices capable of enabling a proper sustenance of the global welfare and healthcare costs is increasing. Sophisticated lower limb wearable robots have been developed over the years in order to prevent and provide a reliable solution to major social and economical issues for people affected by gait disorders. Nevertheless, their acceptability and usability are still limited by several unresolved challenges in terms of physical and cognitive human–robot interactions. The goal of this chapter is to provide an example of the design of the mechatronic architecture of a wearable active pelvis orthosis (APO) for assisting hip flexion–extension movements during activities of daily living (ADL). The device safely complies with the human biomechanics and is adaptive in its mechanical structure and in its control policy to different anthropometries and inter-/intrasubject walking patterns. Starting from a laboratory prototype with off-board control and power supply units to a totally portable version, the design of the active pelvis orthosis followed and advanced the recent trends of the wearable robot development. We expect that in the coming years, people affected by lower limb impairments could take advantage of wearable robots like the APO and experience a reduction in the physical burden of locomotion-related activities, thus increasing their socio-economical engagement and quality of life.

1. Introduction

Lower limb mobility is essential for ADL — walking around, reaching work places, visiting friends, etc. It requires no special thoughts for most persons, but not for the portion of population of those who deal with ambulation difficulties due to various health issues. According to the statistics reported in Ref. [1], up to 35% of people over 70 years old encounter problems in walking, such as slower walking speed and lesser balance control capability. This percentage increases to almost 60% among people aged between 80 and 84 years.[2] Individuals with spinal cord injuries (SCI) may undergo a more severe movement disability. A complete injury can cause a total loss of locomotion functionality. It is estimated that the global incidence of SCI is likely to be from 40 to 80 cases per million people.[3,4] Stroke is another leading cause of disability in all industrialized countries.[5] One of the most common impairments after stroke is hemiplegia which significantly contributes to reduced gait performance. According to the World Health Organization, 15 million people suffer from stroke worldwide each year.[6] The decrease of mobility could also be caused by a limb loss due to amputations. It is estimated that in the US, there are 1.6 million people with amputations in 2005 and this number is expected to reach 3.6 million by 2050.[7] Ambulatory disabilities could bring considerable barriers to the ADL both physically and psychologically. For example, people with decreased walking ability are retrained to walk around, visit friends, or reach walking places. The lack of independency in daily life and isolation from society consequently lead to depression or other psychological disorders.[2,3,6]

Researchers have never stopped exploring approaches to assist the locomotion or restore the lost function. In the recent decades, wearable robotic devices, for instance, assistive exoskeletons and rehabilitation orthoses,[8–10] are attracting great attention. Compared with the traditional assistive devices, like wheel chairs and canes, one of the distinctive features of wearable robotics is their close interaction with the users, the injection of energy in his/her gait pattern and exchange of information between the robot and the person. In Ref. [11], two types of exoskeleton–human interfaces are identified, namely, physical or cognitive interaction. Physical interaction mainly relates to mechanical energy exchanged between the robot and its user, while cognitive interaction mainly involves the information flow between the two entities. These two interfaces are interdependent on each other. A consistent and effective mechanical power transfer is fundamental for the wearer's comfort and for the exoskeleton to rely on correct kinematics and kinetics information. *Vice versa*, the success of this interpretation is fundamental for an exoskeleton to consistently act with natural gait biomechanics, thus restoring more functional and energy-efficient locomotion.

Targeted on various assistive functionalities for different types of users, a great number of state-of-the-art exoskeletons have been designed. For instance, BLEEX,[12] Sarcos-Raytheon "XoS" series (Raytheon, US) and Human Universal Load Carrier (HULC) (Lockheed Martin, US) are developed for the purpose of augmenting the load-carrying capability of the subjects. The force augmentation exoskeletons are mainly aimed at the military field.

In order to help the SCI patients — or people with severely damaged mobility — achieving the aspiration of standing up and walking, research groups or companies from different countries have designed different multi-joint exoskeletons, such as MINDWALKER,[13] ReWalk,[14] Indego Exoskeleton from Vanderbilt University,[15] HAL,[16] Ekso (Ekso Bionics, US), and REX (Rex Bionics, US). Thanks to the body weight support capability of these multi-joint exoskeletons, they could also be used in the gait rehabilitation or training for post-stroke patients in a clinical environment.

In rehabilitation in the robotics field, there are also some treadmill-based exoskeletons for gait training, such as LOPES[17] and Lokomat.[18] Though there are limitations to indoor applications, they can effectively release the therapists from repetitive tasks. In the state of the art, there are also some exoskeletons conceived for assisting the elderly or persons with mild gait impairments. For instance, the HONDA Stride Management Assist (Honda, Tokyo, Japan) and the Active Pelvis Orthosis[19] are specialized in assisting the hip movements in the sagittal plane; the Hyundai Wearable Robotics for walking assistance (Hyundai Motor Company, South Korea) can provide assistance to both knee and hip joints; the unpowered ankle exoskeleton presented in Ref. [20] can reduce the energy consumption during walking; the Exosuit presented in Ref. [21] demonstrated that the compliance of a soft architecture is effective in assisting walking.

The prosperous evolvement of both hardware and software technologies is improving the usability of exoskeletons in assisting ADL. However, how to reduce the weight of the whole system and extend the battery life is still one of the most critical issues in achieving the portability of the exoskeletons. From the software perspective, a challenging goal under exploration is the development of assistive strategies which should act consistently and adapt to specific gait patterns of each user.

2. Current Trends and Approaches

As stated in the introduction section, a possible social scenario for the coming years is that the increasing incidence of gait impairments will lead to an increasing number of individuals needing assistance in ADL, e.g. basic mobility, personal hygiene, and safety awareness. In this scenario, wearable robots could represent effective technologies to improve independency and social participation of people affected by mild lower limb impairments. The reduction of healthcare costs and increment of their productivity would contribute to the sustenance of the global welfare. In order to be useful in daily life scenarios, both physical and cognitive interfaces of a wearable robot should be compliant with natural biomechanics. In other words, it should be able to adapt to continuous variation dictated by the surrounding environment without losing the stability and robustness of its control policy and mechanical structure.[22]

An exoskeleton for gait assistance is generally anthropomorphic in nature. Given the close interaction with the user, the mechanical structure of a wearable robot should be lightweight and integrate several passive adjustable degrees of freedom. This is fundamental for a comfortable physical human–robot interface in order to match the user's joints range of motion (RoM), anthropometric variability, and joints kinematics.[23] For the purpose of being portable, an exoskeleton should be endowed with batteries allowing sufficient power autonomy, still preserving low encumbrances and weights.

The actuation units of the robot should comply with the user's biomechanics with an actuated joint stiffness — similar to one of the anatomical joints they are interfaced with — in order to prevent rigid, uncomfortable and — in the case of high-frequency movements such as spasms or impacts — even painful interactions. In this framework, an elastic approach is required to replace the traditional stiff actuation. The so-called Series Elastic Actuator (SEA) architecture[24] foresees the endowing of a mechanical compliance between the exoskeleton actuators and the user–robot interface and offers many advantages including shock tolerance, love-inflected inertia and accurate and stable closed-loop torque control.

In order to allow the user to perform his/her own movement without hindrance and receive assistance safely and consistently with the performed action, a skilled cognitive interface is needed for the wearable robot. The cognitive interface is expected to be able to decode (i) the intended movement of the user, for instance, ground-level walking, stairs climbing, and (ii) the phase of the periodical high-level locomotion task. On top of the decoding process, the control architecture can switch the desired assistive pattern according to the task keeping the synchronization with its cyclical phase.

3. Active Pelvis Orthosis: Laboratory Prototype

Motivated by the increasing need of technological aids for supporting those who underwent lower limb amputation in the framework of the European project CYBERLEGs (FP7-ICT-2011-2.1 Grant Agreement no 287894), The BioRobotics

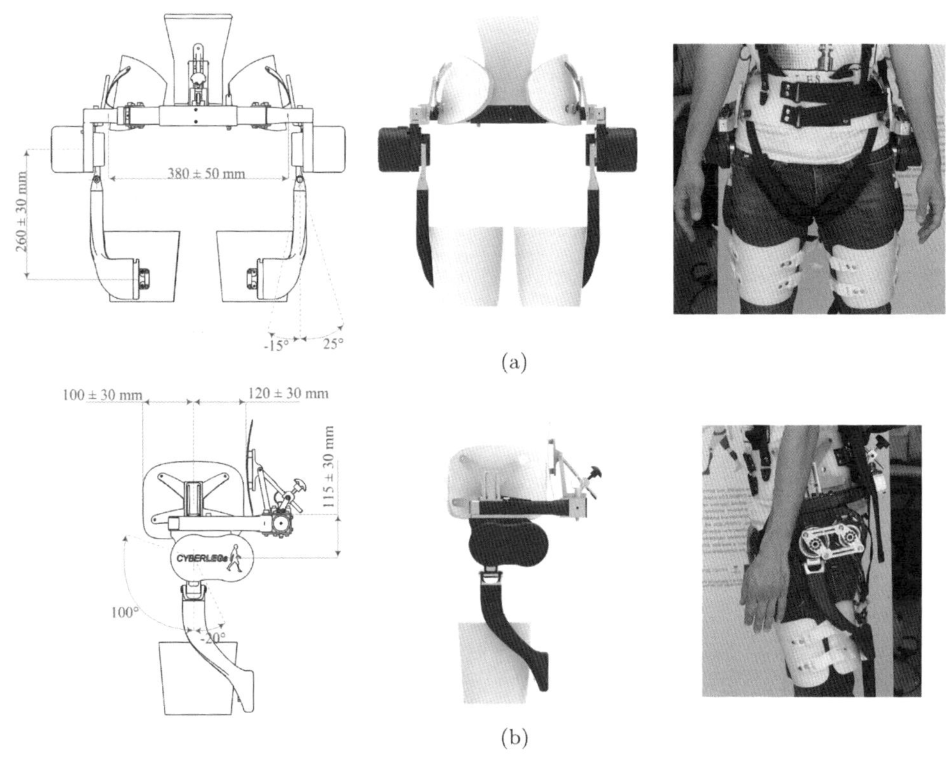

Figure 1. Overview on the α-APO. Frontal (a) and lateral (b) view of APO technical drawings with passive/active DoFs and regulations, CAD model and donned by the user.

Institute (Scuola Superiore Sant'Anna, Pisa, Italy) developed a novel wearable robotic technology for lower limb movement assistance.

The platform, shown in Fig. 1, consists of a lightweight active pelvis orthosis (APO) for assisting hip flexion–extension firstly presented in Ref. [19]. The device was conceived with two innovative solutions. Firstly, it has a novel, compact and lightweight SEA unit which exploits a custom patented torsional spring.[36] Secondly, authors proposed an optimized design based on extremely lightweight carbon fiber linkages, embedding manual adjustment for fitting the orthosis to a wide range of user sizes, and passive DoFs which follow the gait motions out of the flexion–extension plane (pelvis tilting, thigh abduction). The device hence ensures good kinematics compatibility, enhancing the comfort of the human–robot physical interaction, avoiding limitations and constrains to user's gait pattern, and addressing the match of intra- and intersubject anthropometric variability. The mechatronic architecture, i.e. the mechanical structure, the actuation units and the control system, of the α-APO is introduced in the following sections.

3.1. *Mechanical structure*

The device is sustained by a horizontal C-shaped frame, surrounding the user's hips and the back of the pelvis, and interfaced to the trunk by means of three orthotic shells (two lateral and one rear); the frame carries the two actuation units. The structure is realized in two 2.5 mm thickness carbon fiber lateral arms, connected by means of a rear straight bar. The rear bar is composed of an external guide in which two internal rods can slide: the bar length can then be adjusted in order to match the distance between the two lateral shells, ensuring the frame is tightly attached to the upper body in the medial–lateral direction. One of the two sliding rods can be locked by a fast-detach pin (for coarse regulation and fast don-doff procedure) and finely adjusted thanks to a leadscrew mechanism (for a detailed overview, refer to Fig. 2(a). In order to further ease the wearing procedure, the structure can also be completely separated in two parts (right and left).

The human and robot hip flexion–extension axes are aligned in the sagittal plane thanks to the adjustment of the horizontal and vertical positions of the rails in the cuff-frame interface. Furthermore, the back orthotic shell is fixed on the rear bar and adjusted by a screw mechanism to assess a correct and ergonomic pushing

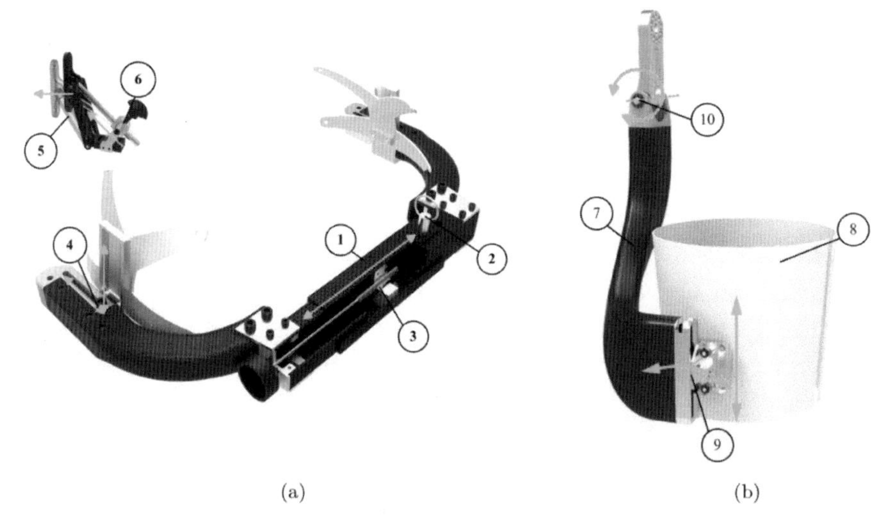

Figure 2. Overview of α-APO sub-systems: (a) C-shaped frame connected to the user's trunk — (1) Rear bar connecting the two carbon fiber arms. (2) Detachable pin for regulation. (3) Leadscrew mechanism for fine adjustment. (4) Rails for flexion–extension axes alignment. (5) Back support interface with the subject's back, namely, lumbar region. (6) Screw mechanism for adjustment. (b) Thigh linkage — (7) Carbon fiber linkage. (8) Orthotic shell interfaced with user's thigh. (9) Sliding and rotational adjustment of the orthotic shells. (10) Passive adduction–abduction rotational axis.

support on the lumbar region of the subject for a correct transmission of the assistive torque (see Fig. 2(a)).

The actuated axes drive two carbon fiber links, molded with a shape sweeping from the lateral to the back side of the thigh. The carbon fiber thickness is 2 mm; this structural optimization leads to the production of lightweight links while the necessary structural stiffness is still preserved. The carbon composites are coupled with the rest of the mechanics by means of aluminium inserts glued to the carbon fiber through a bi-component epoxy resin (Scotch-Weld™9323-3M™, Milan, Italy). The inserts at the interface between carbon fiber and metal components (the thigh links and the trunk support parts) are provided with slots that guarantee the needed regulations toward a comfortable wearing and the human–robot joint axes alignment.

Thigh links are also endowed with a passive rotational DoF for abduction–adduction (as it can be seen in Fig. 2(b)): this joint is located in a distal position with respect to the flexion–extension joint (60 mm below): this choice allows the abduction–adduction passive DoF to not be loaded by the weight of the actuation unit. Although the rotational axis of this passive DoF is not aligned with one of the human joints, it still contributes to provide a comfortable interaction and a non-rigid constraint of the user's leg while walking.

In order to comply with different lower limb lengths, the vertical position of the two plastic orthotic shells, which encircle the user's thigh, is adjustable thanks to lockable sliders situated at the tip of the carbon fiber linkages. These lockable sliders are endowed with a further regulation: it is possible to rotate the shells with respect to the linkage to find the most comfortable position for each user (see Fig. 2(b)).

The α-APO physically interfaces with the user's body in five zones: the three thermo-shaped orthotic trunk shells stabilize the frame over the user's waist, and the two upper leg shells are tightened around the thighs by means of elastic belts. This solution should guarantee a comfortable interaction and a safe transmission of the assistive torque by preventing the human–robot interaction surfaces from slippages. Moreover, the use of a soft orthopedic material and a wide contact area contribute to reduce and distribute the pressure on the user's skin. In addition, two straps allow a portion of the α-APO weight to be supported by the shoulders and thus avoid the trunk from being loaded with an excessive lateral pressure.

All the orthotic shells were custom manufactured with a two-layered structure: a 3 mm-thick internal layer of thermoplastic polyethylene foam (Plastazote® 617S7, Otto Bock, Duderstadt, Germany) for moisture draining and skin transpiration and a 3 mm-thick outer layer of polypropylene (ThermoLyn® Polypropylene

616T20, Otto Bock, Duderstadt, Germany). These shells come in different sizes, and can also be tailor-made for each subject.

3.2. *Actuation units*

α-APO is endowed with two actuation units, one for each hip flexion–extension joint, mounted on the lateral arms. The actuation unit employs an SEA architecture.[24] SEAs have been successfully applied in the field of wearable powered robots mostly to solve safety issues and reduce the inherent output impedance.[25–27] In this case, the actuation is not rigid and allows minimum joint output impedance across the frequency spectrum of gait. Furthermore, variations in the output impedance can still be achieved by means of closed-loop interaction control strategies.[24]

The motor units have been designed taking as reference the hip angle and torque profiles reported by the Winter dataset: in particular, we assumed a natural cadence of 105 steps/min and a user weight of 80 kg.[27] The target amount of assistance was set to 50% of the human torque required during ground-level walking: hence, the actuator was designed in order to provide a maximum torque of 35 Nm.

The SEA in-series elasticity is obtained by means of a custom patented[37] torsional spring with a stiffness of 100 Nm/rad — a value comparable with the human hip average stiffness during ground-level walking[28] — and bears the torsion stress up to the design value without yielding, nor presenting hysteretic or nonlinear behavior. The spring compliance prevents the subject from an uncomfortable (or even painful) interaction with an excessively stiff device in the case of high frequency movements (e.g. sudden spasms, interaction with the ground, etc.). The same spring has been used to design the actuation unit of the NEUROExos elbow exoskeleton developed at The BioRobotics Institute (Scuola Superiore Sant'Anna, Pisa, Italy), and its design and experimental characterization were already presented in Ref. [29].

Each actuation unit (a detailed overview is reported in Fig. 3) is deployed around two parallel axes. One is the axis of the 100 W DC motor (EC60, Maxon Motor®, Sachseln, Switzerland) equipped with an incremental encoder (1024 ppr, MILE, Maxon Motor®, Sachseln, Switzerland) and coupled with a 80:1 Harmonic Drive (HD) (CPL-17A-080-2A, Harmonic Drive®, Limburg, Germany) reduction stage. On the other axis (which is the one actually collocated with the human hip flexion–extension axis), there is the torsional spring in series with a 32-bit absolute encoder (RESOLUTE™, ring: RESA30USA052B, read head: RA32BAA052B30, Renishaw®, Gloucestershire, England), which measures the absolute hip joint angle. Each actuation unit reaches a weight of 1.2 kg. By assuming a RoM of the human hip joint from −20° (minimum extension angle

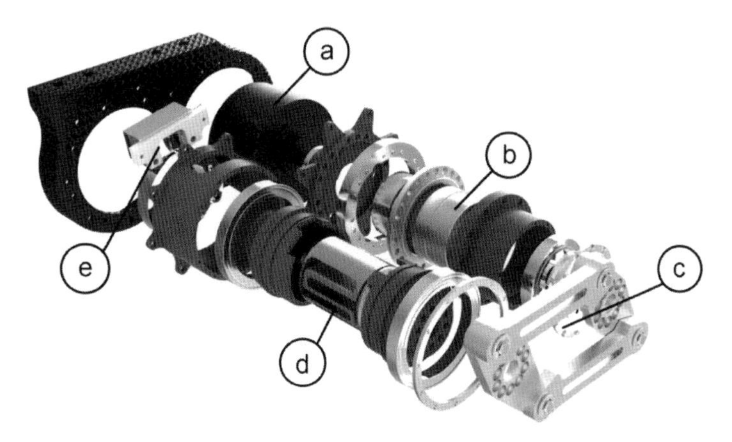

Figure 3. Exploded view of the α-APO series elastic actuation unit: (a) DC motor with embedded incremental encoder, (b) Harmonic drive, (c) 4-bar transmission mechanism, (d) Torsional spring, and (e) Absolute encoder.

during walking) to 90° (maximum flexion angle in a seated position), we opted for a transmission means between the two parallel axes based on a 4-bar mechanism, with a RoM between −30° and 110°, limited by emergency mechanical stops. The two-axis configuration was chosen in order to reduce the overall lateral encumbrance, namely, 110 mm, due to the length of the gear-motor unit and of the torsional spring. Although this encumbrance is relatively small, this solution is a limitation of the current design as it partly prevents the user from swinging his or her arms. However, its encumbrance is comparable to one of other lower limb exoskeletons.[9]

The entire system has a total weight of 4.2 kg (this weight excludes the control unit which is still remotely located in this prototype) and the adjustable DoFs allow the system to comply with a wide range of user's body size.

3.3. *Control system*

The α-APO control system, shown in Fig. 4, is based on a hierarchical architecture that comprises a *low-level torque control* layer (two independent torque controls, one for each actuation unit) and a *high-level* layer implementing an adaptive assistive strategy.

1) *Low-level torque control*: The low-level controller is in charge of managing the actuators in order to track the set torque value to the moving linkage of the exoskeleton. The closed-loop control architecture is that of a classical proportional-integral-derivative (PID) regulator. The PID regulator operates on the error between the desired torque τ_{des} and the measured torque τ, and returns an electrical current

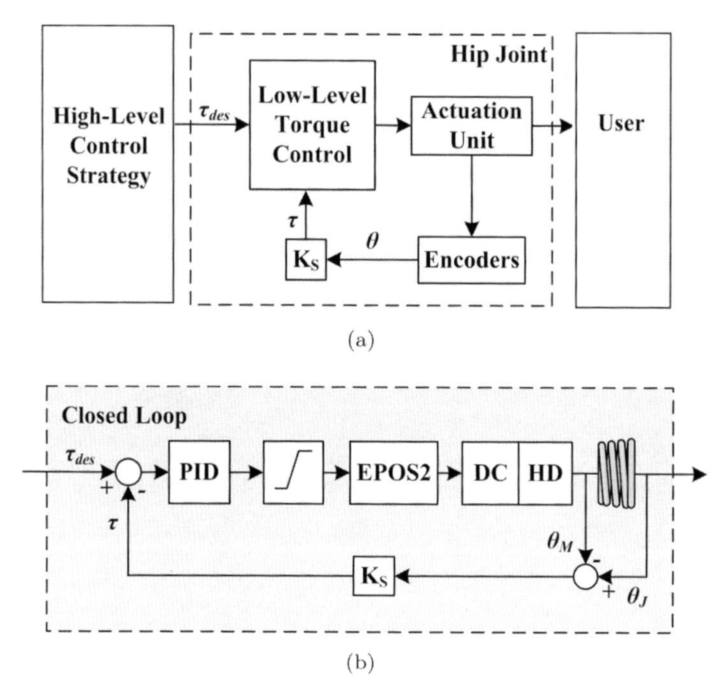

Figure 4. Scheme of the control system of the α-APO: (a) Block diagram of the hierarchical control architecture. (b) Low-level closed-loop torque control.

provided to the motor, within a saturation interval of ± 3.2 A — corresponding to a torque range of ± 35 Nm. The motor current is controlled by means of a commercial servo amplifier (EPOS2 70/10, Maxon Motor®, Sachseln, Switzerland). As it is explained in Ref. [24], the bandwidth of an SEA system controlled by means of a PID compensator can be limited by design. Thus, PID regulator coefficients were tuned manually to achieve the widest closed-loop bandwidth.

The measured torque is estimated from the deformation of the torsional spring by means of the two encoders (respectively measuring the Harmonic Drive output shaft angle θ_M and the joint angle θ_J), being known as the torsional stiffness K_S. Since one of the two encoders is incremental (the one on the motor side), an initializing procedure is needed at the power-on of the system in order to correctly acquire the reference zero value of spring deformation, corresponding to a null transmitted torque: this was achieved through a rigid pin, bypassing the torsional spring (impeding its deformation and then keeping it unloaded), which was then removed after the initialization of the incremental encoder reference value.

2) *High-level assistive control*: In order to be used as a wearable active orthosis for human motion assistance, the torque control should be able to provide the user with the assistive torque with near-zero output impedance, i.e. with minimum

to null joint parasitic stiffness.[29] Aiming at the system usability in a task of gait assistance, we opted for a high-level control strategy, that could provide a desired torque reference variable over the stride. This way, we could assess whether the closed-loop torque control bandwidth was sufficiently large and the parasitic output stiffness sufficiently low to allow the system to track the desired torque with a relatively small error, at different gait speeds. As an assistive control strategy, we selected a model-free (it does not require any *a priori* knowledge about the gait dynamics) algorithm presented in a recent work by Ronsse *et al.*[30] This algorithm has been used to provide users of the LOPES exoskeleton with hip flexion–extension assistance, and it relies on the use of adaptive oscillators (AOs), which are mathematical tools introduced by Righetti *et al.*[31] that — when coupled with a kernel-based nonlinear filter — can constantly track and provide a zero-delay estimate of a non-sinusoidal periodic signal (e.g. hip or knee angle profile during gait), even when it slowly changes its main features such as frequency and envelope over gait cycles.

AOs are a set of nonlinear differential equations capable of synchronizing with an input periodic signal, not by tracking its current value, but rather tracking the signal periodicity characteristics (i.e. amplitude, frequency, and lead phase). Thanks to the capability of this architecture to — instead of doing mere synchronization — learn the frequency (and then the phase) and the envelope of a quasi-periodic teaching signal, we could track and learn the quasi-periodic behavior of each hip joint angle and provide a reliable prediction of the joint angle versus gait phase within the gait cycle. This means that at each gait phase φ, the AO and the nonlinear filter can provide an estimate of both the hip joint angle $\hat{\theta}_J(\varphi)$ and its future value at a phase $\varphi + \Delta\varphi$, namely, $\hat{\theta}_J(\varphi + \Delta\varphi)$, $\Delta\varphi$ being a phase lead tunable by the experimenter. The assistive torque is then computed by setting the $\tau_{\mathrm{des}} = K_v \cdot [\hat{\theta}_J(\varphi + \Delta\varphi) - \hat{\theta}_J(\varphi)]$, K_v being a tunable virtual stiffness. This way, the user's joints are smoothly attracted toward their future positions by means of an attractive virtual stiffness field, while leaving the opportunity to the user to constantly adapt the frequency and shape of his or her gait pattern.

3) *Control unit and safety loop*: The control system runs on a real-time controller, a cRIO-9082 (National Instruments, Austin, Texas, US), endowed with a 1.33 GHz dual-core processor running a NI real-time operating system and a field programmable gate array (FPGA) processor Spartan-6 LX150. Both the high- and low-level layers run at 1 kHz.

The APO control system implements a safety loop that switches off the actuation when the measured torque is higher than 30 Nm or the joint speed is greater than 400°/s. In addition, both the experimenter and the user can turn off the apparatus by means of a red, emergency button.

3.4. *Performance validation*

3.4.1. *Low-level torque controller*

The low-level controller of the α-APO was validated from three points of view: step response to different torque amplitudes, chirp response to a linear chirp torque and output impedance in zero to que mode. The experimental characterization of the low-level control pointed out that the proposed implementation for the SEA and its control system have a suitable dynamic performance to provide an assistive torque with null-to-minimum output impedance.

The step-response experiments pointed out that the tracking capabilities of the device actuator are fast and prompt enough, this feature mainly being a property of the chosen motors and their PID tuning. The chirp response analysis showed that the low-level controller leads to a -3 dB control bandwidth of 15.5 Hz, thus broadly enclosing the typical frequencies of human gait. This result is comparable with those attained with another lower limb device, endowing SEAs and an adaptive-oscillator-based controller, the LOPES platform[17]: the main innovation in this work is that we were able to reach the same performances with a *lightweight and portable* device, while the LOPES is structurally sustained by a treadmill. Finally, within the 0.2–3.2 Hz frequency bandwidth, in zero-torque mode, we measured that the values of parasitic torque and residual stiffness are relatively low and comparable with the ones reported in state-of-the-art robots.[32,33]

3.4.2. *High-level assistive strategy*

In order to evaluate the functionality of the α-APO system, a prototypical task of gait assistance was designed and tested on a healthy volunteer (male, 30 years old, 70 kg). The experiment was carried out at the premises of Don Carlo Gnocchi Foundation (Florence, Italy). The healthy subject was requested to walk on a treadmill for about 2 min at four different velocities (from 2 to 5 km/h) under both the zero-torque and assistive modalities. The usability of the system as an assistive device has been explored by analyzing and comparing the zero-torque and assistive mode experimental session results: in zero-torque mode, we assessed the capability of the α-APO to promptly reject disturbances due to the variability of joint motion, with a peak of resistive torque of 0.4 Nm, while in assistive modality, we observed how the system was able to provide a high amount of net positive power (up to 60 W for a peak torque of 10 Nm) with minimal differences between the joint angle motion profile between zero-torque and assistive condition (apart from the increased variability over different strides), this being a proof that the α-APO in assistive mode does not affect the natural gait cadence.

4. β-APO: Portable Version

Even if highly compliant to human biomechanics and to several anthropometries, as a laboratory prototype, the α-version has the main limitation of a wired power supply and communication with the remote desktop of the operator. As stated in the introduction of this chapter, to be usable and effective in assisting people in ADL, a wearable robot should be portable and battery operated. With the ultimate goal of achieving a totally portable device and updating the requirements derived from the development and the experimental characterization of the α-APO, the β-version of the APO, namely, β-APO, was designed and developed. An overview of the system is provided in Fig. 5.

The design of the β-APO was grounded based on important assumptions highlighted during the preliminary assessment of the usability of the α-version: (i) placement of the actuation units on the back-side of the device in order to minimize the lateral encumbrance, thus allowing the natural arm swinging of the user; (ii) revision of the passive DoFs to allow free hip adduction–abduction and intra extra-rotation; (iii) revision of the actuation unit design in order to have absolute encoders to measure the deformation of the torsional spring without any zeroing procedure at the power on; and (iv) the β-APO should be a fully wearable and portable system: all the components of the electronics and control system being included in a backpack connected with the exoskeleton. This last feature was necessary to allow the use of the device outside the laboratory environment, thus enhancing the possibility to validate the use of the device into scenarios of ADL.

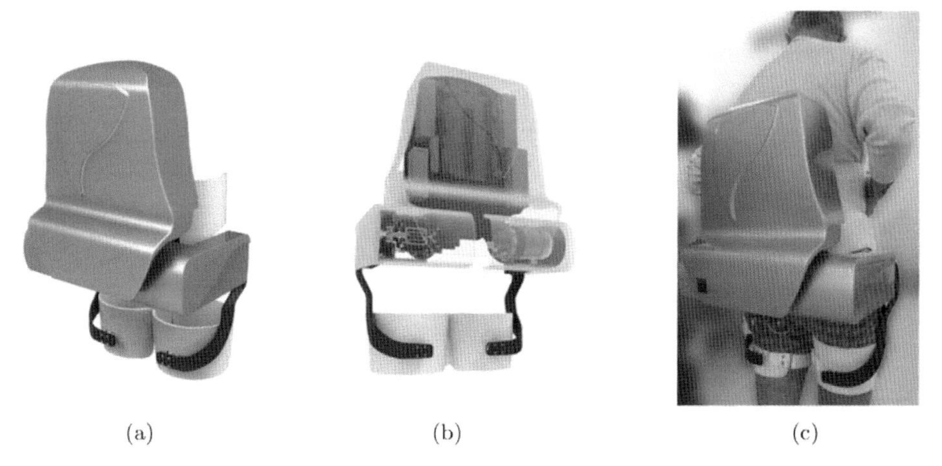

(a) (b) (c)

Figure 5. Overview of the β-APO: (a) CAD model of the system, (b) CAD model of the electronic board, battery packs and actuation units integrated in the mechanical structure, and (c) β-APO donned by an end-user.

In this section, we provide the description of the new mechatronic architecture focusing on the items and solutions which advance the α-version. As it has been done for the α-version, the description will be given for the three sub-systems: mechanical structure, actuation unit, and control system.

4.1. *Mechanical structure*

The mechanical structure of the β-APO is constituted of three main parts: the pelvis frame, the transmission system and the thigh linkages. The pelvis frame structure is constituted of a main carbon fiber plate connecting the exoskeleton to the pelvis cuff and then to the user. Two carbon fiber plates (one for each leg) can slide on it by means of two linear guides. The linear guides allow an easy wearing of the actuation units of the exoskeleton.

Two carbon fiber lateral extensible arms are connected to the central element of the device through a novel chain of passive DoFs. Each lateral arm is endowed with passive regulation mechanisms to guarantee anthropometries matching and proper alignment of actuated and human joint axes. A transmission system based on steel cable is embedded into the carbon fiber lateral arm and transmits the torque from the actuation unit to the flexion extension joint.

A curved carbon fiber link was designed for connecting the β-APO to the thighs through orthotic shells.

The novelty of the designed mechanical structure with respect to the current state of the art on lower limb wearable robotics is the integration of a kinematic chain[38] that allowed to place the actuation units on the rear part of the device, i.e. on the back of the person for maintaining a more natural swing of the arms in the sagittal plane. The kinematics chain allows to have both axes of adduction–abduction and flexion–extension collocated with the anatomical joint axes. Furthermore, the abduction–adduction can be spring loaded for compensating the moment generated by the weight of lateral assembly on the adduction–abduction joint.

4.2. *Actuation units*

The β-APO is endowed with two actuation units, one for each hip flexion–extension joint. Each actuation unit is located on the rear part of the lateral arms.

Following the same assumption given for the α-APO, the actuation unit has the structure of an SEA. In this case, the actuation unit has a single axis configuration connected to the torsional spring whose deformation is directly measured by an absolute encoder. A second absolute encoder placed on the hip axis measures the actual hip angle. Each actuation unit reaches a weight which is slightly higher than 1 kg.

4.3. *Control system*

The β-APO control system is based on the same hierarchical architecture described in the α-APO prototype: closed-loop torque controls are independent for each actuation unit.

1) *Low-level torque control*: The low-level torque control layer relies on a PID compensator designed to achieve the minimum joint output impedance and a relatively high closed-loop bandwidth. The controller still operates on the error between the desired torque reference τ_{des} and the measured torque τ computed being known the stiffness of the torsional spring. The sensory apparatus comprises two absolute encoders recording, respectively, the deformation of the spring and the joint angle: as an advantage with respect to the α-APO prototype, there is no need for the zeroing procedure of the torsional spring deformation.

2) *High-level control strategy*: During the test phase, we used the same high-level layer of the control architecture of the α-APO. It is worth noting that the flexibility of reconfigurable real-time controller allowed for the implementation and validation of several control approaches for assisting people in ADL.

3) *Control Unit and Safety Loop*: The control system runs on a real-time controller, a sbRIO-9632 (National Instruments, Austin, Texas, US), endowed with a FPGA processor. The high-level layer runs at 100 Hz. The low-level layer runs on the FPGA at 1 kHz. Both the experimenter and the user can turn off the apparatus by means of a red, emergency button.

The main advancement of the β-version is given by the portability of the system. The control electronics in the β-APO are embedded inside the backpack of the mechanical structure with the batteries as well. The integration of the controller and power supplies in the device leads to the achievement of not only a wearable but also a completely portable system. Portability allows to overcome the restriction of operating in the laboratory environment and opening the possibility to investigate on the efficacy of the β-APO in ADL.

A Wi-Fi access point is used for data logging and control of the platform via wireless communication. Furthermore, the device can be interfaced by means of 4 ZigBee module to a wearable sensory apparatus composed by a set of seven inertial measurements units and a pair of sensitive insoles, the latter being developed at The BioRobotics Insitute (Scuola Superiore Sant'Anna, Pisa, Italy).[34]

The integration of external wearable sensory apparatus enabled the possibility of designing several experimental activities with the goal of testing the feasibility of assistive strategies in unstructured environment, i.e. not only treadmill walking but also ground-level walking and stair climbing.[35] The ability of a portable wearable robot to reliably intend the desired movement and the performed locomotion-related activities is of fundamental importance for the usability of the device in ADL. The intention detection can be performed without actively involving the person in the decoding process. On top of the intuitiveness of the controller, the reliability of the system enhances its acceptability for end-users who find it easy and safe to be used.

In addition, the system has successfully demonstrated a comfortable and safe usability. The device was indeed worn by an impaired subject, namely, a transfemoral amputee, who was asked to freely walk in an open space wearing the β-APO under zero-torque mode (see Fig. 6). Intentional movement of the subject was not hindered by the parasitic stiffness making it possible to normally walk with no additional effort on the limb. Furthermore, a walking session receiving assistance was tested to assess the effective feasibility of the assistive modality. The device was capable of smoothly providing a safe and reliable assistive torque on the subject without altering his normal kinematics.

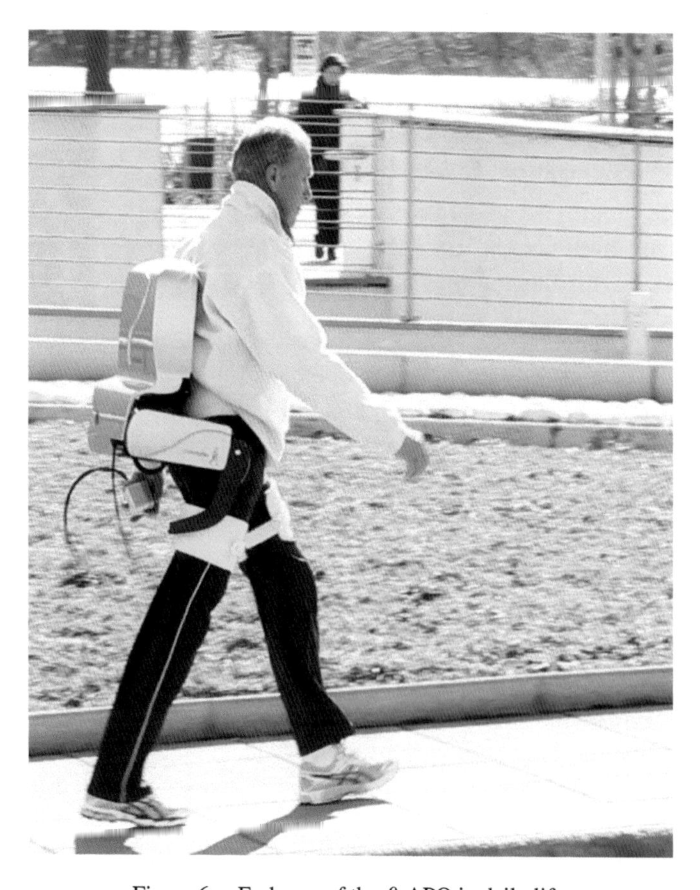

Figure 6. End-user of the β-APO in daily life.

5. γ-APO

5.1. *Mechatronic description*

Despite the great advancement in terms of portability and usability in out-of-lab scenario, the β-version is still redundant in many components, thus in terms of weight — which actually limits its comfort when worn — and dependability. In order to overcome these limitations, the design was steered toward the advancement and optimization of the γ-APO structure in order to achieve a really portable lightweight device (targeted weight <6 kg) while still ensuring the structural features needed for providing effective assistance.

The structure of the γ -APO consists of a carbon fiber frame that embeds one active and one passive DoF for each side, allowing the user to freely perform movements of abduction–adduction at the hip level, while receiving assistance on the flexion–extension. Two SEA units are mounted on the rear part of the device. The overall weight of the device (thanks to a high percentage 40–45% of composite materials) is around 5.0 kg, including batteries and control electronics. γ-APO is a battery-operated fully-autonomous wearable and portable device; its autonomy reaches about 2 hours. On top of the closed-loop torque control, it is possible to conceive/integrate a virtually-infinite number of different assistive strategies, which have the objective to set the assistance, coherently with the intended locomotion task and residual user movement ability. This flexibility is guaranteed by a set of I/Os reconfigurable port which allows to interface the device with an external sensory apparatus.

5.2. *Service scenario*

Prospective main end-users of the APO are as follows: (i) subjects who are affected by weak and cautious gait syndromes; people affected by weak gait syndromes usually exhibit high steppage, dropping foot and waddling, as a consequence of neurological, muscular or vascular diseases, such as stroke, degenerative vascular diseases (e.g. diabetes mellitus), herniated lumbar disk, multiple sclerosis, muscular atrophy, ALS or Parkinson's disease; (ii) elderly users who — albeit not having been diagnosed with a specific syndrome — would highly benefit from a system capable of alleviating the burden of walking, therefore all users showing typical senile gait characteristics; and (iii) all-cause lower limb amputees who may benefit from a system like the APO helping them to recover a more energy-efficient gait pattern. APO will be a bilateral hip orthosis. It will come in three different sizes (to cope with the different range of anthropometries) and will have passive regulations for fine matching the intrasubject variability within the selected range of anthropometries. This device will also be easy to be interfaced with standard harness systems, for a safe use of the device within the clinical environment, with patients suffering from severe to mild gait impairment.

6. Conclusion

The incidence of gait impairments is increasing and in a few years, the amount of people needing healthcare and assistance will overwhelm the number of those who are supposed to deliver such services. Technological advancements in the design of lightweight actuators, flexible electronic boards for general purpose programming and lightweight batteries have opened the frontiers to the design of compact and lightweight wearable robots for assistance and rehabilitation of impaired people. Focusing on lower limb wearable robotics, in the last decade, several commercial devices have reached the market for rehabilitation of post-stroke patients, restoration of locomotion functionality for hemiplegic and paraplegic people and assistance during walking for mildly impaired subjects. Ergonomics of the system's mechanical structure, intuitiveness of the controller and general acceptability of these devices are, nevertheless, unresolved challenges.

In this chapter, we presented a novel robotic platform conceived for assisting people with mild lower limbs impairments in ADL. The mechatronic architecture of the first laboratory prototype was described in detail; a lightweight SEA and a mechanical structure endowed with several passive regulations to match a wide percentile of anthropometries were the main novelty of the lightweight APO. Early usability assessment provided guidelines to advance its limitations in terms of design, including the requirement for its portability. The portable version of the APO came with a novel kinematic chain and a battery-operated cognitive unit; it enabled the feasibility of out-of-lab investigations, ergonomic assessment and design of control policies for effective assistance-as-needed (AAN) in ADL. Finally, following an optimization analysis, an engineered portable version, will be soon delivered. APO will be lightweight and compact — thanks to the high percentage of composite materials — easy to don and doff and capable of assisting people in locomotion-related activities with intuitive and reliable approaches which do not require the help of personnel with relevant expertise.

We expect that people using the APO technology will be able to walk better and faster, safer and steadier, and overall be able to enjoy a reduced physical burden in performing their ADL, enhanced social engagement and quality of life.

Acknowledgments

Andrea Parri and Tingfang Yan are equal contributors. Andrea Parri, Francesco Giovacchini, Mario Cortese, Marco Muscolo, and Nicola Vitiello have commercial interests in IUVO S.r.l, a spin-off company of Scuola Superiore Sant'Anna. Currently, the IP protecting the APO technology has been licensed to IUVO S.r.l. for commercial exploitation.

References

1. U. N. D. of Economic, World Population Ageing (2013).
2. A. B. Schultz. (1992). Mobility impairment sin the elderly: Challenges for biomechanics research, *Journal of Biomechanics* 25(5):519–528.
3. M. Chan. (2013). International Perspectives on Spinal Cord Injury, 4.
4. World Health Organization (2013), Spinal Cord Injury, *Media Centre, Fact Sheets n°384* 1–22.
5. J. -M. Belda-Lois, S. Mena-del Horno, I. Bermejo-Bosch, J. C. Moreno, J. L. Pons, D. Farina, M. Iosa, M. Molinari, F. Tamburella, A. Ramos, A. Caria, T. Solis-Escalante, C. Brunner and M. Rea. (2011). Rehabilitation of gait after stroke: a review towards a top-down approach, *Journal of Neuroengineering Rehabilitation* 8(1):66.
6. A. G. Thrift, D. a. Cadilhac, T. Thayabaranathan, G. Howard, V. J. Howard, P. M. Rothwell and G. a. Donnan. (2014). Global stroke statistics, *International Journal of Stroke* 9(1):6–18.
7. K. Ziegler-Graham, E. J. MacKenzie, P. L. Ephraim, T. G. Travison and R. Brookmeyer. (2008). Estimating the prevalence of limb loss in the United States: 2005 to 2050, *Archives of Physical Medicine and Rehabilitation* 89(3):422–429.
8. T. Yan, M. Cempini, C. M. Oddo and N. Vitiello. (2014). Review of assistive strategies in powered lower-limb orthoses and exoskeletons, *Robotics and Autonomous Systems* 64: 120–136.
9. A. M. Dollar and H. Herr. (2008). Lower extremity exoskeletons and active orthoses: challenges and state-of-the-art, *IEEE Transactions on Robotics* 24(1):144–158.
10. M. R. Tucker, J. Olivier, A. Pagel, H. Bleuler, M. Bouri and O. Lambercy. (2015). Control strategies for active lower extremity prosthetics and orthotics: a review.
11. J. L. Pons. (2008). *Wearable Robots: Biomechatronic Exoskeletons.* John Wiley and Sons.
12. H. Kazerooni, R. Steger and L. Huang. (2006). Hybrid Control of the Berkeley Lower Extremity Exoskeleton (BLEEX), *International Journal of Robotics Research* 25(5–6):561–573.
13. E. S. A. Estec, J. Gancet, M. Ilzkovitz, G. Cheron, Y. Ivanenko, H. van der Kooij, F. van der Helm, F. Zanow and F. Thorsteinsson. (2011). Mindwalker: A brain controlled lower limbs exoskeleton for rehabilitation. Potential applications to space, *11th Symposium on Advanced Space Technologies in Robotics and Automation*, 12–14.
14. A. Esquenazi, M. Talaty, A. Packel and M. Saulino. (2012). The ReWalk powered exoskeleton to restore ambulatory function to individuals with thoracic-level motor-complete spinal cord injury, *American Journal of Physical Medicine and Rehabilitation* 91:911–921.
15. R. J. Farris, H. a Quintero and M. Goldfarb. (2011). Preliminary evaluation of a powered lower limb orthosis to aid walking in paraplegic individuals, *IEEE Transaction on Neural Systems and Rehabilitation Engineering* 19(6):652–659.
16. Y. Sankai. (2010). HAL: Hybrid assistive limb based on cybernics, *Robotics Research*, 25–34.
17. J. F. Veneman, R. Kruidhof, E. E. G. Hekman, R. Ekkelenkamp, E. H. F. Van Asseldonk and H. van der Kooij. (2007). Design and evaluation of the LOPES exoskeleton robot for interactive gait rehabilitation, *IEEE Transaction Neural Systems Rehabilitation Engineering* 15(3): 379–386.
18. M. Drużbicki, W. Rusek, S. Snela, J. Dudek, M. Szczepanik, E. Zak, J. Durmala, A. Czernuszenko, M. Bonikowski and G. Sobota. (2013). Functional effects of robotic-assisted locomotor treadmill therapy in children with cerebral palsy, *Journal of Rehabilitation Medicine* 45(4):358–363.

19. F. Giovacchini, F. Vannetti, M. Fantozzi, M. Cempini, M. Cortese, A. Parri, T. Yan, D. Lefeber and N. Vitiello. (2014). A light-weight active orthosis for hip movement assistance, *Robotics and Autonomous Systems* 73:123–134.
20. S. H. Collins, M. B. Wiggin and G. S. Sawicki. (2015). Reducing the energy cost of human walking using an unpowered exoskeleton. *Nature*, 522(7555):212–215.
21. A. Asbeck, S. M. M. De Rossi, I. Galiana, Y. Ding and C. Walsh. (2014). Stronger, Smarter, Softer, *IEEE Robotics and Automation Magazine* 21(4):22–33.
22. R. E. Cowan, B. J. Fregly, M. L. Boninger, L. Chan, M. M. Rodgers and D. J. Reinkensmeyer. (2012). Recent trends in assistive technology for mobility, *Journal of Neuroengineering and Rehabilitation* 9(1):20.
23. A. Schiele and F. C. T. Van Der Helm. (2006). Kinematic design to improve ergonomics in human machine interaction, *IEEE Transaction on Neural Systems and Rehabilitation Engineering* 14(4):456–469.
24. G. A. Pratt and M. M. Williamson. (1995). Series elastic actuators, in *Proceedings 1995 IEEE/RSJ International Conference on Intelligent Robots and Systems. Human Robot Interaction and Cooperative Robots* 1:399–406.
25. J. F. Veneman, R. Ekkelenkamp, R. Kruidhof, F. C. van der Helm and H. van der Kooij. (2006). A Series Elastic- and Bowden-Cable-Based Actuation System for Use as Torque Actuator in Exoskeleton-Type Robots, *International Journal of Robotics Research* 25(3):261–281.
26. M. Zinn, B. Roth, O. Khatib and J. K. Salisbury. (2004). A new actuation approach for human friendly robot design, *International Journal of Robotics Research* 23(4):379–398.
27. D. A. Winter. (2009). *Biomechanics and Motor Control of Human Movement.* John Wiley and Sons.
28. C. J. Walsh, K. Endo and H. Herr. (2007). A quasi-passive leg exoskeleton for load-carrying augmentation, *International Journal of Humanoid Robotics* 4(3):487–506.
29. N. Vitiello, T. Lenzi, S. Roccella, S. M. M. De Rossi, E. Cattin, F. Giovacchini, F. Vecchi and M. C. Carrozza. (2013). NEUROExos: A powered elbow exoskeleton for physical rehabilitation, *IEEE International Transaction on Robotics* 29(1):220–235.
30. R. Ronsse, T. Lenzi, N. Vitiello, B. Koopman, E. Van Asseldonk, S. M. M. De Rossi, J. Van Den Kieboom, H. Van Der Kooij, M. C. Carrozza and A. J. Ijspeert. (2011). Oscillator-based assistance of cyclical movements: Model-based and model-free approaches, *Medical and Biological Engineering and Computing* 49:1173–1185.
31. L. Righetti, J. Buchli and A. J. Ijspeert. (2009). Adaptive Frequency Oscillators and Applications, *The Open Cybernetics and Systemics Journal* 3:64–69.
32. A. M. Dollar and H. Herr. (2008). Design of a quasi-passive knee exoskeleton to assist running, *IEEE/RSJ International Conference of Intelligent Robotics and System* 747–754.
33. H. Vallery, R. Ekkelenkamp, H. Van Der Kooij and M. Buss. (2007). Passive and accurate torque control of series elastic actuators, *IEEE International Conference on Intelligent Robotics and Systems* 3534–3538.
34. S. Crea, M. Donati, S. M. M. De Rossi, C. M. Oddo and N. Vitiello. (2014). A wireless flexible sensorized insole for gait analysis, *Sensors (Basel).* 14(1):1073–1093.
35. K. Yuan, A. Parri, T. Yan, L. Wang, M. Munih, N. Vitiello and Q. Wang. (2015). Fuzzy-Logic-based hybrid locomotion mode classification for an active pelvis orthosis: preliminary results, *IEEE International Conference on Intelligent Robotics and Systems* 3893–3896.
36. F. Giovacchini, M. Cempini, N. Vitiello, M. C. Carrozza. (2015). Torsional transmission element with elastic response, WO2015001469, International Publication Date: January 8.
37. F. Giovacchini, M. Cempini, N. Vitiello, M.C. Carrozza. (2015). Torsional transmission element with elastic response, WO2015001469, International Publication Date: January 8.
38. N. Vitiello, F. Giovacchini, M. Cempini, M. Fantozzi, M. Moisè, M. Muscolo, M. Cortese. (2015). Sistema di attuazione per ortesi di anca, Application No. FI2015A000025 (Italian Patent), Application Date: February 9. Pending for acceptance.

Chapter 4

USER-ADAPTIVE CONTROL OF ROBOTIC LOWER LIMB PROSTHESES

Tommaso Lenzi and Levi Hargrove

Center for Bionic Medicine, Rehabilitation Institute of Chicago
345 East Superior Street, Chicago, IL, USA 60611

Robotic lower limb prostheses can actively regulate joint torque to restore more natural and efficient ambulation for individuals with leg amputation. Motorized prosthetic joints generate significant amounts of energy, thus allowing amputees to perform activities with active dynamics, such as reciprocal stair climbing and sit-to-stand transitions, that are not possible with conventional passive prostheses. However, to restore physiological ambulation ability with a robotic prosthesis, prosthetic joint movements must be synchronized with the user's movements. This requires the control system to detect the intended ambulation activity and seamlessly adjust the prosthesis movement accordingly. This chapter discusses the challenges in the control of robotic lower limb prostheses, specifically focusing on the most recent approaches to adapting robotic prosthesis movement to the user's intended movement. Examples from our results with a robotic ankle and knee prosthesis will be used to illustrate the potential benefits of using a robotic prosthesis over a conventional passive device. Current limitations and barriers to translating robotic prostheses into clinically viable devices will also be discussed.

1. Introduction: Overview of Lower Limb Prosthesis Technologies

1.1. *Lower limb amputation*

An estimated 1.8 million individuals currently live with amputations in the United States, and an additional 185,000 new amputations occur every year.[1] The majority of amputations occur in the lower limb and are due to vascular disease, frequently a complication of diabetes. Thus, as the population ages and the prevalence of diabetes increases, the number of individuals with lower limb amputation is expected to increase dramatically.[1] Lower limb amputation is a severe condition that affects mobility, independence, and the ability to resume work or leisure-related activities. Despite constant improvements in prosthetic devices and in amputee care, lower limb amputees are still limited in their achievement of normal functions, community mobility, and social activities by current prosthetic options. Most available devices are passive, thus they do not replace the power that would be provided by an intact limb. The individual must compensate for this deficit by increasing the effort of muscles on their residual limb and intact leg. This results in an unnatural, asymmetric, less efficient gait pattern[2] and abnormal body mechanics that can cause further injury, exacerbating the clinical impact of amputation. Even using state-of-the-art prostheses, persons with transfemoral amputations expend far more energy than able-bodied individuals during ambulation.[3] These issues severely affect the quality of life of individuals with lower limb amputation and contribute to secondary complications such as osteoarthritis, back pain, and depression.[4]

1.2. *Passive prostheses*

Most commercially available prosthetic legs are mechanically passive, lightweight devices that can support the body weight of the person and enable basic ambulation abilities. The movement of a passive prosthetic joint relies on the properties of its mechanical components, such as hydraulic or pneumatic valves and sliding joints. Passive prostheses cannot perform net mechanical work, thus these devices do not restore the positive power that would be provided by the intact ankle or knee. More advanced passive prosthetic legs for transfemoral amputees employ sensors and a microcontroller for closed-loop control of joint damping.[5–7] The "intelligent" controller adjusts the damping of the prosthetic joint through a hydraulic damper[8] or by modifying a magnetic field.[9,10] Studies have shown that compared to mechanically passive prostheses, microprocessor-controlled prostheses with variable damping make gait smoother and decrease compensatory strategies used during locomotion.[11–13] However, like mechanically passive devices, microprocessor-controlled prostheses lack the ability to generate energy during locomotion.

1.3. *Limitations of passive prostheses*

Significant positive energy is needed to perform activities that require vertical mobility of the body center of mass, such as ascending stairs or walking up a hill,[14] and, to a lesser extent, to propel the body during ground-level walking.[15] Able-bodied individuals generate the positive energy needed to ambulate by optimally coordinating activation of the leg muscles. Loss of a leg through amputation disrupts this coordination, thus when the biological leg is replaced with a passive prosthesis that cannot generate positive energy, the muscles on the residual limb and the contralateral leg must supply extra energy to perform the intended activity. This compensatory mechanism produces an unnatural, inefficient, and less stable gait pattern.[16,17] As a consequence, passive devices, including microprocessor-controlled devices, provide significantly limited function, especially for individuals with amputations at or above the knee. Individuals with transfemoral amputation using a passive device walk at half the speed of able-bodied persons, while expending twice the metabolic effort.[18] Additionally, everyday activities, such as ascending stairs using reciprocal gait, are almost impossible to perform with a passive device. Thus, passive devices cannot fully replicate the biomechanical function of intact legs or fully restore natural ambulation. The inability of conventional passive prostheses to generate energy severely limits the community mobility and participation of individuals with transfemoral amputation.[4]

1.4. *Powered prostheses*

Powered devices can actively control joint torque and generate energy, potentially enabling individuals with amputation to walk more naturally and to perform activities such as ascending stairs and hills.[19,20] To accomplish this goal, powered prostheses must be capable of contributing biomechanically significant levels of net power output — in the order of 100 W continuously at the joint — while providing approximately 100 Nm of joint torque.[15] This is commonly achieved by powering the prosthetic joint continually throughout the day using battery-operated servomotors. Providing this range of power and torque requires fairly large actuators and batteries,[21] thus powered prostheses are generally heavier than passive devices. Although the weight is comparable to that of the missing limb for the 50th percentile male, this makes them too heavy for 50% of the male population and for a much higher percentage of the female or elderly populations.

Examples of fully powered ankle joints are the BiOM, SPARKy, and Vanderbilt powered ankles.[22–24] Examples of fully powered knee joints are the MIT CSEA,[25] the ETH knee,[26] the Vanderbilt leg,[27] and the Ossur POWER KNEE™.[9] Most recently, the RIC Hybrid Knee Prosthesis, a device with both powered and passive operation modes has been developed at the Rehabilitation Institute of Chicago.[28] Hybrid prostheses focus on restoring vertical mobility tasks rather than improving walking efficiency and thus can be significantly lighter than fully powered devices.

1.5. *Control systems for powered prostheses*

Although powered prostheses have the potential to fully replace the biomechanical function of intact legs, accomplishing this goal requires the controller to synchronize movement of the prosthetic joints with user movement, based on the user's intended ambulation activity. In stance-phase, when the foot is on the ground, the prosthesis joint torque must be regulated to provide physiological body support and propulsion,[29] generating sufficient energy for the intended ambulation activity. In swing-phase, when the foot is off the ground, the prosthesis must synchronize with the movement of the residual limb in order to achieve foot clearance and timely placement of the foot in preparation for the subsequent step. Although these generic control goals are true for stance and swing-phases for all ambulation activities, optimal prosthesis action in each phase changes significantly with different intended ambulation activities.[30] As a consequence, in addition to modulating prosthesis operation within the ambulation cycle, the controller must decipher the intended ambulation activity (e.g. ground-level walking or stair ascent) and seamlessly adjust prosthesis movement to provide biomechanically appropriate function. Such user-adaptive control is necessary to provide biologically appropriate mechanics during ambulation and to enable the full potential of robotic prostheses to be realized clinically.[31]

2. Part 1: Synchronizing the Prosthesis With The User Movement Within The Gait Cycle

2.1. *State of the art*

Early prosthesis controllers[5] used a position-feedback loop to replay pre-planned joint trajectories recorded from able-bodied individuals during walking. Using this controller, amputees were fully responsible for synchronizing their movement with movement of the prosthesis, which lacked any capacity to adapt to the user. This limitation motivated the development of Complementary Limb Motion Estimation control (CLME).[32,33] Rather than using a fixed position trajectory, CLME adapted the position of the prosthetic joints in real time based on the position of the contralateral, intact leg using statistical processing techniques to process data from joint position sensors — e.g. goniometers — placed on the user's intact leg. CLME controllers provided users with a basic ability to modulate prosthesis movement through their intact leg. However, this control approach proved very hard to learn, while also adding the complication of instrumenting the contralateral leg. Most important, CLME control could not restore natural gait dynamics — i.e. joint torque and power — as the inner position-feedback loop did not accommodate the interaction between the prosthesis and the environment. With a position-feedback loop, an active prosthesis responds with the same position trajectory independent of the physical interaction of the prosthesis with the user or the ground. Thus, unlike an intact leg, the position trajectory of the prosthesis would not be affected by bearing more or less body weight on the prosthesis. Notably, CLME was implemented and tested on the first generation of the Ossur POWER KNEE,[34] the first robotic prosthesis to reach the market.

Approaches based on an impedance control framework were proposed to provide users with more natural gait dynamics. Impedance-inspired controllers define the prosthesis torque based on joint angle position and speed. Thus, gait kinematics are not fixed or defined *a priori*, but change based on the dynamic interaction between the prosthesis and the user — e.g. bearing more load on the prosthesis would lead to greater joint displacement. Impedance-inspired controllers are generally used in combination with finite-state machines[35] that divide the gait cycle into discrete parts, also called phases, during which prosthesis joint stiffness, damping, and equilibrium point are kept constant. By changing the virtual impedance of the prosthetic joint only at the transition between defined gait phases, the use of finite-state machines simplifies the control problem by limiting energy generation to known boundary conditions,[21] thus ensuring stability. Although the impedance parameters for different gait phases can theoretically be extracted from intact-leg biomechanics, experiments with amputee subjects showed that subject and speed-specific tuning are required.[36] Tuning is usually performed by engineers based on qualitative reactions from the user and visual feedback from therapists. Most recently, machine-based tuning has been proposed,[37] although it is not yet clear if this would either improve prosthesis performance or simplify the tuning problem. Impedance-inspired controllers address the need for a natural, dynamic interaction with the environment during ambulation while ensuring stability, but the need for subject-specific tuning severely limits their clinical viability.

A further limitation of impedance-inspired controllers is that tuning requirements depend on walking speed and cadence. With fixed impedance parameters, walking at a speed other than that used for tuning does not provide biologically appropriate energetics or kinematics, which are primary goals for a robotic prosthesis. To address this limitation, Goldfarb's group at Vanderbilt University proposed to tune the prosthesis controller for each subject at three speeds — slow, normal, fast — and then to transition between the three discrete tuning sets based on an extrinsic measure of walking speed.[38] Fey *et al.*[39] proposed instead to modulate impedance parameters, such as joint stiffness and equilibrium position, online based on prosthesis kinematics or the axial load on the prosthesis shank, thus attempting to achieve intrinsic speed adaptation — i.e. without an explicit measure of walking speed. This control approach improved prosthesis function across walking speeds and inclines, although it was limited to late stance-phase and thus did not allow adaptation during swing-phase, which is critical to restoring physiological gait symmetry. Despite the ability to produce more natural gait dynamics, the lack of ability to seamlessly adapt to different walking speeds further limits the clinical viability of such impedance-inspired controllers.

Several alternative strategies have been proposed to overcome the limitations of impedance-inspired controllers. In an attempt to achieve intrinsic adaptation to walking speed and cadence, control strategies based on human neuromuscular models were evaluated — both in simulations and experimentally with a robotic ankle–foot prosthesis.[40,41] Neuromuscular model-based control systems were able to adapt online prosthesis ankle push-off (PO) based on walking speed and incline. However, as no tests have yet been performed on knee prostheses, swing-phase adaptation is still lacking. Sugar *et al.*[42] proposed instead to map prosthesis joint torque with a continuous estimate of gait cycle phase, obtained from shank orientation and rotational speed. This approach was again limited to ankle–foot prostheses only. More recently, virtual-constraints approaches have been suggested to render the natural foot roll-over shape arc[43] with a powered ankle and knee prosthesis.[44] However, experiments showed that the virtual-constraints controller requires manual tuning,[45] which strongly limits clinical viability. As for many other approaches, virtual-constraints control is limited to stance-phase only, leaving the challenge of swing-phase adaptation unresolved. Despite significant progress on robotic prosthesis controllers, there remains a need for a user-adaptive strategy that provides biologically accurate function in both stance- and swing phases to enable natural gait efficiency and stability without requiring user- or speed-specific tuning.

2.2. *Experimental results with a powered ankle and knee prosthesis*

Analysis of gait biomechanics at different speeds and cadences[46,47] can provide significant insights on building a user-adaptive controller that does not require tuning. For able-bodied subjects, walking speed greatly affects joint torque demand during both stance- and swing-phases,[15] although different speed-adaptation mechanisms seem to be involved in each phase. In stance-phase, a complex torque modulation takes place, resulting in an overall net energy increase that is linearly proportional to the walking speed. This speed-adaptation mechanism is well described by the trend of quasi-stiffness[48] (i.e. the derivative of the torque–angle relationship with respect to the angle during the execution of the gait cycle). Quasi-stiffness changes consistently as a function of walking speed[47,49,50] resulting in speed-specific torque–angle curves. In swing-phase, fairly invariant angle trajectories are observed across different walking speeds after time normalization. When walking speed increases, swing-phase duration decreases proportionally to stride duration, maintaining an almost constant ratio between stance- and swing-phase duration. As expected for a ballistic position task, joint torques increase proportionally with walking speed during swing-phase.[51] Based on these observations of natural gait biomechanics, we developed a prosthesis controller that enforces physiological quasi-stiffness profiles in stance-phase and ballistic position control in swing-phase.

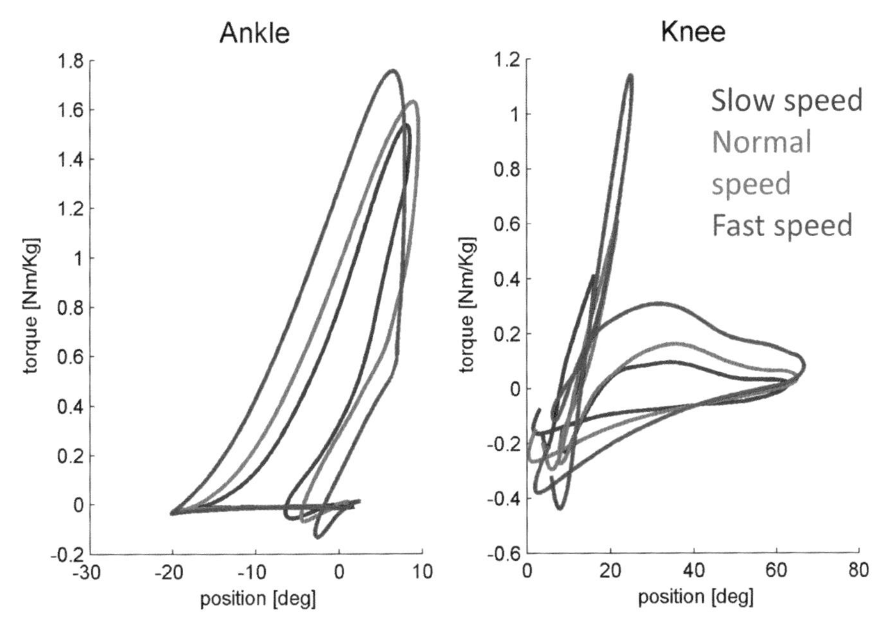

Figure 1. Ankle and knee joint quasi-stiffness curve trends observed in able-bodied subjects walking at three different speeds.[47]

By directly encoding the quasi-stiffness profiles of an intact leg in the stance controller, we eliminated the need to explicitly tune stance-phase control parameters. Most importantly, biologically accurate torque–angle curves can be obtained for any walking speed by encoding a few speed-specific curves from able-bodied studies (Fig. 1)[47] and interpolating based on measured walking speed. Moreover, quasi-stiffness profiles define desired torque solely as a function of the current angle. So we can enforce the desired torque–angle relationship independently from joint velocity, which differs for each subject while walking at the same speed, thus avoiding the need for user-specific tuning.

In swing-phase, we used a minimum-jerk trajectory generator to obtain biologically accurate movement of the prosthesis joints across walking speeds and users. Using this approach, we can obtain a physiological swing movement trajectory and duration at each step without subject- or speed-specific tuning. Figure 2 shows the knee joint position trajectories extracted from able-bodied subjects at three different walking speeds during swing-phase (solid lines); position trajectories estimated with the proposed minimum-jerk trajectory generator are superimposed (dashed lines). As shown in Fig. 2, the minimum-jerk trajectory generator can automatically take the starting swing angle and velocity at each step and smoothly drive the prosthesis through a biomechanically appropriate trajectory in the desired time (which we defined proportionally to the stance-phase duration), thus generalizing

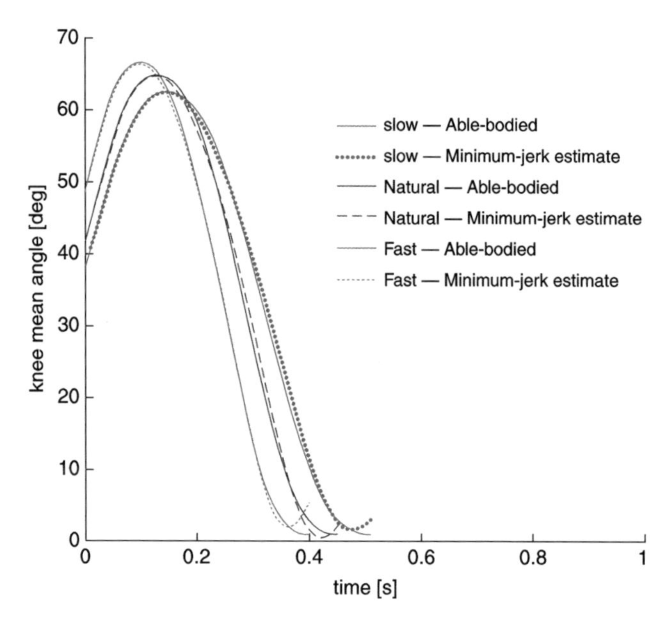

Figure 2. Knee joint position trajectories for three different walking speeds in able-bodied individuals.[47]

across walking speeds and users. In addition, the minimum-jerk approach provides an analytical solution for the position trajectory and its time derivatives, thus simplifying the low-level control problem.

Due to the inherent invariance of quasi-stiffness in the stance-phase and minimum jerk in the swing-phase with respect to speed, these are ideal control variables to achieve speed adaptability in robotic transfemoral prostheses. To test this approach, we implemented the proposed controller on a self-contained ankle and knee prosthesis developed at Vanderbilt University.[52–54] This prosthesis[24] is capable of producing biomechanically appropriate torque, power, and range-of-motion at the ankle and knee joints. It is battery operated and uses brushless DC motors controlled by custom servo amplifiers that are integrated into the embedded control system. The proposed user-adaptive controller was tested by three amputee subjects walking on a treadmill at continuously varying speeds with either their prescribed passive prosthesis or the robotic ankle and knee prosthesis. Specifically, we asked amputee subjects to walk on a treadmill while a therapist increased the treadmill speed progressively from 0.50 m/s to their maximum comfortable speed. Gait kinematics and kinetics were recorded using embedded sensors on the prosthesis. The duration of stride, stance-, and swing-phases were computed offline based on the axial load on the prosthesis.

As a representative example, Fig. 3 shows the ankle (a) and knee (c) joint kinematics profiles recorded during the experimental session performed at variable

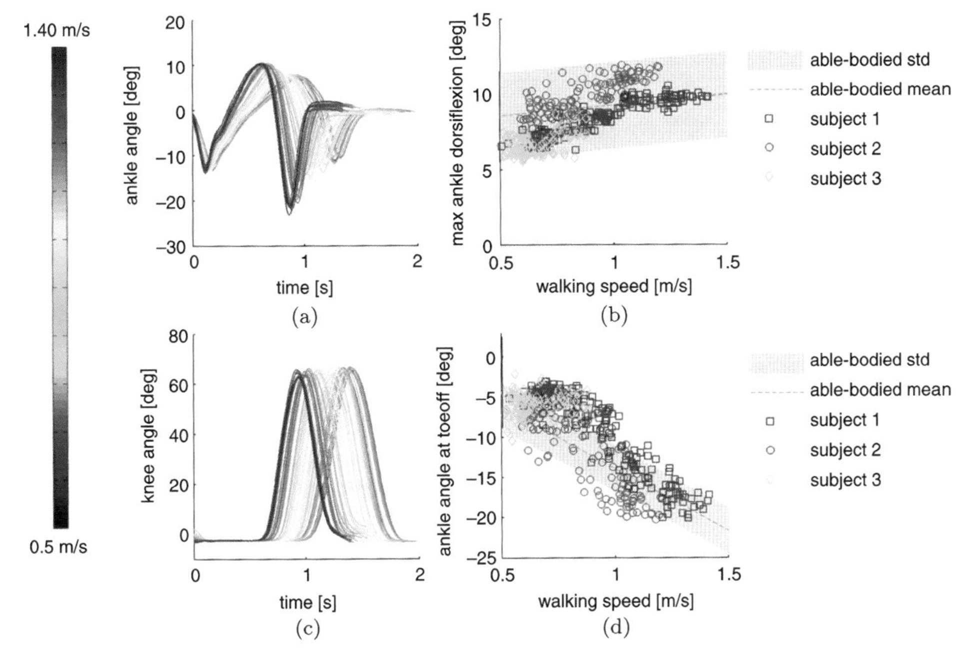

Figure 3. Ankle (a) and knee (c) kinematics of the robotic prosthesis during the variable walking-speed test for one subject; time is zeroed at the beginning of each gait cycle. Ankle angle at the transition between (b) mid-stance to late stance and (d) at late stance to swing-phase. The grey shaded areas in (b) and (d) indicate equivalent data extracted from able-bodied biomechanics.

walking speeds by one of the subjects while using the robotic prosthesis. Different colors indicate different speeds, as indicated by the key on the left side of the figure. The measured ankle angle at the transition between mid-stance to late stance (b) and late stance- to swing-phase (d) are superimposed on the equivalent values extracted from able-bodied data (grey-shaded areas) as a function of the walking speed for the amputee patients (shown with different markers and colors). Although subjects selected different maximum speeds, the measured ankle angle at the transition from mid-stance to late stance (Fig. 3(b)) and from late stance- to swing-phase (Fig. 3(d)) approximated to the trend of able-bodied data as a function of walking speeds (grey-shaded areas, Figs. 3(b) and (d)). This result is significant because we did not impose a position trajectory; rather, we programmed the leg to reproduce the physiological trend of quasi-stiffness, as shown in Fig. 4. Therefore, a biologically accurate trajectory resulted from a natural dynamic interaction between the user, the robotic prosthesis, and the ground.

The analysis of stride-, stance-, and swing-phase durations with the robotic prosthesis is shown in Fig. 5(a). As walking speed increased in the variable-speed test, stride-, stance-phase, and swing-phase duration decreased, indicating an increase in gait cadence. Notably, the prosthesis and intact sides showed very

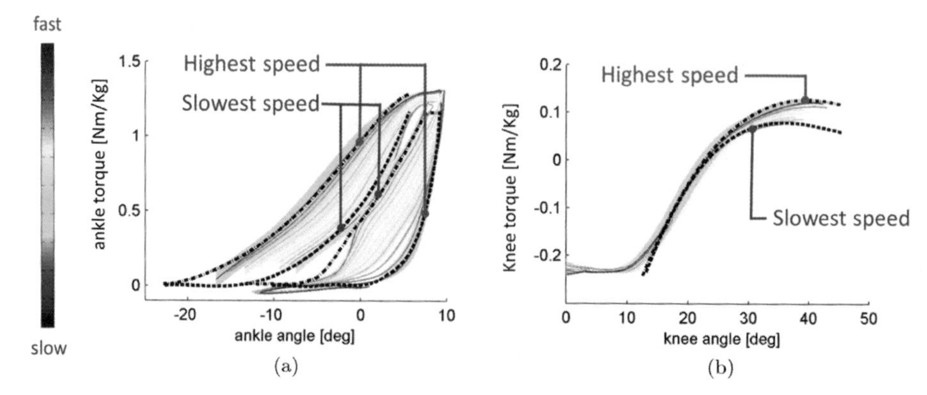

Figure 4. (a) Ankle and (b) knee joint quasi-stiffness curves measured using onboard sensors on the Vanderbilt Leg during the continuously variable speed experiments (solid lines). Superimposed dashed lines represent the quasi-stiffness curves measured on able-bodied subjects and implemented in our stance controller.

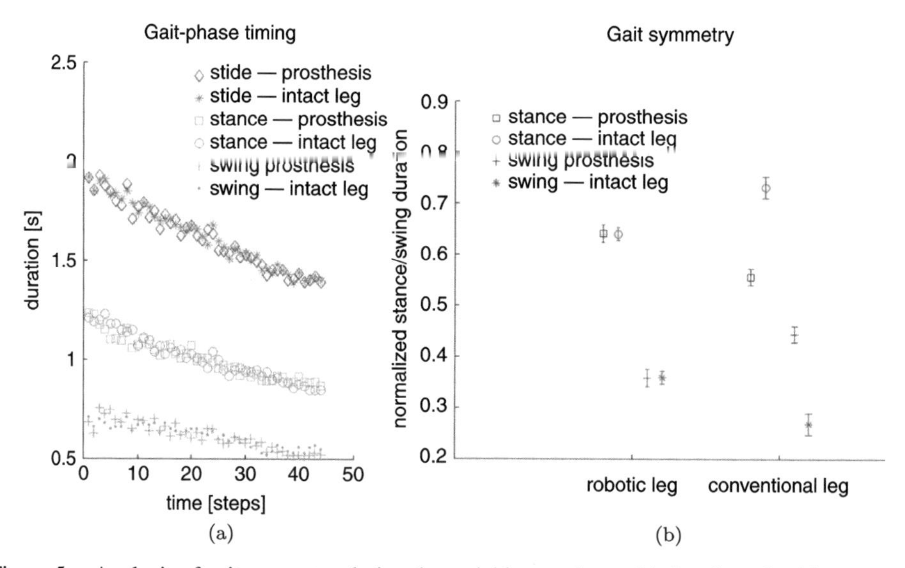

Figure 5. Analysis of gait symmetry during the variable-speed test; (a) duration of stride-, stance-, and swing-phase for the robotic prosthesis and intact leg for each step measured on the variable-speed test by subject 3. (b) Average duration of stance- and swing-phase normalized by stride duration for all three patients for the prosthesis and intact leg; robotic leg on the left, passive prosthesis on the right.

similar timing throughout the test. To quantify gait symmetry, we computed the duration of stance- and swing-phases normalized by stride duration for all the strides recorded during the variable-speed test, and averaged across all subjects. The gait symmetry analysis was performed for both the robotic prosthesis and the conventional passive prosthesis; results are shown in Fig. 5(b). Notably, the proposed swing-phase controller restored physiological gait symmetry independent of walking speed — the root-mean-square difference between the prosthesis and intact leg ranged between 0.039 and 0.089 s. By contrast, the conventional passive prosthesis showed a marked temporal gait asymmetry (Fig. 5(b)). This is very important as gait symmetry has been shown to greatly affect gait stability and efficiency.[55] This result is also significant because the effective swing-phase duration depends not only on swing movement duration but also on the volition of the patient. If patients had waited too long at the end of the swing movement before loading their body weight on the prosthesis, physiological gait symmetry would not have been achieved. Our results indicate not only that swing movement duration was properly adapted at each step but also that patients trusted the variable cadence control and moved in synchrony with the robotic prosthesis.

Proper synchronization of prosthesis movement with user movement is fundamental to support walking at variable speed and cadence, which in turn allows for tuning-free adaptation to the preferred walking pattern of any user. For the first time, our controller enabled a robotic ankle and knee prosthesis to restore biomechanically accurate torque over a wide range of walking speeds without any subject- or speed-specific tuning. In addition, the proposed swing controller enabled the robotic prosthesis to provide a smooth swing movement that drove the prosthetic leg through a physiologically appropriate trajectory independent of the stance-phase controller. By timing the swing movement based on the duration of the previous stance-phase, the robotic prosthesis was able to restore physiological gait symmetry, which is fundamental to restoring gait stability and efficiency to persons with transfemoral amputations.[55] Notably, the benefits of the proposed control framework can be extended beyond ground-level walking. By analyzing the biomechanics of other ambulation activities, such as climbing stairs with a reciprocal gait pattern,[56] we can obtain specific quasi-stiffness curves for any ambulation activity and use them to control the prosthesis during stance-phase. At the same time, the minimum-jerk controller can reproduce the position trajectories of intact limb joints during the swing-phase, by using specific kinematic landmarks for the intended activity, such as the joint position at the end of swing-phase, or the maximum joint position within swing-phase.

We validated the ability of our control approach to enable ambulation activities beyond ground-level walking by testing reciprocal stair climbing with the RIC Hybrid knee prosthesis in an able-bodied subject using a bypass prosthesis.[28] To this end, we first extracted quasi-stiffness curves from able-bodied subjects as they climbed stairs using reciprocal gait[14] and implemented these data in the stance-phase controller. Then, we extracted the maximum knee flexion position and ending position in swing-phase and used these two reference points in the minimum-jerk controller. Finally, the subjects climbed the stairs using reciprocal gait, using the powered knee by-pass RIC Hybrid Knee prosthesis. Experimental results are shown

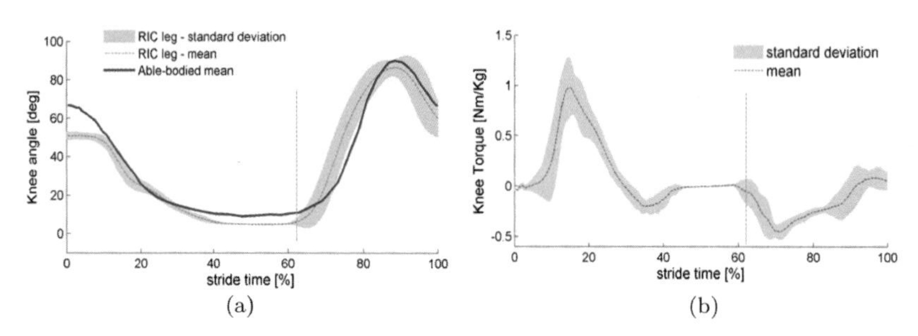

Figure 6. Reciprocal stair climbing. (a) Average knee position trajectory of the prosthesis (solid lines) superimposed to that of able-bodied subjects (dashed line). (b) Average knee prosthesis torque.

in Fig. 6. The prosthesis knee joint position trajectory averaged across 20 gait cycles of reciprocal stair climbing (dashed red line) is superimposed over the data extracted from able-bodied subjects (solid blue line) in Fig. 6. Prosthesis torque profiles are shown in Fig. 6(b). Our control strategy allowed the subject to climb stairs with a reciprocal pattern without the need for user- or cadence-specific tuning.

2.3. *Open challenges, future directions*

Novel user-adaptive control strategies for robotic prostheses hold significant promise to restore more natural ambulation for individuals with lower limb amputation. The ability to synchronize online with the user movement, without requiring subject-specific tuning, is a significant step toward clinical viability for these novel robotic technologies. However, further significant improvements are still needed, including the ability to accommodate non-periodic tasks, such as starting, stopping, turning, and cutting, as well as reacting to unexpected environmental constraints or disturbances.

Synchronizing the action of a robotic leg prosthesis with the user movement intention during non-periodic, non-steady state tasks requires a better cognitive and physical integration of the mechanical and biological systems. Not only must the robotic prosthesis understand the user's intent and generate appropriate movements instantaneously, but it must also minimize the cognitive load on the user so that the movement adaptation would be perceived as natural. Three key research areas are expected to make an important impact in the near future to achieve a truly symbiotic human–robot interaction. First, advanced neural interfaces could favor the integration between the users central nervous system and the robotic prosthesis. On one hand, they could improve the robotic accuracy in detecting the user movement intention. On the other, they could provide a novel way to give users a real-time feedback on the prosthesis state, both in terms of exteroception (e.g. physical contact with the external environment) and proprioception (e.g. position and torque applied by the prosthesis). Second, robotic environmental awareness could be achieved by using novel bi- and tri-dimensional imaging sensors in combination with sensory fusion algorithm, giving the robotic leg controller the information needed to autonomously adapt to environmental constraints. Finally, shared control policy are expected to advance the performance of powered prostheses by allowing users to retain the high-level control of movements, without incurring high cognitive burden or safety issues.

3. Part 2: Adapting the Prosthesis Action to the User-intended Ambulation Activity

3.1. *State of the art*

Users may complete many different ambulation modes using passive mechanical prostheses; however, this often results in abnormal biomechanics as they make compensatory movements. For example, during sit-to-stand activities, unilateral above-knee amputees must rely on their sound limb. During stair climbing activities, the users often have exaggerated hip flexion during swing so that the prosthetic toe clears the upcoming step. Using powered prosthesis can reduce or eliminate many of these compensatory actions provided the prosthesis is controlled properly.

As noted in Sec. 1, several approaches are suitable for controlling the prosthesis within the gait cycle. Many of these approaches are suitable regardless of the type of ambulation activity being performed and only require different tuning parameters.[21,31,39] It is even possible to combine different fundamental approaches based on the activity being performed or phase of gait. For example, impedance control may be used during stance-phase and position control may be used during swing-phase. The key to allowing flexible user adaptive control is to know where you are in the gait cycle and what activity you are intending to perform. Ideally, this should be achieved naturally, seamlessly, and automatically.

Several approaches have been successfully used to signal to the prosthesis what activity the user intends to perform. The most straightforward approach is to use a key-fob, and it has been successfully used to program activity-specific control modes, such as a “cycling” mode into a prosthesis. The drawback of this approach is that it requires a secondary component (the fob) and is not well-suited for seamless and automatic transitions. Complementary Limb Motion Estimation control (CLME), as discussed previously, can also be used to inform the prosthesis what activity is desired to be performed. Again, limitations of this approach are that it requires secondary componentry to instrument the sound limb, and it also enforces some degree of symmetry in the activities that need to be performed. A third approach is to require the user to make an exaggerated body movement which is measured by a sensor, for example an inertial measurement unit, on the prosthesis. While safe, effective, and robust, this approach still requires some degree of compensatory movement. This can even be accomplished using electromyographic (EMG) signals, where an explicit dorsi-flexion or plantar-flexion contraction can be used to change modes of operation.

Recently, several groups have used supervised machine learning approaches to perform "user intent recognition" by interpreting signals measured from sensors within the prosthesis,[57] attached to the user or their socket,[58,59] or in combination.[60,61] This is accomplished by collecting a set of algorithm training data to teach the algorithm to recognize steady-state activities and seamless transitions between activities. Collecting the algorithm training data is not trivial because it must be representative of realistic conditions encountered during daily life activities, and the user must be operating in cooperation with the prosthesis during its collection. A practical method for collecting such data is to perform a set of challenging ambulation circuits where the prosthesis is remotely controlled by an experimenter or clinician.[62] After the data has been collected and the structure of the data has been learned, the system compares patterns in real time to those stored in memory to form high-level control decisions.

3.2. *Experimental results with a powered ankle and knee prosthesis*

To demonstrate the feasibility of using both EMG and mechanical sensors, we performed a set of experiments using the same self-contained ankle and knee prosthesis described in Sec. 2.2.[52–54] We configured a finite-state machine to allow for the following activities, standing, walking, walking up and down slopes/ramps, and walking up and down stairs (Fig. 7). Impedance parameters were empirically hand-tuned for each individual for each of the states within the finite-state machine.[63] State transitions within an activity were governed by thresholds applied to simple mechanical sensors. For example, the transition between stance and swing were controlled by comparing a load-cell sensor to a hand-set threshold value. State transition between ambulation modes were learned using a pattern recognition system and were allowed to occur at the heel-contact and toe-off timings in gait.

Seven subjects with transfemoral amputation or knee disarticulation were recruited for ambulation using the prosthesis. Data were recorded from 13 mechanical sensors (relative position and velocity of the knee and ankle joints, load in the vertical axis, current to the knee motor, current to the ankle motor, from a 6-DOF inertial measurement unit mounted on the shank), and nine EMG control locations (semitendinosus, biceps femoris, tensor fasciae latae, rectus femoris, vastus lateralis, vastus medialis, sartorius, adductor magnus, and gracilis). Representative data from selected sensors is shown in Fig. 8.

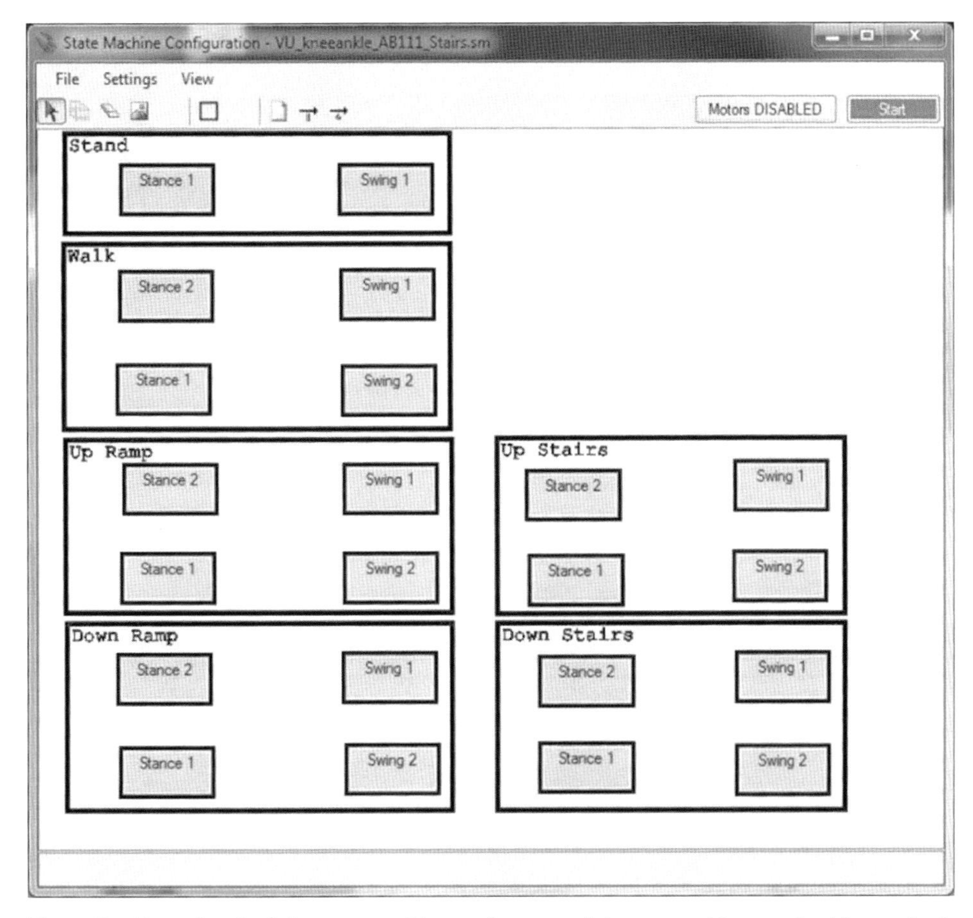

Figure 7. Example of a finite-state machine used to control the powered knee and ankle prosthesis across multiple activities.

Patients completed 20 ambulation circuits within the laboratory when a researcher controlled the operations of the device for the patient using a remote control.[62] It was visually confirmed that the prosthesis was behaving as the user intended and data were labelled by the state-machine so that supervised machine learning algorithms could be used to map the signal patterns to the corresponding activity. After the intent recognition system was trained, the users attempted 10 additional ambulation circuits to evaluate the overall system performance when using two different real-time pattern recognition controllers.

Features were extracted from each signal to reveal discriminatory information. For mechanical sensors, the feature set included the mean, standard deviation, maximum, and minimum from each analysis window. For EMG signals (mean absolute value, slope-sign changes, zero-crossings, and waveform length), four time domain and two autoregressive features were extracted.[61] In one real-time

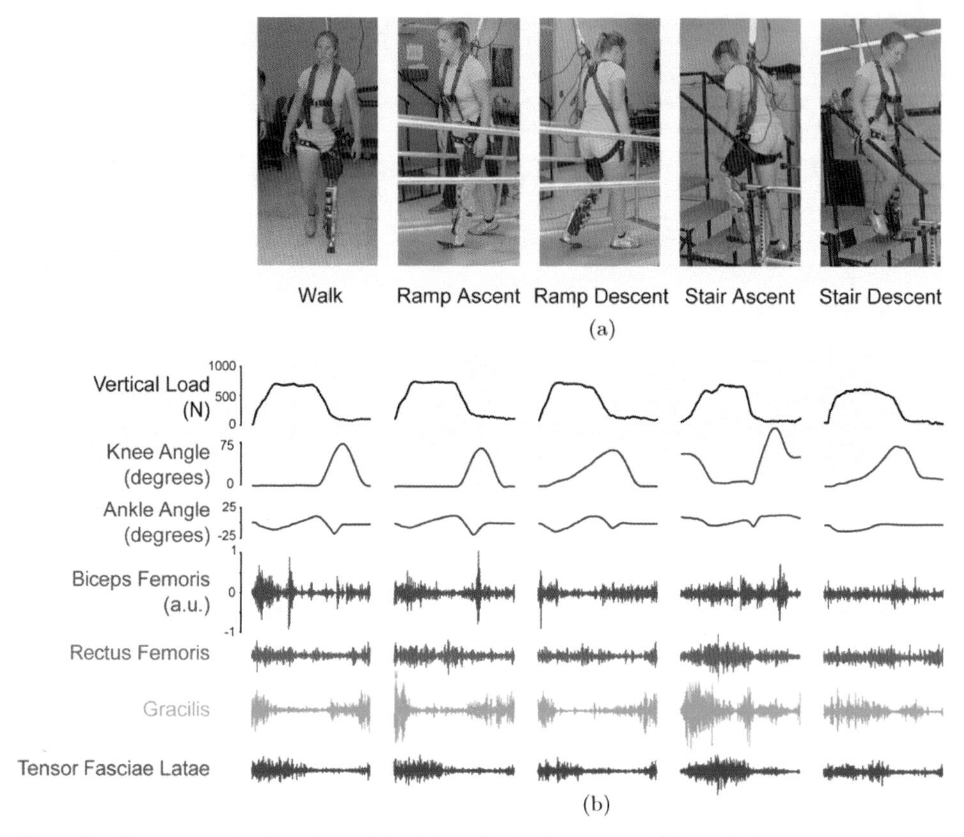

Figure 8. Representative data three of the 13 mechanical sensors and four of nine EMG control site locations for different ambulation activities.

control configuration, all features were then classified using a two time-slice Dynamic Bayesian Network (DBN), whereas in the other control configuration, only mechanical sensor features were classified using a phase-dependent linear discriminant analysis (LDA) classifier. Results are quantified in terms of classification error. This is defined as the percentage of steps that are misclassified by the intent recognition system. Classification errors may be computed using leave-one-out-cross-validation using steps from the offline ambulation trials or by observation when using the real-time control system (i.e. inspecting the output of the control system and verifying that it predicted what the person was actually trying to do) (Fig. 9).

The results of the offline analysis showed (1) that adding information extracted from EMG recordings reduced classification error rates, which is consistent with prior results obtained using passive prostheses[60] and (2) that using a DBN provided further reductions in classification error rates compared to a LDA classifier. This is expected because the DBN is capable of integrating temporal patterns which are

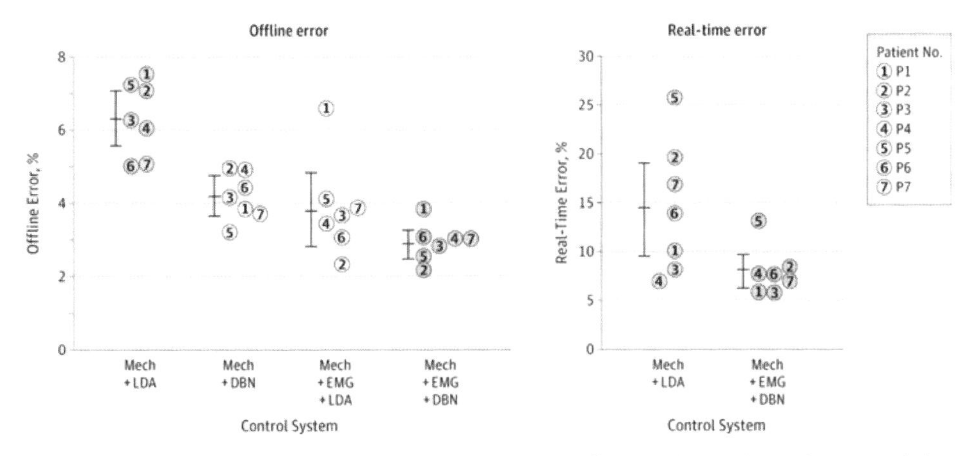

Figure 9. The classification error results obtained from offline testing and real-time ambulation using different intent recognition systems. The activities trained in this experiment were walking, walking up and down ramps, and walking up and down stairs.

inherent in cyclic gait into the intent recognition decisions. The results were also consistent for the real-time testing results, where an embedded system completely governed the operation of the prosthesis.

Completing the previously described experiments are costly and require a diverse team of scientists, engineers, and clinicians. Furthermore, the developed systems clearly still produce classification errors. The impact of these areas depends on when it occurs, how long it lasts for, and what activity the user was trying to complete.[64] In fact, the lower-level controller can filter the response of the error in some cases such that it is not noticeable to the user, whereas in other cases it may cause a moderate or even a substantial perturbation.[65]

In many circumstances, it is easier to perform offline analyses of data collected when the prosthesis was always programmed to operate within the correct mode. Correlating the relationship between offline performance and online performance in the case of upper limb prosthetics have proven to be very challenging with only weak correlations having been reported. However, using the previously described data, we have found a strong correlation between offline and online performance for lower limb prostheses (Fig. 10). Using this relationship, we can infer what impact improvements an algorithm might provide to real-time control without actually performing the real-time testing which is challenging, costly, and poses some safety risks to subjects when the control system makes an error.

3.3. *Open challenges, future directions*

Most intent recognition experiments, particularly those investigating possible use of EMG signals, have been performed within a single experimental session. Limited

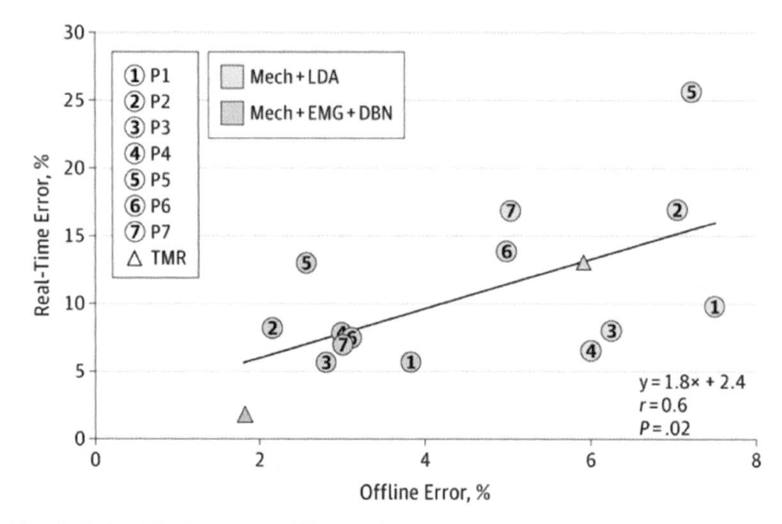

Figure 10. Relationship between offline and online performance for a powered lower limb prosthesis. Note that the slope of the line-of-best-fit is nearly 2. This implies that a 1 percentage point change in offline-error corresponds to a 2 percentage point change in real-time control.

work has been completed to determine how well these systems might perform over the course of days, weeks, or months.[57,66] Changes in electrode positioning with respect to underlying muscles may cause corresponding changes in signal patterns each time the patient dons the device. Alternatively, changes in weight may result in changes measured from mechanical sensors. More sophisticated intent recognition systems that incorporate real-time user adaptation may be required.

Developing adaptive control systems for upper limb prosthetics has been very challenging and clinically unsuccessful. This is least partially attributed to using upper limb prosthesis in a largely unconstrained workspace making it difficult to find a suitable error signal to supervise adaptation. For the lower limb application, we can use prior knowledge of expected gait profiles to help generate an error signal and supervise adaptation. This is an emerging area of exciting research possibilities.

Wearable sensors are becoming small, robust, and unobtrusive. Implantable sensors allowing for chronic and stable electrophysiological recordings have now been demonstrated in humans. It is likely that it will be feasible to instrument the contralateral limb, trunk, or even the head in the near future. This opens the possibility of using camera-based computer vision, gaze detection, or algorithms that rely on EEG signals to supplement information in other sensors that are currently used. Whatever input signals are used, it will be necessary to have robust and efficient sensor fusion algorithms to process the data and communicate seamlessly with the leg prosthesis.

References

1. K. Ziegler-Graham, E. J. MacKenzie, P. L. Ephraim, T. G. Travison and R. Brookmeyer. (2008). Estimating the prevalence of limb loss in the United States: 2005 to 2050, *Archives of Physical Medicine and Rehabilitation* 89(3):422–429.
2. R. Seroussi and A. Gitter. (1996). Mechanical work adaptations of above-knee amputee ambulation, *Archives of Physical Medicine and Rehabilitation* 77, November.
3. M. Grimm, C. GuÉnard and S. MesplÉ-Somps. (2002). Energy storage and return prostheses: Does patient perception correlate with biomechanical analysis? *Clinical Biomechanics* 17(5):325–344.
4. J. P. Pell, P. T. Donnan, F. G. Fowkes and C. V Ruckley. (1993). Quality of life following lower limb amputation for peripheral arterial disease, *European Journal of Vascular and Endovascular Surgery* 7:448–451.
5. D. L. Grimes and W. C. Flowers. (1977). Feasibility of an active control scheme for above knee prostheses, *Journal of Biomechanical Engineering* 215–221.
6. D. Popović, M. N. Oğuztöreli and R. B. Stein. (1995). Optimal control for an above-knee prosthesis with two degrees of freedom, *Journal of Biomechanics* 28(1):89–98.
7. L. Peeraer, B. Aeyels and G. Van der Perre. (1990). Development of EMG-based mode and intent recognition algorithms for a computer-controlled above-knee prosthesis, *Journal of Biomedical Engineering* 12(3):178–182.
8. I. Otto Bock. (1998). Orthopedic Industry, Manual for the 3c100 Otto Bock C-LEG. Duderstadt, Germany.
9. OSSUR, The POWER KNEE, The POWER KNEE http://bionics.ossur.com/Products/POWER-KNEE/SENSE.
10. B. Aeyels, L. Peeraer, J. Vander Sloten and G. Van der Perre. (1992). Development of an above-knee prosthesis equipped with a microcomputer-controlled knee joint: first test results, *Journal of Biomedical Engineering* 14:199–202.
11. M. B. Taylor, E. Clark, E. a Offord and C. Baxter. (1996). A comparison of energy expenditure by a high level trans-femoral amputee using the intelligent prosthesis and conventionally damped prosthetic limbs, *Prosthetics and Orthotics International* 20(2):116–121.
12. T. Schmalz, S. Blumentritt and R. Jarasch. (2002). Energy expenditure and biomechanical characteristics of lower limb amputee gait: the influence of prosthetic alignment and different prosthetic components, *Gait Posture* 16(3):255–263.
13. J. L. Johansson, D. M. Sherrill, P. O. Riley, P. Bonato and H. Herr. (2005). A clinical comparison of variable-damping and mechanically passive prosthetic knee devices, *American Journal of Physical Medicine and Rehabilitation* 84(8):563–575.
14. B. J. McFadyen and D. A. Winter. (1988). An integrated biomechanical analysis of normal stair ascent and descent, *Journal of Biomechanics* 21(9):733–744.
15. D. a Winter. (1983). Energy generation and absorption at the ankle and knee during fast, natural, and slow cadences, *Clinical Orthopaedics and Related Research* 175:147–154.
16. R. Seroussi and A. Gitter. (1996). Mechanical work adaptations of above-knee amputee ambulation, *Archives of Physical Medicine and Rehabilitation* 77 November.
17. S. F. Donker and P. J. Beek. (2002). Interlimb coordination in prosthetic walking: effects of asymmetry and walking velocity, *Acta Psychologica (Amst).* 110(2–3):265–288.
18. R. L. Waters, J. Perry, D. Antonclli and H. Hislop. (1976). Energy cost of walking of amputees: the influence of level of amputation, *Journal of Bone and Joint Surgery, America* 58(1): 42–46.
19. B. E. Lawson, H. A. Varol, A. Huff, E. Erdemir and M. Goldfarb. (2013). Control of stair ascent and descent with a powered transfemoral prosthesis, *IEEE Transactions on Neural Systems and Rehabilitation Engineering* 21(3):466–473.

20. M. Goldfarb, E. J. Barth, M. a. Gogola and J. a. Wehrmeyer. (2003). Design and energetic characterization of a liquid-propellant-powered actuator for self-powered robots, *IEEE/ASME Transactions on Mechatronics* 8(2):254–262.
21. F. Sup, A. Bohara and M. Goldfarb. (2008). Design and control of a powered transfemoral prosthesis, *International Journal of Robotics Research* 27(2):263–273.
22. S. K. Au, J. Weber and H. Herr. (2009). Powered ankle–foot prosthesis improves walking metabolic economy, *IEEE Transactions on Robotics* 25(1):51–66.
23. J. K. Hitt, T. G. Sugar, M. Holgate and R. Bellman. (2010). An active foot–ankle prosthesis with biomechanical energy regeneration, *Journal of Medical Devices* 4(1):011003.
24. F. Sup, H. A. Varol, J. Mitchell, T. J. Withrow and M. Goldfarb. (2009). Preliminary evaluations of a self-contained anthropomorphic transfemoral prosthesis, *IEEE ASME Transactions on Mechatronics* 14(6):667–676.
25. E. J. Rouse, L. M. Mooney and H. M. Herr. (2014). Clutchable series-elastic actuator: Implications for prosthetic knee design, *International Journal of Robotics Research* 33: 1611–1625.
26. S. Pfeifer, A. Pagel, R. Riener and H. Vallery, (2015). Actuator with angle-dependent elasticity for biomimetic transfemoral prostheses, *IEEE/ASME Transactions on Mechatronics* 20(3): 1384–1394.
27. B. Lawson, J. Mitchell, D. Truex, A. Shultz, E. Ledoux and M. Goldfarb. (2014). A robotic leg prosthesis: design, control, and implementation, *Robotics and Automation Magazine* 21(4): 70–81.
28. T. Lenzi, J. Sensinger, J. Lipsey, L. Hargrove and T. Kuiken. (2015). Design and preliminary testing of the RIC hybrid knee prosthesis, in *37th Annual International Conference of the IEEE Engineering in Medicine and Biology Society (EMBC)* 1683–1686.
29. J. Markowitz, P. Krishnaswamy, M. F. Eilenberg, K. Endo, C. Barnhart and H. Herr. (2011). Speed adaptation in a powered transtibial prosthesis controlled with a neuromuscular model, *Philosophical Transactions of the Royal Society B* 366(1570):1621–1631.
30. M. Goldfarb. (2013). Consideration of Powered Prosthetic Components as They Relate to Microprocessor Knee Systems, *Journal of Prosthetics and Orthotics* 25:P65–P75.
31. H. M. Herr and A. M. Grabowski. (2012). Bionic ankle–foot prosthesis normalizes walking gait for persons with leg amputation, *Proceedings of the Royal Society B* 279(1728):457–464.
32. H. Vallery and M. Buss. (2006). Complementary limb motion estimation based on interjoint coordination using principal components analysis, *Proceedings of the International Conference on Control Applications*, 933–938.
33. H. Vallery, R. Ekkelenkamp, M. Buss and H. van der Kooij. (2007). Complementary limb motion estimation based on interjoint coordination: Experimental evaluation, in *IEEE 10th International Conference on Rehabilitation Robotics (ICORR)*, 798–803.
34. P. F. Pasquina, P. R. Bryant, M. E. Huang, T. L. Roberts, V. S. Nelson and K. M. Flood. (2006). Advances in amputee care, *Archives of Physical Medicine and Rehabilitation* 87(3): 34–43.
35. F. Sup, A. Bohara and M. Goldfarb. (2008). Design and control of a powered transfemoral prosthesis, *International Journal of Robotics Research* 27(2):263–273.
36. A. M. Simon, N. P. Fey, S. B. Finucane, R. D. Lipschutz and L. J. Hargrove. (2013). Strategies to reduce the configuration time for a powered knee and ankle prosthesis across multiple ambulation modes, in *2013 IEEE International Conference on Rehabilitation Robotics (ICORR)* 1–6.
37. D. Wang, M. Liu, F. Zhang and H. Huang. (2013). Design of an expert system to automatically calibrate impedance control for powered knee prostheses, in *IEEE International Conference on Rehabilitation Robotics* 1–5.

38. F. Sup, H. A. Varol, J. Mitchell, T. J. Withrow and M. Goldfarb. (2009). Self-contained powered knee and ankle prosthesis: Initial evaluation on a transfemoral amputee, in *IEEE International Conference on Rehabilitation Robotics (ICORR, 2009)* 638–644.
39. N. P. Fey, a M. Simon, a J. Young and L. J. Hargrove. (2014). Controlling knee swing initiation and ankle plantarflexion with an active prosthesis on level and inclined surfaces at variable walking speeds, *IEEE Journal of Translational Engineering in Health and Medicine* 1–12.
40. H. Geyer and H. Herr. (2010). A muscle-reflex model that encodes principles of legged mechanics produces human walking dynamics and muscle activities, *IEEE International Transactions on Neural Systems and Rehabilitation Engineering* 18(3):263–273.
41. M. F. Eilenberg, H. Geyer and H. Herr. (2010). Control of a powered ankle–foot prosthesis based on a neuromuscular model, *IEEE Transactions on Neural Systems and Rehabilitation Engineering* 18(2):164–173.
42. M. A. Holgate, W. B. Alexander and T. G. Sugar. (2008). Control algorithms for ankle robots? a reflection on the state-of-the-art and presentation of two novel algorithms, *International Conference on Biomedical Robots and Biomechatronics* 97–102.
43. A. H. Hansen and D. S. Childress. (2010). Investigations of roll-over shape: implications for design, alignment, and evaluation of ankle–foot prostheses and orthoses, *Disability and Rehabilitation* 32(26):2201–2209.
44. R. D. Gregg, T. Lenzi, N. P. Fey, L. J. Hargrove and J. W. Sensinger. (2013). Experimental effective shape control of a powered transfemoral prosthesis, in *2013 IEEE International Conference on Rehabilitation Robotics (ICORR)*, 1–7.
45. R. D. Gregg, T. Lenzi, L. J. Hargrove and J. W. Sensinger. (2014). Virtual constraint control of a powered prosthetic leg: from simulation to experiments with transfemoral amputees, *IEEE Transactions on Robotics* in press.
46. A. H. Hansen, D. S. Childress, S. C. Miff, S. A. Gard and K. P. Mesplay. (2004). The human ankle during walking: implications for design of biomimetic ankle prostheses, *Journal of Biomechanics* 37(10):1467–1474.
47. D. A. Winter. (1990). *Biomechanics and Motor Control of Human Movement* 2.
48. R. Davis and P. DeLuca. (1996). Gait characterization via dynamic joint stiffness, *Gait Posture.*
49. K. Shamaei, G. S. Sawicki and A. M. Dollar. (2013). Estimation of Quasi-Stiffness of the human knee in the stance phase of walking, *PLoS One* 8(3):e59993.
50. K. Shamaei, G. S. Sawicki and A. M. Dollar. (2013). Estimation of quasi-stiffness and propulsive work of the human ankle in the stance phase of walking, *PLoS One* 8(3): e59935.
51. D. A. Winter and D. G. E. Robertson. (1978). Joint torque and energy patterns in normal gait, *Biological Cybernetis* 29(3):137–142.
52. T. Lenzi, L. Hargrove and J. W. Sensinger. (2014). Speed-adaptation mechanism: robotic prostheses can actively regulate joint torque, *Robotics* 21(4):94–107.
53. T. Lenzi, L. J. Hargrove and J. W. Sensinger. (2014). Minimum jerk swing control allows variable cadence in powered transfemoral prostheses, in *Engineering in Medicine and Biology Society (EMBC), 2014 36th Annual International Conference of the IEEE*, 2492–2495.
54. T. Lenzi, L. Hargrove and J. W. Sensinger. (2014). Preliminary evaluation of a new control approach to achieve speed adaptation in robotic transfemoral prostheses, in *IEEE/RSJ International Conference on Intelligent Robots and System*, 2049–2054.
55. L. Nolan, A. Wit, K. Dudziñski, A. Lees, M. Lake and M. Wychowañski. (2003). Adjustments in gait symmetry with walking speed in trans-femoral and trans-tibial amputees, *Gait Posture* 17:142–151.
56. R. Riener, M. Rabuffetti and C. Frigo. (2002). Stair ascent and descent at different inclinations, *Gait Posture* 15(1):32–44.

57. H. A. Varol, F. Sup and M. Goldfarb. (2010). Multiclass real-time intent recognition of a powered lower limb prosthesis, *IEEE Transactions on Biomedical Engineering* 57(3):542–551.
58. H. Huang, T. a Kuiken and R. D. Lipschutz. (2009). A strategy for identifying locomotion modes using surface electromyography, *IEEE Transactions on Biomedical Engineering* 56(1):65–73.
59. S. Au, M. Berniker and H. Herr. (2008). Powered ankle–foot prosthesis to assist ground-level and stair-descent gaits, *Neural Networks* 21(4):654–666.
60. H. Huang, F. Zhang, L. J. Hargrove, Z. Dou, D. R. Rogers and K. B. Englehart. (2011). Continuous locomotion-mode identification for prosthetic legs based on neuromuscular-mechanical fusion, *IEEE Transactions on Biomedical Engineering* 58(10):2867–2875.
61. A. J. Young, T. A. Kuiken and L. J. Hargrove. (2014). Analysis of using EMG and mechanical sensors to enhance intent recognition in powered lower limb prostheses, *Journal of Neural Engineering* 11(5):056021.
62. A. J. Young, A. M. Simon and L. J. Hargrove. (2014). A training method for locomotion mode prediction using powered lower limb prostheses, *IEEE Transactions on Neural Systems and Rehabilitation Engineering* 22(3):671–677.
63. A. M. Simon, K. a Ingraham, N. P. Fey, S. B. Finucane, R. D. Lipschutz, A. J. Young and L. J. Hargrove. (2014). Configuring a powered knee and ankle prosthesis for transfemoral amputees within five specific ambulation modes, *PLoS One* 9(6):e99387.
64. F. Zhang, M. Liu and H. Huang. (2015). Effects of locomotion mode recognition errors on volitional control of powered above-knee prostheses, *IEEE Transactions on Neural Systems and Rehabilitation Engineering* 23:64–72.
65. L. J. Hargrove, A. J. Young, A. M. Simon, N. P. Fey, R. D. Lipschutz, S. B. Finucane, E. G. Halsne, K. A. Ingraham and T. A. Kuiken. (2015). Intuitive control of a powered prosthetic leg during ambulation: a randomized clinical trial, *JAMA* 313(22):2244–2252.
66. J. Spanias, E. Perreault and L. Hargrove. (2015). Detection of and Compensation for EMG Disturbances for Powered Lower Limb Prosthesis Control, *IEEE Transactions on Neural Systems and Rehabilitation Engineering* 4320:1–1.

Chapter 5

ANKLE PROSTHETICS AND ORTHOTICS: TRENDS FROM PASSIVE TO ACTIVE SYSTEMS

Thomas G. Sugar[*,†], Jeffrey A. Ward[†], and Martin Grimmer[‡]

[*]*Arizona State University, The Polytechnic School,*
6075 S. Innovation Way West, Mesa, AZ 85212
[†]*SpringActive, Inc, 2414 W 12th St #4, Tempe, AZ 85281*
[‡]*Technical University of Darmstadt,*
Magdalenenstraße 27, 64289 Darmstadt, Germany

Great strides have been made over the last two decades to develop powered, active, ankle–foot orthoses and prostheses. Lightweight, powerful systems return gait movements and torques (kinematics and kinetics) to the user. An explosion of research in the areas of biomechanics, control, and mechanical design has allowed systems to assist and enhance the user's ambulatory pattern. This review will discuss the trends in the development of wearable robotic systems enhancing ankle gait. Trends in passive systems include the development of lightweight carbon fiber systems for drop foot. Trends in active systems include the development of lightweight, battery-powered, motorized ankle–foot orthoses to aid in rehabilitation of stroke survivors. Similar systems are being built to assist transtibial and transfemoral amputees. Many new systems are quasi-passive and use minimal control techniques to tune the device during the gait cycle. Lastly, there has been a trend to develop soft-actuation techniques that do not rely on rigid exoskeletal structures. The trend is for smarter, more lightweight, powerful systems that return better gait kinematics and kinetics reducing metabolic cost.

1. Introduction

The confluence of robotics, biomechanics, control, and design has allowed for the development of exciting new powered/active prosthetics and orthotics. New powered systems allow users to regain their functions to walk, run, and jump after an amputation.

This chapter will focus on lower limb orthotic and prosthetic systems. New energy storing passive orthoses and prostheses allow users to regain function. Active systems improve function by lifting the toe in swing-phase and making it easier to walk. New, quasi-active systems are being developed that use a small amount of energy to change the characteristics of the device to enhance gait. These systems are finding a niche where limited amounts of actuation and battery power are needed.

The article will end with a discussion of soft robotic systems where non-rigid exoskeletal structures are being used. These systems offer the possibilities of larger freedom of movement, reduced weight, and enhanced comfort.

This article will not focus on control algorithms for prosthetic systems. A systematic review article on controllers has been written in Ref. [1]. Other review articles on prosthetic systems can be found as well in Refs. [2–7].

2. Orthotic Systems

Many stroke survivors, people with frailty, and others are in need of some type of bracing system at the ankle to enhance stability, strength and/or to raise the toe. Powered orthoses allow users to regain more function by enhancing push-off (PO) at the end of stance and picking the toe up in the swing-phase of the gait cycle. This section will be divided to explain passive, active, and quasi-active systems.

2.1. *Passive orthotic systems*

New passive carbon fiber bracing systems are lightweight and robust, see Fig. 1. These systems allow a user to store energy as the leg rolls over the ankle and use this energy to assist PO. For users with drop-foot, the brace keeps the toe from scuffing the floor and reduces hip circumduction.

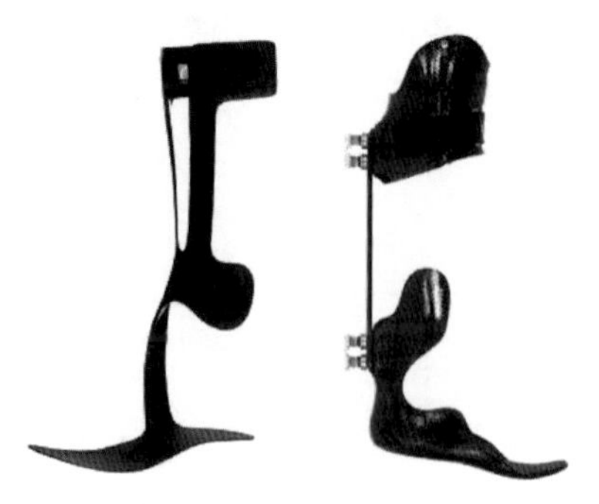

Figure 1. Carbon fiber brace used to increase balance and strength at the ankle, courtesy of www.ossur.com. On the right, an IDEO^{TM} brace with a heel cup, strut, and calf strap. It allows the angular stiffness to be adjusted quickly.[8,9]

Researchers at Brooke Army Medical Center are developing a brace, IDEO™, to allow users to walk and run.[8,9] The IDEO™ (Intrepid Dynamic Exoskeletal Orthosis) consists of a heel cup connected to a cuff at the shank by support links. The stiffness of the support links can be tuned and designed for the individual user. Also, as the user regains strength or performs more active functions, the support links or struts can be adjusted by changing the geometry of the link or adding and subtracting links. The adjustment allows for the tuning of the angular stiffness. As the user rolls over the ankle, energy is stored and returned to allow more function. The device can be used by people that have had ankle fusion, nerve loss, and/or muscle loss.

2.2. *Active orthotic systems*

Active orthotic systems for stroke survivors have been developed by many researchers in Refs. [10–21]. These systems use a motor and spring or a pneumatic muscle to store energy as the leg rolls over the ankle and use this energy for PO, see Fig. 2. Secondly, the angular stiffness of the brace can be tuned to the user by adjusting the stiffness of the spring. Thirdly, these systems can raise the toe for users with drop foot. van der Kooij developed a spring-based system to provide PO power as well,[22] see Fig. 3. In this system, the compliant lever arm is able to store and release energy. Durfee and his group have developed a hydraulic brace.[23–25] The virtual stiffness of the device can be altered to determine the best fit and comfort for the user, see Fig. 3.

Powered orthoses have also been developed that allow for inversion and eversion as well, see Fig. 4. These systems use two actuators to push and pull to plantarflex and dorsiflex the ankle. The actuators are used in counter-motion to invert and evert the ankle.[11,12,26] In a design by Mooney *et al.*, they were able to

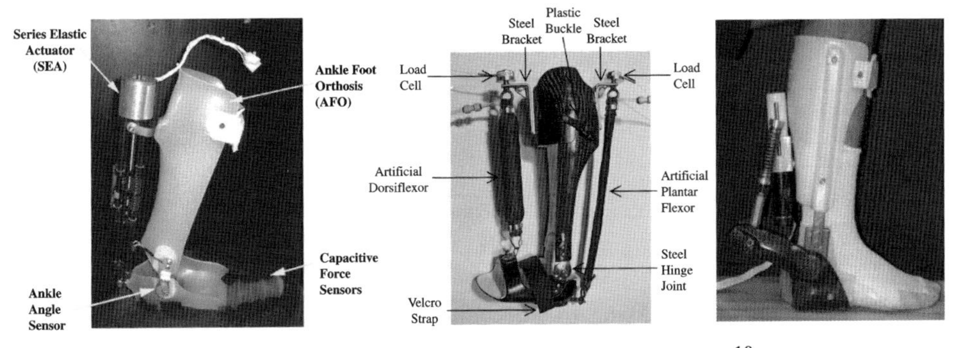

Figure 2. Herr developed an orthosis powered by a series elastic actuator.[10] Ferris developed an EMG-controlled orthosis powered by pneumatic muscles.[19] Sugar developed a Robotic Tendon that stored and released energy in a spring.[13,14]

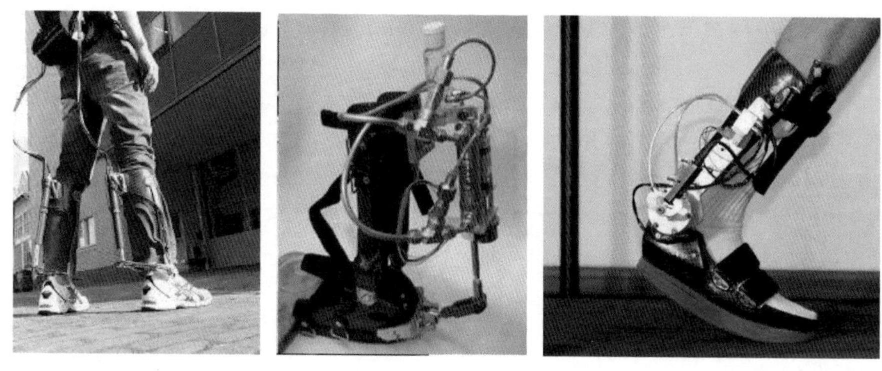

Figure 3. The Achilles ankle exoskeleton uses a flexible lever arm to store and release energy.[22] Hydraulic and pneumatic orthoses by Durfee are shown in the middle and to the right.[23–25]

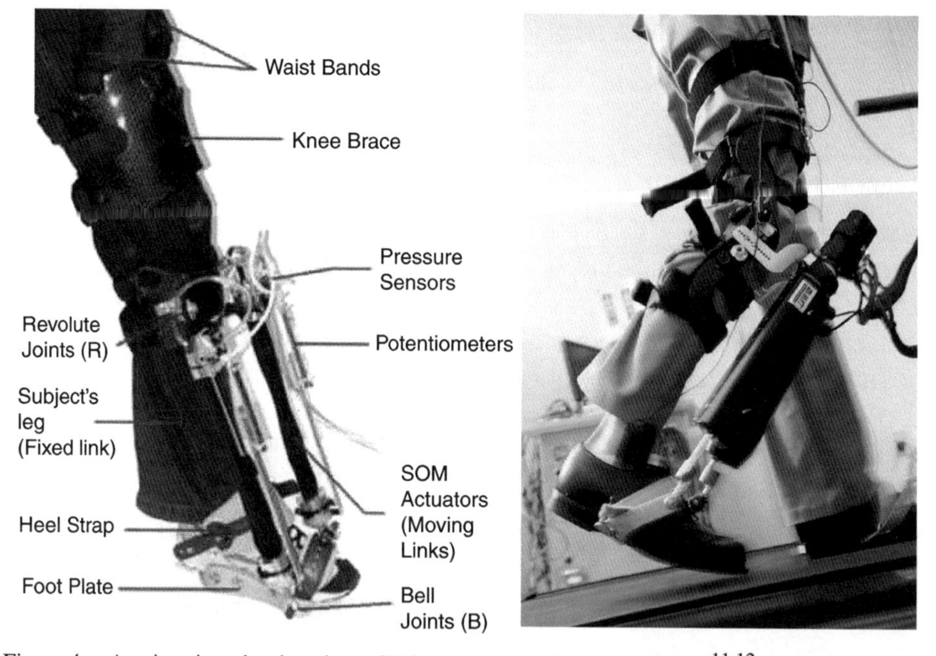

Figure 4. A gait trainer developed at ASU is based on a tripod mechanism.[11,12] The anklebot uses two series elastic actuators.[26]

design a system that reduced metabolic cost,[27,28] see Fig. 5. Hollander developed a joint torque augmentation robot (JTAR) that used a spring-based, Bowden cable system to assist PO at the ankle,[29] see Fig. 6.

2.3. *Quasi-active orthotic systems*

Collins and Sawicki developed a passive orthosis with a clutching mechanism that augmented metabolic cost reducing it to below normal.[30] As the foot rolls over the ankle, the clutch is engaged and the spring is stretched, see Fig. 7. The spring

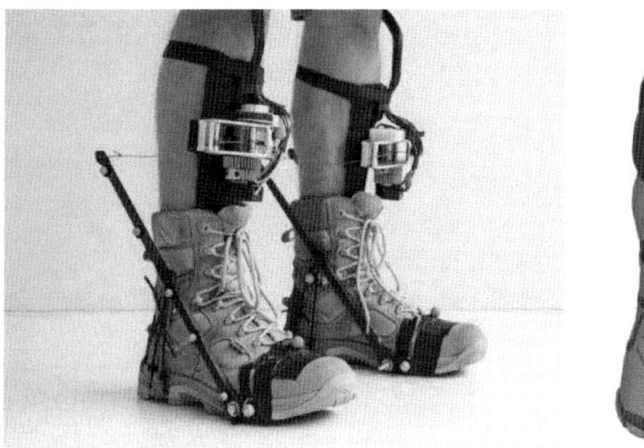

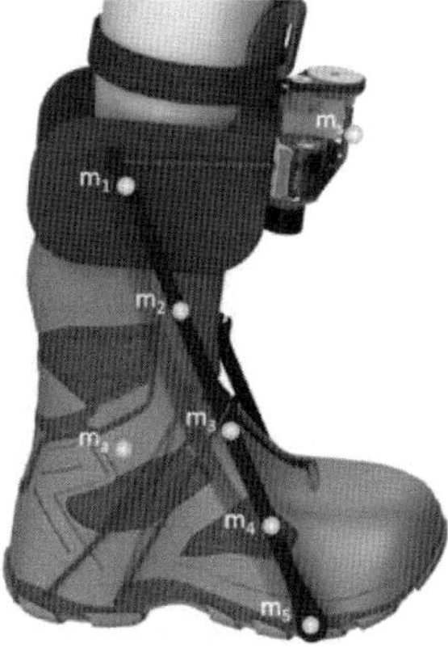

Figure 5. A DC moto/gearbox was used to pull a cable at the shank to create a PO at late stance.[27,28]

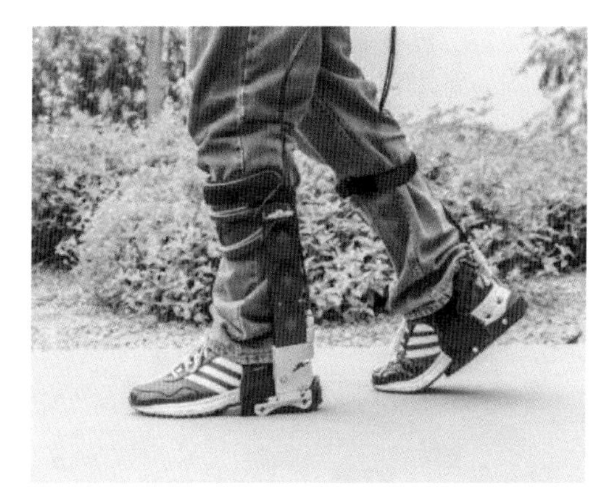

Figure 6. A Bowden cable pulled on a spring at the ankle to assist PO.[29]

releases its energy to aid in PO. The spring reduces the breaking effort of the muscle as the leg rolls over the ankle. The clutch is then released so that the foot can move freely during the swing-phase.

Svensson *et al.* designed an orthosis that can accommodate inclines and stairs.[31] A magnetorheological damper is used to adjust the foot when ascending and descending stairs, see Fig. 8.

3. Prosthetic Systems

Over the last two decades, there is increased focus on developing prosthetic systems that better mimic the kinematics and kinetics of able-bodied gait. In the early 2000s, research into powered lower limb prostheses began rapidly expanding in the United States. The expansion was largely driven by government investment toward the goal of assisting wounded soldiers. These devices are able to give the user a powerful

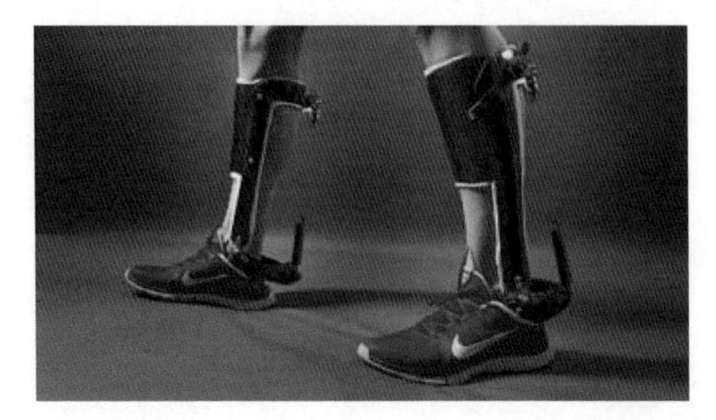

Figure 7. A spring is mounted in parallel with the Achilles tendon.[30]

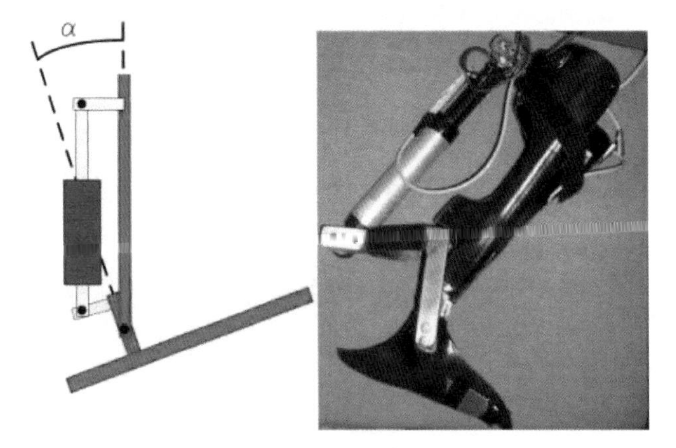

Figure 8. A quasi-active orthosis prototype was designed that can adjust the ankle angle to allow for ascending and descending stairs.[31]

PO as well as lift the toe during the swing-phase. Powered prostheses are being developed and commercialized. This section will focus on passive, powered, and quasi-active systems. Better passive prosthetic systems are being designed with carbon fiber energy storage devices. Lastly, quasi-active systems tune the prosthetic device with minimal power.

3.1. *Passive prosthetic systems*

Before the 1980s, prosthetic feet were dominated by simple non-energy storing feet such as the solid ankle, cushioned heel (SACH) foot. Because users wanted to be more active, energy storage and release (ESAR) feet were developed. The first EASR foot was the Seattle foot which used a spring-based keel to store some of the braking energy of the user as the leg rolls over the ankle. The next innovation was the Flex foot. The all-carbon fiber foot allowed for a lightweight foot that could

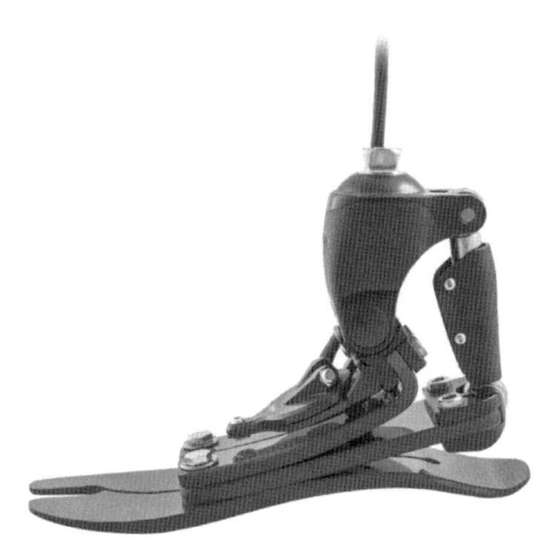

Figure 9. The ProFlex foot by Ossur, courtesy https://www.ossur.com/prosthetic-solutions/products/dynamic-solutions/pro-flex.

store and release energy. A very good review article was written by Lefeber's group outlining the progress of prosthetic feet from passive systems to active systems.[3,7] New prosthetic feet include the ProFlex by Ossur which uses a four-bar linkage and a passive foot. The foot has greater peak power and range of motion as compared to standard feet, see Fig. 9.

3.2. *Active prosthetic systems*

With the advent of better motors, batteries, sensors, and microprocessors, powerful, active systems were developed in the 2000s. (Earliest work dates to the 1970s and 1980s at MIT and Belgrade.[32]) Some of the newer active systems were developed by Herr, Sugar, and Goldfarb.[33–43] The first commercial ankle, the Proprio foot by Ossur, could actively position the keel during gait, but it did not store any additional energy in the spring.

Herr developed a series of powered ankles that were based on a series elastic actuator with an additional parallel spring used in the stance-phase.[33] The parallel spring allowed for a second load path reducing the torque that the motor must supply. He used a reflex controller to give an additional push as the user pushed against the keel.[34] His ankle was commercialized under IWalk, BIOM, and then under the brand BionX, see Fig. 10.

At the Human Machine Integration Laboratory, Sugar developed the SPARKy ankle (Spring Ankle with Regenerative Kinetics),[35–38] see Fig. 11. This ankle used a much softer spring to store and release energy. It was based on a Robotic Tendon concept, an actuator that mimics the biological muscle tendon complex.[13,14] In the robotic tendon concept, the proximal side of the spring was positioned and

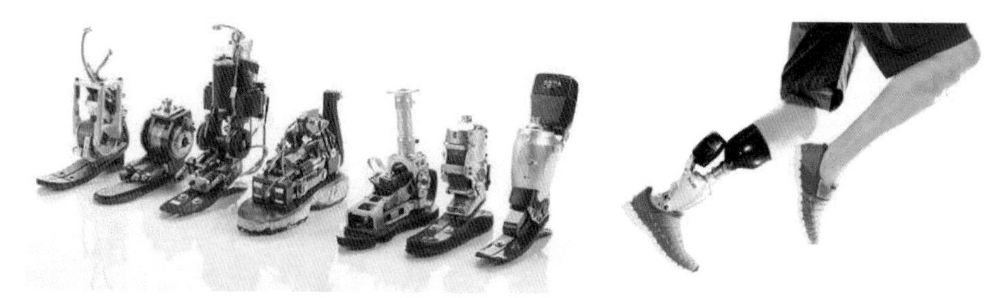

Figure 10. Herr developed a series of prototype ankles that used a series elastic actuator with an additional spring parallel to the load path.[33] The ankle was commercialized under the BionX brand, courtesy www.bionx.com.

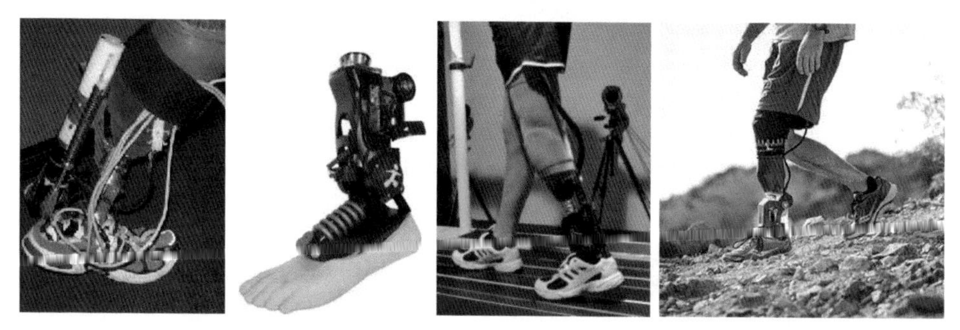

Figure 11. The SPARKy ankle allowed users to walk, run, jump, and walk up and down mountains.[35–38]

controlled to obtain correct angles and moments, and the distal side of the spring was not controlled. They used a continuous controller based on the phase angle of the tibia to adjust the proximal side of the spring.[39,44,45] Holgate designed an active, compliant parallel mechanism, see Fig. 12. In a three link mechanism, one link was powered with a motor, a spring was used in the second link, and the keel was attached to the third link.[46]

Goldfarb's research team initially focused on a transfemoral prosthesis that powered both the knee and ankle.[40–43] Their work focused on the development of a full system that allowed walking, running, and upslope walking,[47] see Fig. 13. The controller typically used a set of impedance gains that were gain scheduled by a state controller for the different phases of gait. Current research focused on fall prevention and perturbations.[48,49] The team has also developed a transtibial prosthesis as well.[50]

Lefeber's group developed the AMP 2 and AMP 3 devices.[3,7,51–53] These devices used unique spring and clutch mechanisms to store and release energy, see Fig. 14. One clutch system stored energy in the PO (push-off) spring just after heel strike to be used later to assist push-off. In the AMP 3 device, a second clutch (locking mechanism 1) allowed the system to set the "home position" as the heel

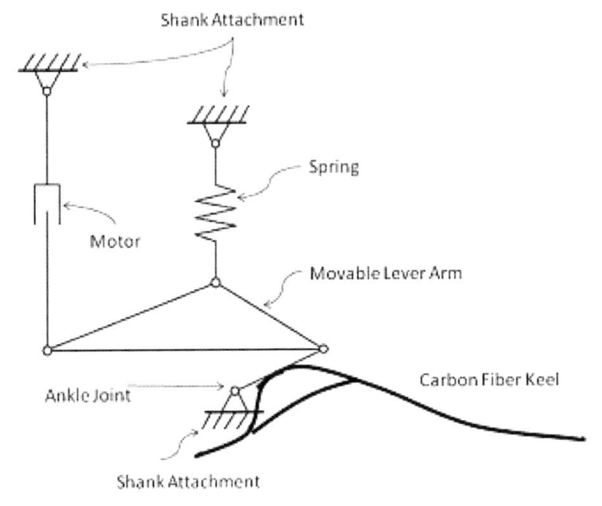

Figure 12. In a compliant, parallel mechanism, the energy and forces are shared by the motor and spring.[46]

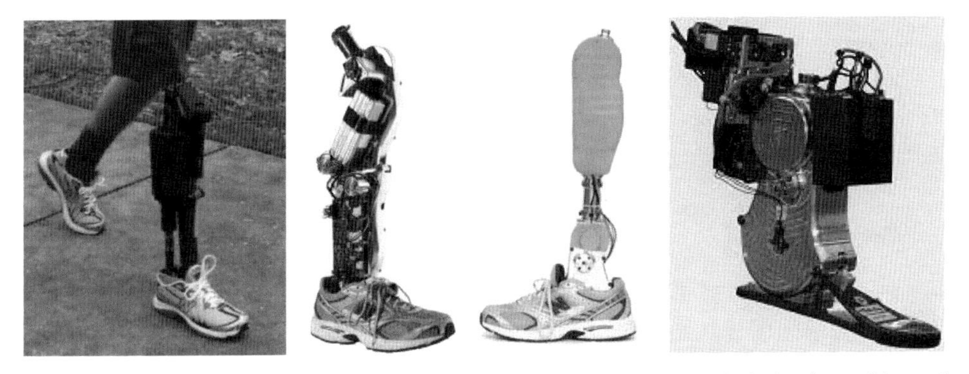

Figure 13. A transfemoral prosthesis was developed that powered both the ankle and knee.[40–43,48,49] Current research has focused on an ankle device as well.[50]

touched the ground. In this way, the starting angle of the device can be adjusted up or down depending on the slope of the terrain.

The group also developed a method to store energy in springs in the new type of transmission. A series of springs are stretched one by one to store energy when needed.[54]

Multi-joint ankle systems have been developed as well, see Fig. 15.

Vogelwede developed a novel four bar linkage with a torsional spring to achieve push-off power in a powered ankle prosthesis,[58] see Fig. 16. The linkage was tailored for a walking profile.

Instead of using a spring in series with the motor, a new ankle was designed that is based on a parallel elastic actuator.[59] If the position of the parallel spring

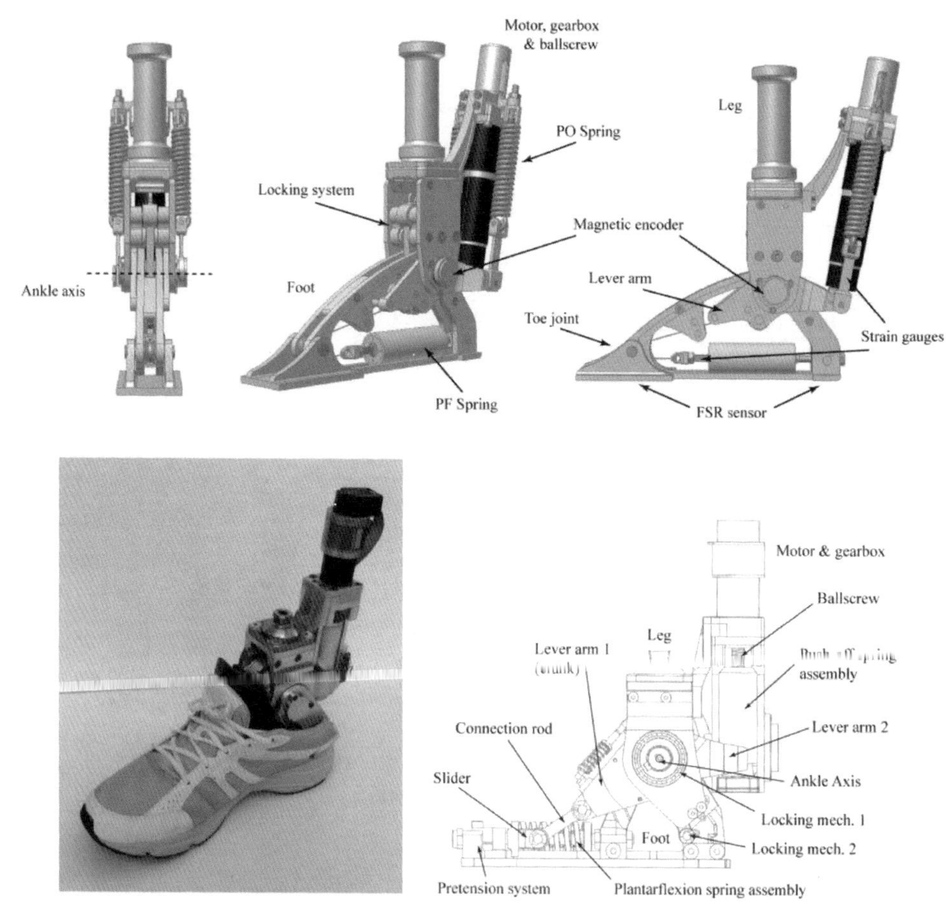

Figure 14. The AMP 2 device used a locking clutch to store energy in the PO (push-off) spring.[7,51,52] The AMP 3 device used a resettable, overrunning clutch at the ankle axis to adjust the starting angle of the device.[53]

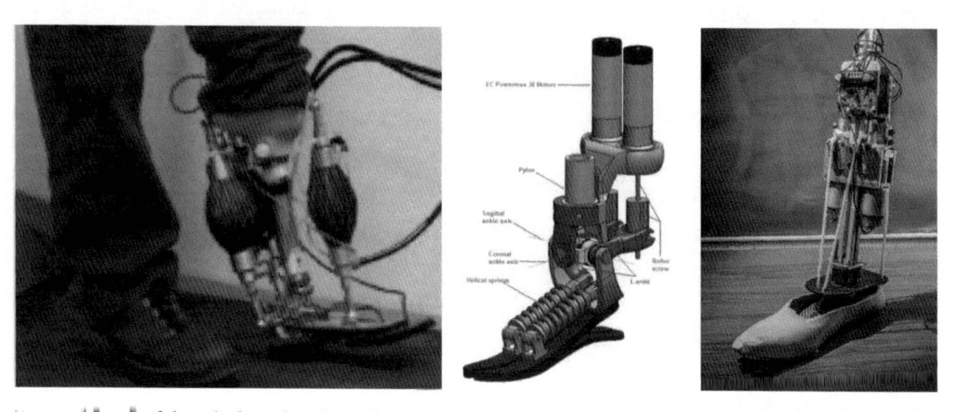

Figure 15. Lefeber designed a pleated, pneumatic muscle prosthesis with two degrees of freedom; Bellman designed a multi-joint SPARKy ankle; Rastgaar designed a two degrees of freedom ankle based on cable joints.[55–57]

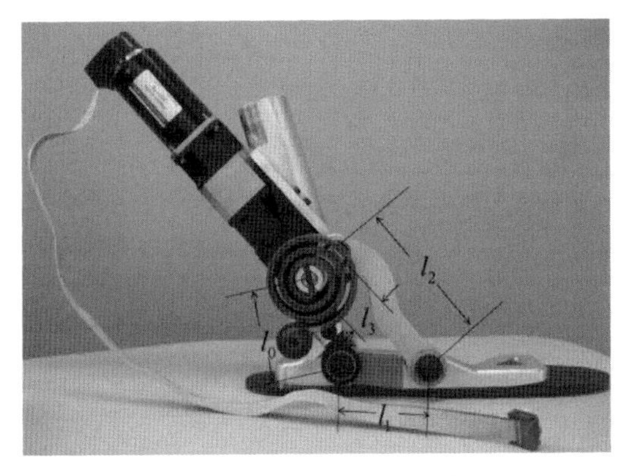

Figure 16. A torsional spring and four-bar linkage are used to create a moment about the ankle joint.[58]

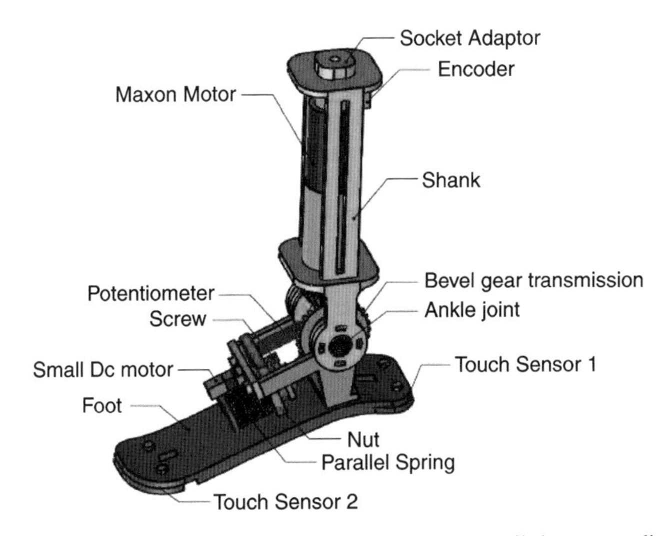

Figure 17. A spring is mounted in parallel with the motor. A small dc motor adjusts the parallel spring.[59]

can be dynamically adjusted, peak required motor torque can be reduced and total input energy requirements can be reduced as well, see Fig. 17. This concept was first mentioned by Lefeber.[3,7]

Wang developed a powered ankle prosthesis that can create a moment about the ankle joint and the toe,[7] see Fig. 18.

A non-anthropomorphic ankle design was created by Sup *et al.*[60] The goal is to reduce the socket interface moments while still injecting power into the gait cycle, see Fig. 19.

The CamWalk ankle has two degrees of freedom that are coupled by springs, see Fig. 20. At heel strike, the leg pushes down on the leg pylon compressing

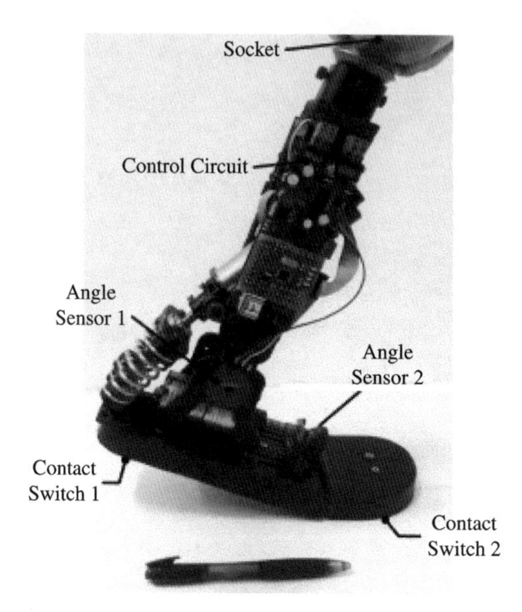

Figure 18. Series, elastic actuators are used to control the moments about the ankle and toe.[7]

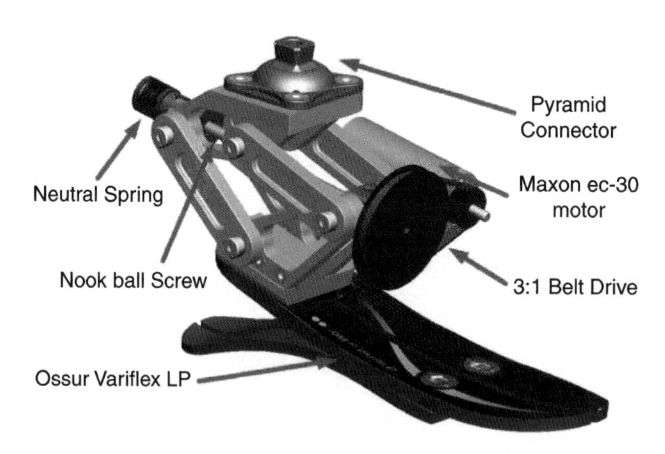

Figure 19. A non-anthropomorphic design to reduce socket forces.[60]

springs to generate propulsive power used later in the gait cycle.[61] The rotational joint is coupled to the leg compression.

Klute designed a transtibial prosthesis that was able to control the torque in the transverse plane,[62] see Fig. 21. They argue that controlling the transverse torque is needed because turning composes a large fraction of steps during the day. The group also developed a cam-based transtibial prosthesis that can control the torque

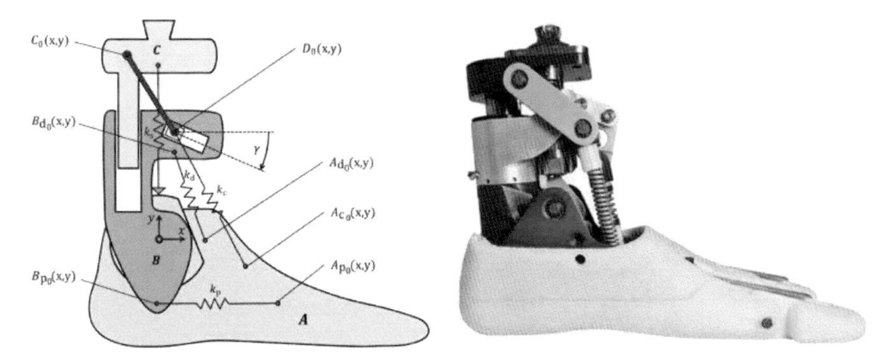

Figure 20. As the pylon is compressed, the stored energy is used later for PO power.[61]

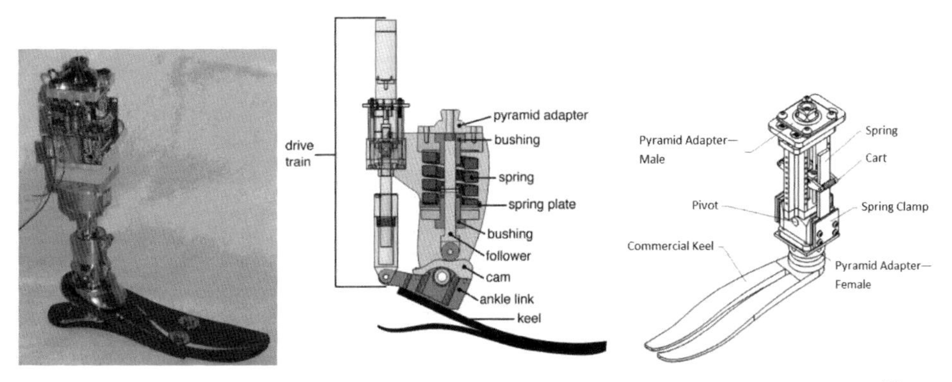

Figure 21. A powered ankle prosthesis was developed that can control the transverse torque.[62] The ankle in the middle can control the torque in the sagittal plane based on a motor, spring, and cam.[63] The ankle on the right can control the stiffness in the coronal plane.[65]

in the sagittal plane.[63] They show that the addition of the cam and parallel spring both reduce the peak actuator torque by 74%. The parallel spring is compressed at the neutral position when the pylon is vertical. They are also designing a variable stiffness prostheses.[64] Lastly, they are designing a foot that can adjust the stiffness in the coronal plane,[65] see Fig. 21. A cart moves up and down a leaf spring adjusting the stiffness of the beam.

Reiner and Vallery designed a transfemoral prosthesis based on a nonlinear transmission and parallel springs.[66] The goal was to develop a method where the actuator's stiffness is a function of joint angle, see Fig. 22.

A powered prosthesis was designed by Grimmer and Seyfarth that can be used to evaluate elastic designs and control concepts. The Powered Ankle Knee Orthoprosthesis (PAKO) uses series springs with changeable stiffness to power the ankle,[67] see Fig. 23.

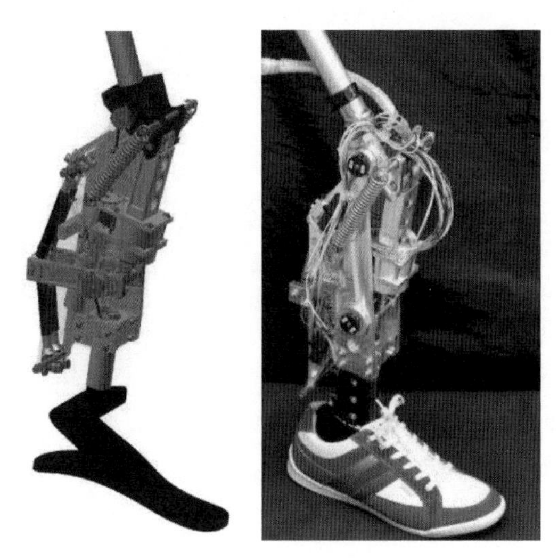

Figure 22. A series elastic actuator is combined with parallel springs and a nonlinear transmission in a transfemoral prosthesis.[66]

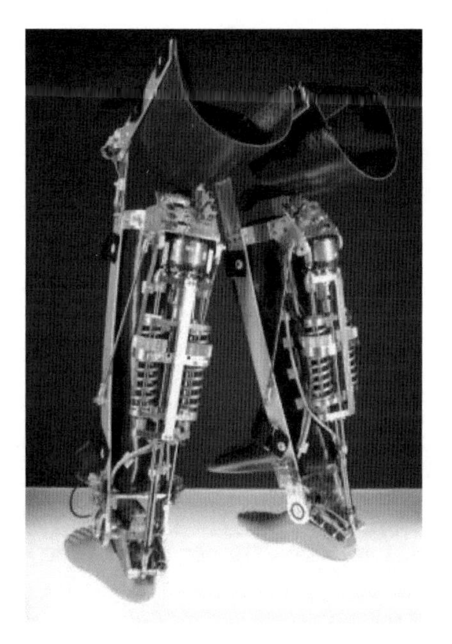

Figure 23. A powered transfemoral prosthesis simulator to test mono-articular springs.[67]

A spring-based ankle was developed at the Catholic University at Louvain, Belgium,[68] see Fig. 24. They used adaptive oscillators to control the movement.

There are many active systems being designed by companies such as Basic[2]Bionics, Ossur, BionX, SpringActive, and Freedom Innovations. Research is being done in Japan on a transtibial prosthesis.[69] In China, a pneumatic

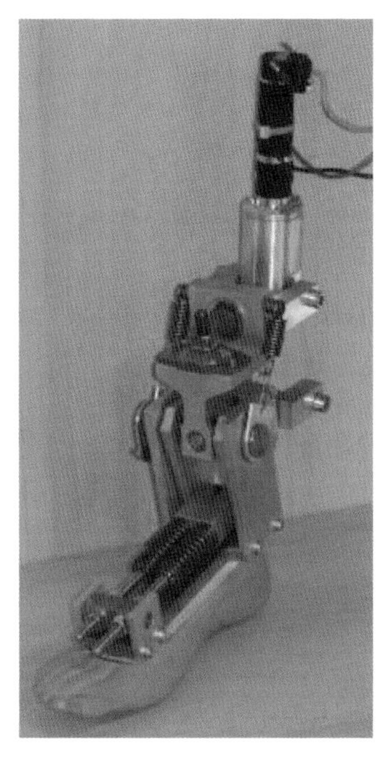

Figure 24. A spring-based ankle was controlled using adaptive oscillators.[68]

muscle-based transfemoral prosthesis has been built.[70] Nonlinear-based controllers are being developed for a transfemoral prosthesis.[71]

In summary, there has been an explosion of the development of powered ankle systems. Series springs reduce the required motor velocity during push-off (PO) reducing the required motor peak-power. Parallel springs add an additional load path, reducing the required motor torque and again reducing the required motor peak-power. Most groups use an impedance control scheme while a couple of groups use a reflex controller or phase-based controller.

3.3. *Quasi-active prosthetic systems*

The goal of quasi-active systems is to use a small motor or clutch to adjust the properties of the device during the gait cycle. Because these systems use a small amount of energy, they should be more cost effective and last longer before the need of a battery charge

A method was developed to capture energy in a spring and delay the release of the energy until other times in the gait cycle,[72] see Fig. 25. As the carbon fiber foot is bent, the string or fiber is shortened and held by the brake motor. The motor can then release the energy at other times.

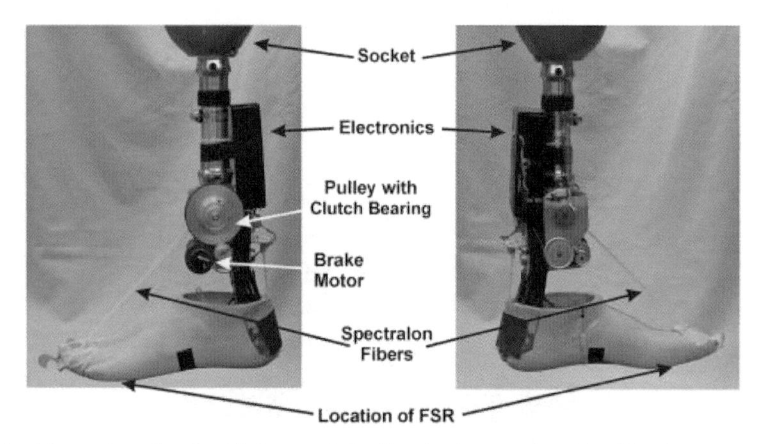

Figure 25. The carbon fiber keel is bent and the fiber is shortened and held by the brake motor. The energy can be released later in the cycle.[72]

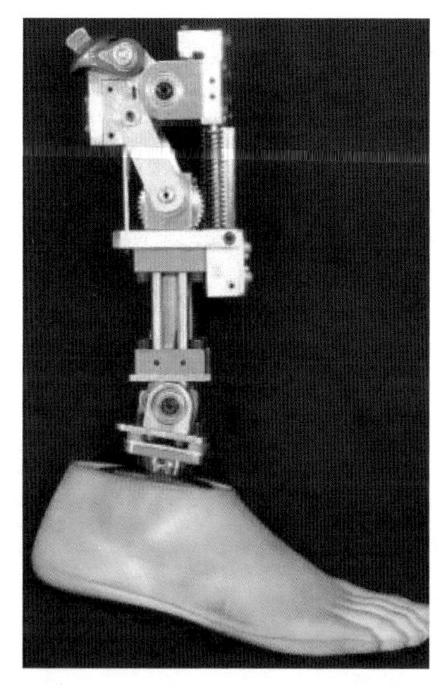

Figure 26. The knee and ankle are coupled to make it easier to climb stairs.[73]

A passive mechanism was designed to allow knee movement to adjust the ankle movement to make stair ascension easier,[73] see Fig. 26.

A microprocessor ankle is used to control the damping behavior of the ankle.[74,75] In ground-level walking, a motor is used to generate a nonlinear braking torque. The motor controls the angle of the foot during the swing-phase, see Fig. 27.

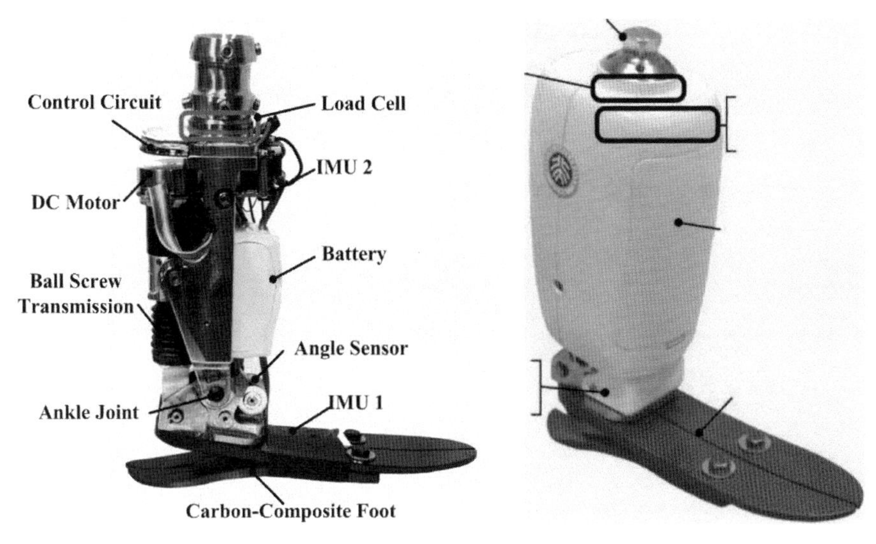

Figure 27. A motor/ball screw transmission is used to control the damping about the ankle joint during the stance-phase.[74,75]

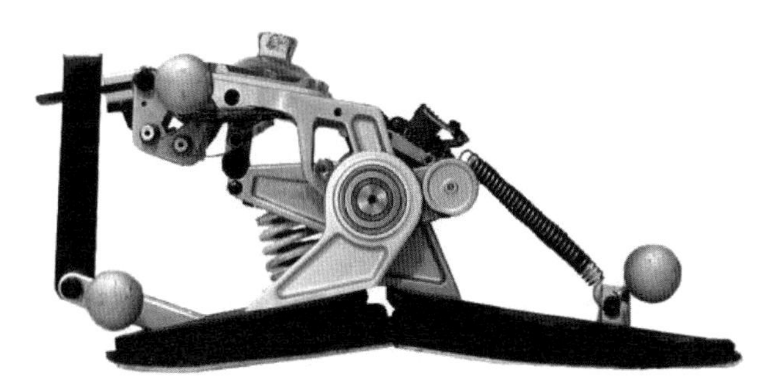

Figure 28. The prosthesis was able to store energy at heel stroke and release the energy later in the gait cycle.[76]

A prosthesis was designed that can capture energy at heel strike and store the energy until PO, see Fig. 28. The foot was called a Controlled Energy Storage and Return prosthetic foot (CESR).[76]

Hansen developed a passive ankle that can adjust to slopes.[77] A cam-based clutch was designed and tested, see Fig. 29. A user's comfort and exertion was reduced when walking downhill. The torque angle curve was shifted toward plantarflexion when walking downhill.

Svensson also designed an ankle that can accommodate slopes.[78] The angle of the foot blade is adjusted by a small DC motor when the foot is in the air in an unloaded state, see Fig. 30.

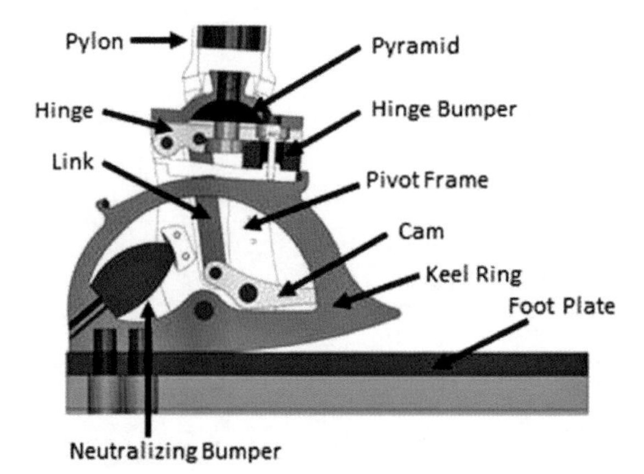

Figure 29. A passive cam system was developed to shift the torque angle curve when walking on slopes.[77]

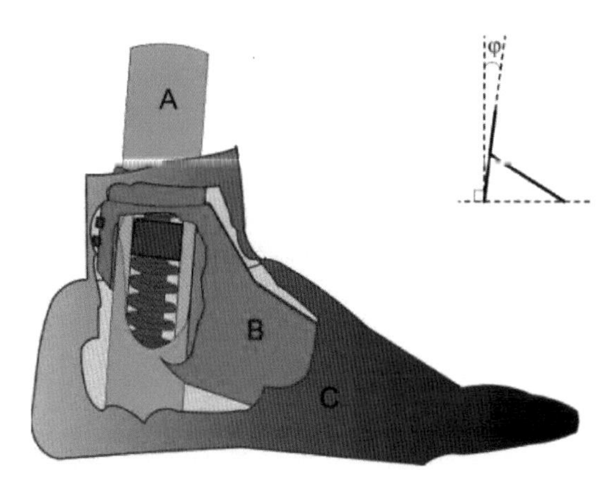

Figure 30. The keel B is adjusted up or down by the motor/screw at A. As the motor moves up and down, the vertical axis at A is tilted by an amount ϕ.[78]

4. Soft Wearable Robotics

Researchers are starting to develop actuation systems based on flexible joints and non-rigid structures.[79,80] The advantage of these systems includes increased freedom of movement, reduced weight, and increased comfort. Walsh *et al.* designed a spring-cable system that can be worn on the leg, see Fig. 31. During the stance, the cable is stretched by the leg and additional motor power stretches the cable more. The energy stored in the spring is used in late stance for PO.

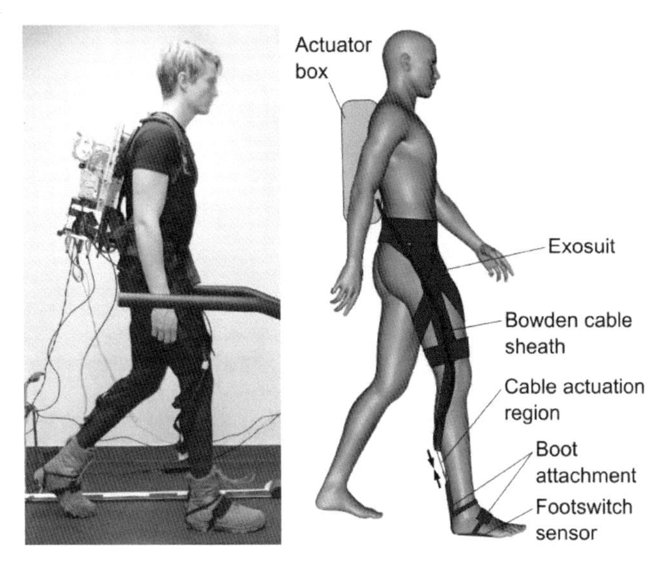

Figure 31. A soft exosuit is designed to be worn tightly on the leg. The cable is pulled during stance to aid POs.[79,80]

5. Conclusion

The confluence of robotics, biomechanics, and design allow researchers to develop exciting legged devices, orthoses, prostheses, and soft exosuit systems. As actuation, embedded microprocessors and sensors, and controllers improve, more sophisticated devices will be worn.

Even though sophisticated systems are being designed, the understanding of how active wearable systems affect human physiology, disease recovery, and pathological gait is still in its infancy. More research into control systems that seamlessly interact with users is needed. Research is just starting to show that autonomous systems can reduce metabolic cost. Only a few systems have been able to overcome their weight penalty and actually augment the user.[28,30,81–83]

Another question is: how sophisticated can a powered prosthetic system become? Is it possible to use two motors to change ankle position and stiffness even though the system might be too heavy and complicated? Is it possible to use two motors to power both plantarflexion and dorsiflexion as well as inversion and eversion. Prototypes have been designed, but the cost, complexity and weight might be too high. Lastly, is it possible to design a complete ankle that can adjust stiffness in the sagittal, transverse, and coronal planes? Hopefully, with new technological improvements, it will be possible to build even more sophisticated systems.

Future research must be into giving the user a feeling of proprioception back. It is hoped that peripheral nerve interfaces will allow the user volitional control of an ankle as well as feedback of ground reaction forces.

We envision the day that these systems will be worn to assist, enhance and replace human limbs to allow people to function with peak performance.

References

1. T. Yan, M. Cempini, M. O. Cologero and N. Vitiello. (2015). Review of Assistive Strategies in Powered Lower-Limb Orthoses and Exoskeletons, *Robotics and Autonomous Systems* 64.
2. M. Grimmer and A. Seyfarth. (2014). Mimicking human-like leg function in prosthetic limbs, *Neuro-Robotics* Springer, 105–155.
3. R. Versluys, P. Beyl, M. Van Damme, A. Desomer, R. Van Ham and D. Lefeber. (2009). Prosthetic feet: State-of-the-art review and the importance of mimicking human ankle–foot biomechanics, *Disability and Rehabilitation: Assistive Technology* 4:65–75.
4. I. Diaz, J. J. Gil and E. Sanchez. (2011). Lower limb robotic rehabilitation: literature review and challenges, *Journal of Robotics*.
5. S. Viteckova, P. Kutilek and M. Jirina. (2013). Wearable Lower Limb Robotics: A Review, *Biocybernetics and Biomedical Engineering* 33:96–105.
6. M. Zhang, T. C. Davies and S. Xie. (2013). Effectiveness of robot-assisted therapy on ankle rehabilitation — A systematic review, *Journal of NeuroEngineering and Rehabilitation* 10.
7. P. Cherelle, G. Mathijssen, Q. Wang, B. Vanderborght and D. Lefeber. (2014). Advances in propulsive bionic feet and their actuation principles, *Advances in Mechanical Engineering* 6:984046.
8. E. R. Esposito, R. V. Blanck, N. G. Harper, J. R. Hsu and J. M. Wilken. (2014). How does ankle-foot orthosis stiffness affect gait in patients with lower limb salvage?, *Clinical Orthopaedics and Related Research®* 472:3026–3035.
9. J. C. Patzkowski, R. V. Blanck, J. G. Owens, J. M. Wilken, K. L. Kirk, J. C. Wenke, J. R. Hsu and S. T. R. Consortium. (2012). Comparative effect of orthosis design on functional performance, *The Journal of Bone and Joint Surgery* 94:507–515.
10. J. A. Blaya and H. Herr. (2004). Adaptive control of a variable-impedance ankle–foot orthosis to assist drop-foot gait, *IEEE Transactions on Neural Systems and Rehabilitation Engineering* 12.
11. K. Bharadwaj, K. W. Hollander, C. A. Mathis and T. G. Sugar. (2004). Spring over muscle (SOM) actuator for rehabilitation devices, *26th Annual International Conference on IEMBS '04: IEEE.*
12. K. Bharadwaj, T. G. Sugar, J. B. Koeneman and E. J. Koeneman. (2005). Design of a robotic gait trainer using spring over muscle actuators for ankle stroke rehabilitation, *ASME Journal of Biomechanical Engineering* 127:1009–1013.
13. K. W. Hollander, R. Ilg and T. G. Sugar. (2005). Design of the Robotic Tendon, *Design of Medical Devices*.
14. K. W. Hollander, R. Ilg, T. G. Sugar and D. E. Herring. (2006). An Efficient Robotic Tendon for Gait Assistance, *ASME Journal of Biomechanical Engineering* 128:788–791.
15. J. Ward, A. Boehler, D. Shin, K. Hollander and T. Sugar. (2008). Control Architectures for a Powered Ankle Foot Orthsosis, *International Journal of Assistive Robotics and Mechatronics* 9:2–13.
16. J. Ward, T. Sugar, A. Boehler, J. Standeven and J. R. Engsberg. (2011). Stroke survivors' gait adaptations to a powered ankle foot orthosis, *Advanced Robotics* 25: 1879–1901.

17. J. A. Ward, S. Balasubramanian, T. Sugar and J. He. (2007). Robotic gait trainer reliability and stroke patient case study, in *IEEE 10th International Conference on Rehabilitation Robotics, ICORR*, 554–561.
18. D. P. Ferris. (2009). The exoskeletons are here, *Journal of NeuroEngineering and Rehabilitation* 6.
19. D. P. Ferris, K. E. Gordon, G. S. Sawicki and A. Peethambaran. (2006). An improved powered ankle–foot orthosis using proportional myoelectric control, *Gait & Posture* 23:425–428.
20. D. P. Ferris, G. S. Sawicki and M. A. Daley. (2007). A Physiologist's Perspective on Robotic Exoskeletons for Human Locomotion, *International Journal of Humanoid Robotics* 4:507–528.
21. G. Sawicki, K. Gordon and D. P. Ferris. (2005). Powered Lower Limb Orthoses: Applications in Motor Adaptation and Rehabilitation, in *IEEE 9th International Conference on Rehabilitation Robotics*, 206–211.
22. C. Meijneke, W. van Dijk and H. van der Kooij. (2014). Achilles: an autonomous lightweight ankle exoskeleton to provide push-off power, in *5th IEEE RAS & EMBS International Conference on Biomedical Robotics and Biomechatronics* 12–15.
23. K. A. Shorter, G. F. Kogler, E. Loth, W. K. Durfee and E. T. Hsiao-Wecksler. (2011). A portable powered ankle-foot orthosis for rehabilitation, 48:459–472.
24. K. A. Shorter, J. Xia, E. T. Hsiao-Wecksler, W. K. Durfee and G. F. Kogler. (2013). Technologies for powered ankle-foot orthotic systems: Possibilities and challenges, *IEEE/ASME Transactions on Mechatronics* 18:337–347.
25. W. Durfee, J. Xia and E. Hsiao-Wecksler. (2011). Tiny hydraulics for powered orthotics, in *2011 IEEE International Conference on Rehabilitation Robotics (ICORR)* 1–6.
26. J. W. Wheeler, H. I. Krebs and N. Hogan. (2004). An ankle robot for a modular gait rehabilitation system, presented at the Proceedings. 2004 IEEE/RSJ International Conference on Intelligent Robots and Systems (IROS 2004).
27. L. M. Mooney and H. M. Herr. (2016). Biomechanical walking mechanisms underlying the metabolic reduction caused by an autonomous exoskeleton, *Journal of NeuroEngineering and Rehabilitation* 13:1.
28. L. M. Mooney, E. J. Rouse and H. Herr. (2014). Autonomous exoskeleton reduces metabolic cost of human walking, *Journal of NeuroEngineering and Rehabilitation* 11.
29. K. W. Hollander, N. Cahill, R. Holgate, R. Churchwell, P. Clouse, D. Kinney and A. Boehler. (2014). A Passive and Active Joint Torque Augmentation Robot (JTAR) for Hip Gait Assistance, in *ASME 2014 International Design Engineering Technical Conferences and Computers and Information in Engineering Conference*, V05AT08A079–V05AT08A079.
30. S. H. Collins, M. B. Wiggin and G. S. Sawicki. (2015). Reducing the energy cost of human walking using an unpowered exoskeleton, *Nature* 522.
31. W. Svensson and U. Holmberg. (2008). Ankle-foot-orthosis control in inclinations and stairs, in *2008 IEEE Conference on Robotics, Automation and Mechatronics*, 301–306.
32. F. Sup, H. A. Varol, J. Mitchell, T. J. Withrow and M. Goldfarb. (2009). Self-contained powered knee and ankle prosthesis: initial evaluation on a transfemoral amputee, in *IEEE International Conference on Rehabilitation Robotics (ICORR, 2009)*, 638–644.
33. S. Au, M. Berniker and H. Herr. (2008). Powered ankle-foot prosthesis to assist level-ground and stair-descent gaits, *Neural Networks* 21.
34. H. Geyer and H. Herr. (2010). A muscle-reflex model that encodes principles of legged mechanics produces human walking dynamics and muscle activities, *IEEE Transactions on Neural Systems and Rehabilitation Engineering* 18:263–273.
35. J. Hitt and T. Sugar. (2010). Load carriage effects on a robotic transtibial prosthesis, in *2010 International Conference on Control Automation and Systems (ICCAS)* 139–142.
36. J. K. Hitt, R. Bellman, M. Holgate, T. G. Sugar and K. W. Hollander. (2007). The SPARKy (spring ankle with regenerative kinetics) project: Design and analysis of a robotic transtibial

prosthesis with regenerative kinetics, in *ASME 2007 International Design Engineering Technical Conferences and Computers and Information in Engineering Conference* 1587–1596.
37. J. K. Hitt, M. Holgate, R. Bellman, T. G. Sugar and K. W. Hollander. (2009). Robotic Transtibial Prosthesis with Biomechanical Energy Regeneration, *Industrial Robot: An International Journal* 36:441–447.
38. J. K. Hitt, T. G. Sugar, M. Holgate and R. Bellman. (2010). An active foot–ankle prosthesis with biomechanical energy regeneration, *Journal of Medical Devices* 4:011003.
39. M. A. Holgate, J. K. Hitt, R. D. Bellman, T. G. Sugar and K. W. Hollander. (2008). The SPARKy (Spring Ankle with Regenerative kinetics) project: Choosing a DC motor based actuation method, in *2nd IEEE RAS & EMBS International Conference on Biomedical Robotics and Biomechatronics, BioRob 2008* 163–168.
40. F. Sup, H. A. Varol and M. Goldfarb. (2011). Upslope Walking With a Powered Knee and Ankle Prosthesis: Initial Results With an Amputee Subject, *IEEE Transactions on Neural Systems and Rehabilitation Engineering* 19:71–78.
41. F. Sup, A. Bohara and M. Goldfarb. (2008). Design and control of a powered transfemoral prosthesis, *The International Journal of Robotics Research* 27:263–273.
42. F. Sup, H. A. Varol, J. Mitchell, T. J. Withrow and M. Goldfarb. (2009). Preliminary evaluations of a self-contained anthropomorphic transfemoral prosthesis, *IEEE/ASME Transactions on Mechatronics* 14:667–676.
43. K. Fite, J. Mitchell, F. Sup and M. Goldfarb. (2007). Design and control of an electrically powered knee prosthesis, in *IEEE 10th International Conference on Rehabilitation Robotics (ICORR, 2007)* 902–905.
44. M. A. Holgate, A. W. Böhler and T. G. Sugar. (2008). Control algorithms for ankle robots: A reflection on the state-of-the-art and presentation of two novel algorithms, in *2nd IEEE RAS & EMBS International Conference on Biomedical Robotics and Biomechatronics, 2008. BioRob 2008* 97–102.
45. M. A. Holgate, T. G. Sugar and A. W. Böhler. (2009) A novel control algorithm for wearable robotics using phase plane invariants, in *IEEE International Conference on Robotics and Automation, 2009. ICRA'09* 3845–3850.
46. M. Holgate and T. G. Sugar. (2014). Active Compliant Parallel Mechanisms, in *ASME 2014 International Design Engineering Technical Conferences and Computers and Information in Engineering Conference*, V05AT08A080–V05AT08A080.
47. A. H. Shultz, B. E. Lawson and M. Goldfarb. (2015). Running with a powered knee and ankle prosthesis, *IEEE Transactions on Neural Systems and Rehabilitation Engineering* 23:403–412.
48. B. E. Lawson, H. A. Varol, F. Sup and M. Goldfarb. (2010). Stumble detection and classification for an intelligent transfemoral prosthesis, in *2010 Annual International Conference of the IEEE Engineering in Medicine and Biology Society (EMBC)* 511–514.
49. B. E. Lawson, H. A. Varol and M. Goldfarb. (2011). Standing stability enhancement with an intelligent powered transfemoral prosthesis, *IEEE Transactions on Biomedical Engineering* 58:2617–2624.
50. A. H. Shultz, J. E. Mitchell, D. Truex, B. E. Lawson and M. Goldfarb. (2013). Preliminary evaluation of a walking controller for a powered ankle prosthesis, in *2013 IEEE International Conference on Robotics and Automation (ICRA)* 4838–4843.
51. P. Cherelle, A. Matthys, V. Grosu, B. Vanderborght and D. Lefeber. (2012). The amp-foot 2.0: Mimicking intact ankle behavior with a powered transtibial prosthesis, in *4th IEEE RAS & EMBS International Conference on Biomedical Robotics and Biomechatronics (BioRob)* 544–549.
52. P. Cherelle, V. Grosu, A. Matthys, B. Vanderborght and D. Lefeber. (2014). Design and validation of the ankle mimicking prosthetic (AMP-) foot 2.0, *IEEE Transactions on Neural Systems and Rehabilitation Engineering* 22:138–148.

53. P. Cherelle, V. Grosu, M. Cestari, B. Vanderborght and D. Lefeber. (2014). The amp-foot 3-new generation propulsive prosthetic feet with explosive motion characteristics: design and validation, *Under Review*.
54. G. Mathijssen, P. Cherelle, D. Lefeber and B. Vanderborght. (2013). Concept of a series-parallel elastic actuator for a powered transtibial prosthesis, *Actuators* 59–73.
55. R. Versluys, A. Desomer, G. Lenaerts, O. Pareit, B. Vanderborght, G. Perre, L. Peeraer, and D. Lefeber. (2008). A biomechatronical transtibial prosthesis powered by pleated pneumatic artificial muscles, *International Journal of Modelling, Identification and Control* 4:394–405.
56. R. D. Bellman, M. A. Holgate and T. G. Sugar. (2008). SPARKy 3: Design of an active robotic ankle prosthesis with two actuated degrees of freedom using regenerative kinetics, in *2nd IEEE RAS & EMBS International Conference on Biomedical Robotics and Biomechatronics, BioRob 2008* 6.
57. E. M. Ficanha, M. Rastgaar and K. R. Kaufman. (2014). A two-axis cable-driven ankle-foot mechanism, *Robotics and Biomimetics* 1:1–13.
58. J. Sun and P. A. Voglewede. (2014). Powered transtibial prosthetic device control system design, implementation, and bench testing, *Journal of Medical Devices* 8:011004.
59. F. Gao, H. Ma, W.-H. Liao, L.-y. Qin and B. Chen. (2015) Design of powered ankle-foot prosthesis driven by parallel elastic actuator, in *2015 IEEE International Conference on Rehabilitation Robotics (ICORR)*, 374–379.
60. A. LaPre and F. Sup. (2013). Redefining Prosthetic Ankle Mechanics, in *IEEE International Conference on Rehabilitation Robotics*.
61. J. J. Rice and J. M. Schimmels. (2014). Design and Evaluation of a Passive Ankle Prosthesis With Rotational Power Generation by a Compliant Coupling Between Leg Deflection and Ankle Rotation, in *ASME 2014 International Design Engineering Technical Conferences and Computers and Information in Engineering Conference*, V05AT08A047–V05AT08A047.
62. N. M. Olson, and G. K. Klute. (2015) Design of a transtibial prosthesis with active transverse plane control, *Journal of Medical Devices* 9:045002.
63. J. Realmuto, G. Klute and S. Devasia. (2015). Nonlinear passive cam-based springs for powered ankle prostheses, *Journal of Medical Devices* 9:011007.
64. G. K. Klute, J. C. Perry and J. M. Czernicki. Variable stiffness prosthesis for transtibial amputees, *Dept of Veteran Affairs, Seattle, WA USA* 2.
65. G. K. Klute, J. Gorges, K. Yeates and A. D. Segal. (2015). Variable Stiffness Prosthesis to Improve Amputee Coronal Plane Balance, in *American Academy of Orthotists and Prosthetists, 41st Academy Annual Meeting & Scientific Symposium*.
66. S. Pfeifer, A. Pagel, R. Riener and H. Vallery. (2015). Actuator with angle-dependent elasticity for biomimetic transfemoral prostheses, *IEEE/ASME Transactions on Mechatronics* 20: 1384–1394.
67. M. Grimmer. (2015). Powered Lower Limb Prostheses, University of TU-Darmstadt.
68. C. Everarts, A. Thissen, B. Dehez, A. J. Ijspeert and R. Ronsse. (2011). Control and design of an active prosthesis based on adaptive oscillators, in *10 Belgian Day on Biomedical Engineering — Joint Meeting with IEEE EMBS Benelux Chapter* 1–2.
69. R. Suzuki, T. Sawada, N. Kobayashi and E. P. Hofer. (2011). Control method for powered ankle prosthesis via internal model control design, in *2011 IEEE International Conference on Mechatronics and Automation*.
70. M. Wu, T. Driver, S.-K. Wu and X. Shen. (2014). Design and preliminary testing of a pneumatic muscle-actuated transfemoral prosthesis, *Journal of Medical Devices* 8:044502.
71. H. Zhao, J. Reher, J. Horn, V. Paredes and A. D. Ames. (2015). Realization of nonlinear real-time optimization based controllers on self-contained transfemoral prosthesis, in *Proceedings of the ACM/IEEE Sixth International Conference on Cyber-Physical Systems*, 130–138.

72. M. Mitchell, K. Craig, P. Kyberd, E. Biden and G. Bush. (2013). Design and development of ankle-foot prosthesis with delayed release of plantarflexion, *Journal of Rehabilitation Research and Development* 50:409–422.
73. S. Yoshida, T. Wada and K. Inoue. (2015). A passive transfemoral prosthesis with movable ankle for stair ascent, in *2015 IEEE International Conference on Rehabilitation Robotics (ICORR)*, 7–12.
74. Q. Wang, K. Yuan, J. Zhu and L. Wang. (2014). Finite-state control of a robotic transtibial prosthesis with motor-driven nonlinear damping behaviors for level ground walking, in *2014 IEEE 13th international workshop on Advanced motion control (AMC)*, 155–160.
75. Q. Wang, K. Yuan, J. Zhu and L. Wang. (2015). Walk the Walk: A lightweight active transtibial prosthesis, *IEEE Robotics & Automation Magazine* 22:80–89.
76. A. D. Segal, K. E. Zelik, G. K. Klute, D. C. Morgenroth, M. E. Hahn, M. S. Orendurff, P. G. Adamczyk, S. H. Collins, A. D. Kuo and J. M. Czerniecki. (2012). The effects of a controlled energy storage and return prototype prosthetic foot on transtibial amputee ambulation, *Human Movement Science* 31:918–931.
77. E. Nickel. (2014). Passive prosthetic ankle–foot mechanism for automatic adaptation to sloped surfaces, *Journal of Rehabilitation Research and Development* 51:803.
78. W. Svensson and U. Holmberg. (2006). An autonomous control system for a prosthetic foot ankle, in *4th IFAC Symposium on Mechatronic Systems, 12–14 September, 2006, Ruprecht-Karls-University, Germany* 856–861.
79. A. T. Asbeck, R. J. Dyer, A. F. Larusson and C. J. Walsh. (2013). Biologically-inspired soft exosuit, in *2013 IEEE International Conference on Rehabilitation Robotics (ICORR)* 1–8.
80. A. T. Asbeck, S. M. De Rossi, K. G. Holt and C. J. Walsh. (2015). A biologically inspired soft exosuit for walking assistance, *International Journal of Robotics Research* 0278364914562476.
81. J. Kerestes, T. G. Sugar and M. Holgate. (2014). Adding and subtracting energy to body motion — phase oscillator, in *Proceedings of the ASME 2014 International Design Engineering Technical Conferences & Computers and Information in Engineering Conference*, Buffalo, NY.
82. P. Malcolm, W. Derave, S. Galle and D. De Clercq. (2013). A simple exoskeleton that assists plantarflexion can reduce the metabolic cost of human walking, *PLoS ONE* 8.
83. J. A. Norris, K. P. Granata, M. R. Mitros, E. M. Byrne and A. P. Marsh. (2007). Effect of augmented plantarflexion power on preferred walking speed and economy in young and older adults, *Gait & Posture* 25:620–627.

Chapter 6

SOFT ROBOTIC GLOVE FOR COMBINED ASSISTANCE AND REHABILITATION DURING ACTIVITIES OF DAILY LIVING

Kevin C. Galloway*, Panagiotis Polygerinos†,
Robert J. Wood‡,§, and Conor J. Walsh‡,§

*Vanderbilt School of Engineering, Nashville, TN, USA, 37212
†Ira A. Fulton Schools of Engineering, Arizona State University, Mesa, AZ, USA, 85212
‡Wyss Institute for Biologically Inspired Engineering, Harvard University, Cambridge, MA, USA, 02138
§Harvard John A. Paulson School of Engineering and Applied Sciences, Cambridge, MA, USA, 02138

The human hand plays an important role in the manipulation and exploration of the environment. Unfortunately, when disease or injury impedes hand function, the consequences are numerous including disrupting quality of life, independence, and financial stability. In this chapter, we present the development of a soft robotic glove designed to support basic hand function. The glove uses soft fluidic actuators programmed to apply assistive forces to support the range of motion of a human hand. More specifically, we present a method of fabrication and characterization of these soft actuators as well as consider an approach for controlling the glove. This analysis concludes with results from preliminary human subjects testing where glove performance was evaluated on a healthy and an impaired subject.

1. Introduction

Hand function plays an important role in performing activities of daily living (ADL) and maintaining an independent and healthy quality of life. However, people afflicted by stroke, cerebral palsy, muscular dystrophy, spinal cord injury (SCI), or traumatic brain injury may lose the ability to actively and accurately control the wrist, thumb, and fingers. If left untreated, these impairments contribute to the loss of advanced grasps[1,2] such as the ability to perform many fundamental activities of daily living.

Physical therapy has been shown to be beneficial for recovering hand function in patients with acute conditions; however, current practice is labor intensive, costly, and limited to clinical environments.[3,4] Individuals with degenerate conditions often suffer from deficits and require assistance to compensate for loss of muscle strength. Therefore, an assistive device that can safely interface with soft tissue and provide grasp assistance for ADL, or task-specific training, could play a critical role in returning independence to users over the course of their life.

A variety of wearable robotic hand devices have been developed for rehabilitation purposes and primarily consist of rigid exoskeleton designs.[5,6] These devices are typically designed for use in a clinical setting and are often not well suited for use as an assistive device or task-specific training. They include the Box-and-Block test, the Nine-Hole Peg test, or the Jebsen hand function test. Recently, new approaches using soft robotic technology have emerged with designs for assistive hand devices that utilize flexible and soft materials such as cable-driven or fluidic soft actuators for supporting finger motion.[7–16] These soft systems are engineered using low-cost fabrication techniques, provide adaptable morphology in response to environmental changes and are ideally suited for gripping and manipulating delicate objects and wearable applications.

A soft wearable robotic device could lead to greater advances in at-home assistive activity and rehabilitation by providing: (a) safe human-robotic interaction due to the soft and compliant materials used for their fabrication, (b) low component cost due to inexpensive materials (e.g. fabrics, elastomers, etc.) and single actuation source to actuate all fingers (i.e. pump), (c) ability to provide customizable actuation based on patient anatomy, and (d) suitability to provide combined assistance and rehabilitation during ADL. This chapter presents such a device that utilizes inexpensive hydraulic soft actuators made from elastomeric materials with fiber reinforcements to control the fingers. The hydraulic soft actuators are mounted to the dorsal side of the hand, resulting in an open-palm design (see concept application in Fig. 1).

This chapter begins with describing the features and capabilities of a specific type of soft robotic actuator that is suitable for integration into a soft robotic glove. We describe the principle of operation of these actuators and the steps required to fabricate them. This is followed by a description of the design approach that can be followed to create actuators that can match the motion of the fingers or thumb during a grasping operation. The overall system, including the textile design that enables an open-palm glove and portable power/control unit that supports controlled pressurization of the actuators. The level of assistance provided by the soft robotic glove is characterized using an array of pressure sensors affixed to a cylinder demonstrating a force level suitable for assistance during ADL. We present a control system to detect the intent of the wearer that is based on surface

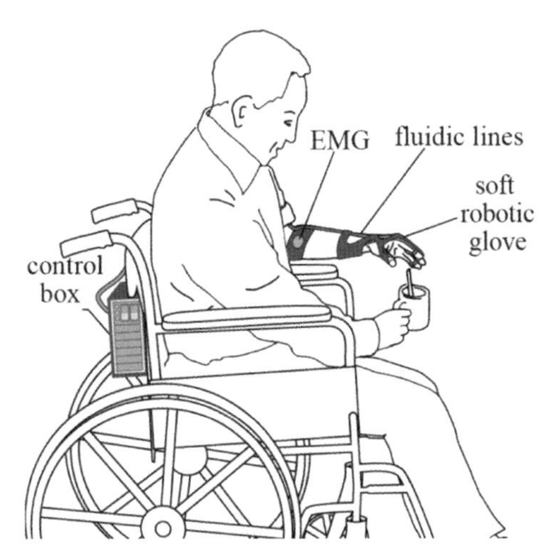

Figure 1. Concept of a soft robotic glove providing assistance in ADL to individuals with hand impairments through the use of a soft robotic glove that detects user intent through EMG signals in the forearm (reprinted from Ref. [33]).

electromyography of the muscles in the forearm and demonstrate its operation on a healthy subject and a patient with muscular dystrophy. Finally, we present some pilot testing demonstrating the ability of the proposed soft robotic glove to improve grasping during simulated functional tasks.

2. Fiber-reinforced Soft Actuators

2.1. *Overview*

A fundamental component of soft robotics is the soft fluidic actuator, a deformable shell that converts potential energy of a pressurized fluid into a mechanical force that can be used to create motion.[17] Pneumatic and hydraulic powered soft actuators are promising candidates for robotics applications because of their lightweight, high power-to-weight ratio, low material cost, ease of fabrication with emerging digital fabrication techniques and controllability with single inputs that can produce complex motions. There is a long history of soft actuator designs including bellow-type designs that unfold shell material to support bending, rotary and linear motions, and Mckibben actuators, which elastically strain a shell material within an anisotropic fiber reinforcement to create linear contraction coupled with radial expansion.[17,18] Most relevant to the present discussion is the pioneering work by Koichi Suzumori where he embedded radial and axial fiber reinforcements into elastomeric materials to control the elastic deformation of multi-lumen, multi-degree of soft bending actuators.[19] Recent work by a number of groups has also focused on developing analytical and computational models for predicting the motion and forces produced by this class of actuator as a function of their material properties and geometry.[20–23]

2.2. *Fabricating a fiber-reinforced soft actuator*

The soft actuators presented in this work[a] consist of an elastomeric, tubular bladder that deforms in response to fluid pressurization and anisotropic reinforcements in its wall that determine the deformation.[24–28] These actuators can operate at high pressures (up to 80 psi) and are highly compliant (i.e. able to fully bend with less than 1 N of force when unactuated), but can exert significant force (~20 N at the tip) when pressurized.

Fiber-reinforced soft actuators are fabricated in a multi-step molding process. This approach offers complete control over every aspect of the assembled soft actuator including geometry, fiber reinforcements, and material properties. The actuators presented in this work are constructed from a silicone rubber compound (Elastosil M4601, Wacker Chemie AG, Germany) that offers high elongation before failure (~700%), good tear strength (~30 N/mm), and a Shore A hardness of 28. The first step begins with defining the shape of the bladder or the portion of the actuator that will contain the pressurized fluid. For the purpose of illustration, Fig. 2(a) illustrates a half-round steel rod that defines the inner shape of the bladder with a 3D printed two-part mold that defines the outer geometry. Raised features on the inside of the mold define paths for fiber reinforcements and are transferred to the rubber body during molding. Alignment features at either end of the mold support axial alignment of the rod. It should be noted that bladder geometry can be of many different shapes. For example, the bladder can be molded with a rectangular cross-section by changing the rod cross-section and the mold. After molding the bladder, fiber reinforcements are added to the bladder's surface (Figs. 2(b)–2(c)). Woven fiberglass (S2-6522 plain weave 4 oz. weight) is glued to the flat face to serve as the strain-limiting layer that promotes bending during fluid pressurization (Fig. 2(b)). A single Kevlar thread (0.38 mm diameter) wound around the length of the actuator body secures the strain-limiting layer and helps constrain the bladder from radial swelling during pressurization (Fig. 2(c)). The entire assembly is then placed into another mold to encapsulate the actuator body in a 1 mm thick silicone layer to secure the reinforcements during operation (Fig. 2(d)). Once cured, the actuator body can be removed from the mold and the half round steel rod. The ends of the actuator can be closed by placing one end into a small cup of uncured silicone. Once this end has cured, a 10–32 vented screw can be fed through the silicone cap to serve as the mechanical connection for the pneumatic tubes. The other open end

[a]Additional fabrication resources available at www.softroboticstoolkit.com.

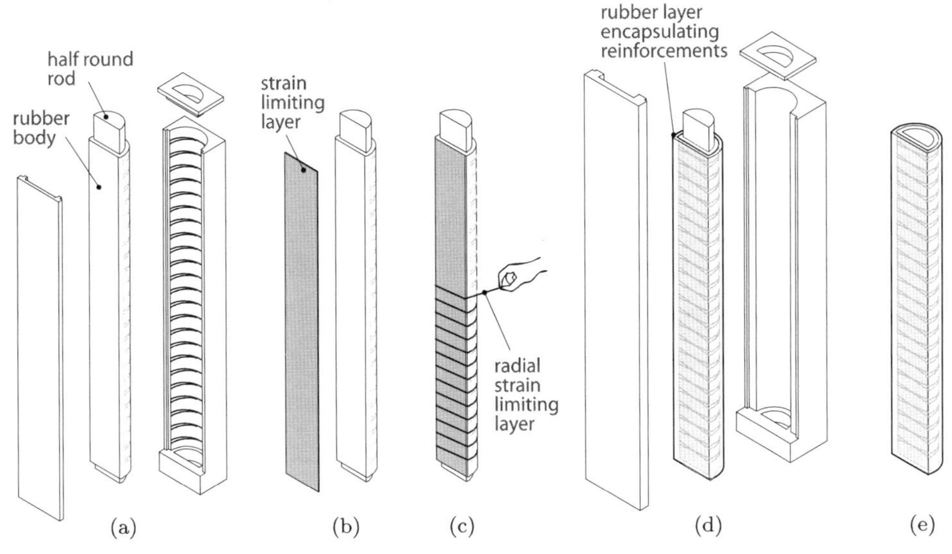

Figure 2. Schematic outlining stages of the soft fiber-reinforced bending actuator fabrication process: (a) the first molding step using a 3D printed part, (b) the strain-limiting layer (woven fiberglass) is attached to the flat face of the actuator, (c) fiber reinforcing thread is wound along the length of the actuator, (d) the second molding step, the entire actuator is encapsulated in a layer of silicone to anchor all reinforcements, and (e) the steel rod is removed and both ends of the actuator are capped allowing one end to have a port for the inflow/outflow of fluid (reprinted from Ref. [26]).

can be closed in the same manner. When a pressurized fluid is applied to the interior of this actuator, it produces a bending motion (Fig. 3(a)). In this example, the strain-limiting layer (e.g. woven fiberglass) constrains one face of the bladder from stretching, and a symmetric arrangement of helical fiber threads constrains radial swelling. Upon pressurization, the wall of the actuator with the strain limited layer can be approximated as flexible, yet inextensible (i.e. fixed length), whereas all the other portions of the actuator are allowed to grow lengthwise. This asymmetrical strain along the length of the actuator causes it to bend or curl in the direction of the strain limiting layer.

2.3. *Programming single motions*

Using the same molds, a soft actuator can be constructed so as to produce other motions (Fig. 3) by altering the fiber reinforcement scheme in steps b and c of Fig. 2. Some of the classes of mechanically programmable motions include bend, bend–twist, extend, contract, and extend–twist. Figure 3 outlines some of these fiber reinforcement recipes. For example, a bend–twist actuator — an actuator that bends and twists as it is pressurized to form a helical shape — follows the same reinforcement steps of a bending actuator with the exception that one helical radial

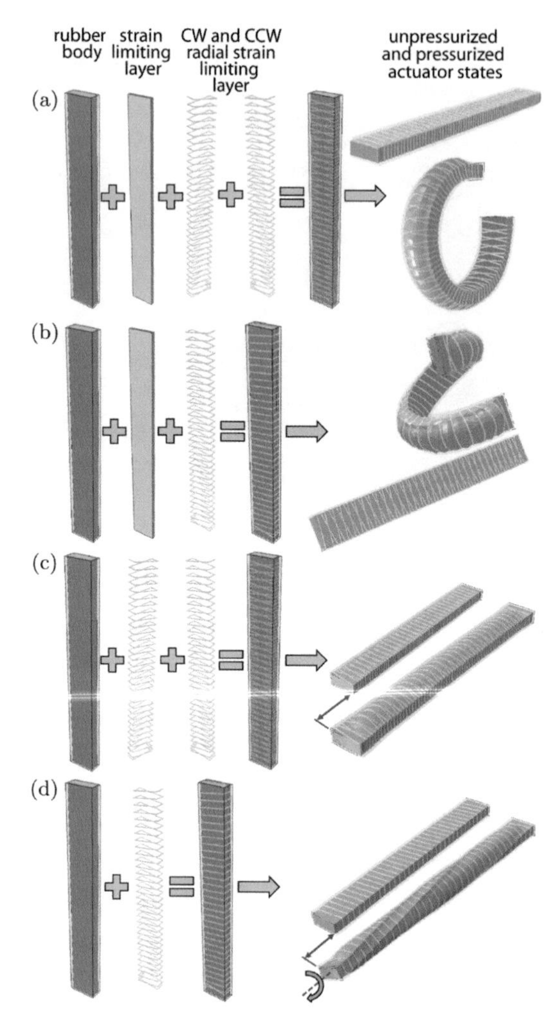

Figure 3. Exploded and assembled view of soft actuator components of the inactive and active states: (a) soft bending actuator, (b) Bend–twist soft actuator, (c) Linearly extending soft actuator, and (d) Twisting soft actuator (reprinted from Ref. [27]).

strain limiting is applied (CW or CCW) and not a symmetric one. Similarly, a linearly extending soft actuator is a symmetric winding of a radial strain-limiting layer (CW and CCW) without a strain-limiting layer (e.g. woven fiberglass).

2.4. *Principles of programming complex motions*

The range of motion of a single actuator can be further expanded by combining the motion classes in series or segments to create multi-segment soft actuators (e.g. separate bending and extending sections in one actuator). Specific to the assistive glove application, two types of multi-segment soft actuators are needed

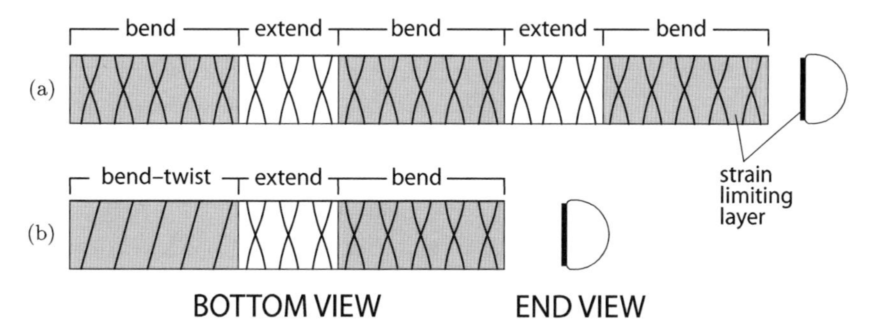

Figure 4. Segmented fiber reinforcement configurations to generate multiple forms of motion in a single soft actuator: (a) illustrates the lower layer of a soft actuator with alternating bending and extending segments which is achieved by selective addition or elimination of the strain limiting layer and (b) illustrates a soft actuator with bend twist, extend, and bend segments, which is achieved by modifying strain fiber reinforcements (reprinted from Ref. [26]).

to support complete hand closure. The first multi-segment actuator was designed to support the fingers (i.e. index, middle, ring, and small finger) closing in the sagittal plane by combining bending and extending fiber reinforcement strategies (Fig. 4(a)). Actuators that incorporate extension are more compatible with the finger skeletal kinematics by compensating for the distance between the soft actuator lying on the dorsal side of the finger and the finger joint axes. The second multi-segment actuator adds a bend–twist motion for the thumb to support opposition grasp motion (Fig. 4(b)). The length of each extending, bending, and twisting actuator segment was empirically estimated such that when pressurized up to 345 kPa (50 psi), the actuator's motion analogously corresponded to the individual skin extension, joint angle, and twisting joint angle of biological fingers.

3. Soft Robotic Glove

3.1. *Motion requirements*

Matching the range of motion of the actuator to the hand is important for comfort and force distribution. Several hand studies quantify the degrees of freedom and biomechanics of the hand.[7,29,30] Based on these studies and empirical observation, the soft actuators should have three bending degrees of freedom for each finger (i.e. index, middle, ring, and little fingers). Similarly, at least two bending DOFs and a rotating one (combination of flexion and abduction) around the carpometacarpal (CMC) joint of the thumb are required to support opposition grasping.

As part of our evaluation, we conducted a benchmark range of motion hand study with a healthy participant. Motion data were collected with an electromagnetic (EM) tracking system (TrakSTAR, Ascension Tech. Corp., Milton, VT) where small EM tracking sensors were attached to a stretchable, thin silicone strip mounted above the fingers. This arrangement was designed to capture the range of motion of the fingers with a stretchable framework that would not impede the range of motion of the hand. For the fingers, three EM tracking sensors tracked the position of each finger joint — metacarpophalangeal (MCP), proximal interphalangeal (PIP) and distal interphalangeal (DIP). A fourth sensor was placed at the fingertip and the fifth at the wrist (carpal level) to act as a reference point for all the other sensors. For the thumb, two sensors tracked the interphalangeal (IP) and MCP joints, another tracked the thumb tip, and a last sensor was positioned on the wrist, at the CMC joint. Each finger was individually flexed five times while the position coordinates of the EM tracking sensors were recorded relative to the reference tracker located at the wrist (numbered as 1 in Fig. 5(a)). Figures 5(b) and 5(c) show the trajectory of each fingertip and the location of each joint in the final flexed position in space. Furthermore, these results also capture the thumb flexion at the IP and MCP joints as well as the rotation at the CMC joint resulting from the opposition. The sum of joint angles for this participant was measured to be approximately 250 and 160 degrees for the middle finger and the thumb, respectively. These results were found to be within the range of motion of joints reported in the literature,[7,29,30] therefore making these a fair representation of average hand range of motion and generalizable to other hand sizes. Furthermore, this experimental method can be applied to measure the range of motion of the soft robotic glove and used to evaluate its ability to match and support the range of motion of a human hand.

3.2. *Actuator output force requirements*

Healthy adult females and males can generate grip forces up to 300 and 450 N, respectively.[9,31,32] For an impaired hand, these force values can be much smaller[9] or non-existent depending on the condition. With this in mind, we propose that any assistive hand technology solution does not need to restore complete hand strength, but rather return enough to support most activities of daily living. A study from Matheus *et al.* benchmarked grasping and manipulating forces (e.g. grasping a glass of water or a fruit, picking up a wallet or telephone, stirring a pot, etc.) and found that most objects of daily living do not weigh more than 1.5 kg.[33] Taking this into account, we estimate that to support a 1.5 kg load with a palmar grasp (four fingers against the palm of the hand) and assuming a conservative coefficient of friction of 0.255 (determined by Ref. [33]), each soft actuator would need to exert a distal tip force of around 7.3 N. While this is an approximation that does not take into account the distribution of the hand's forces on an object, it does offer guidance for actuator performance criteria.

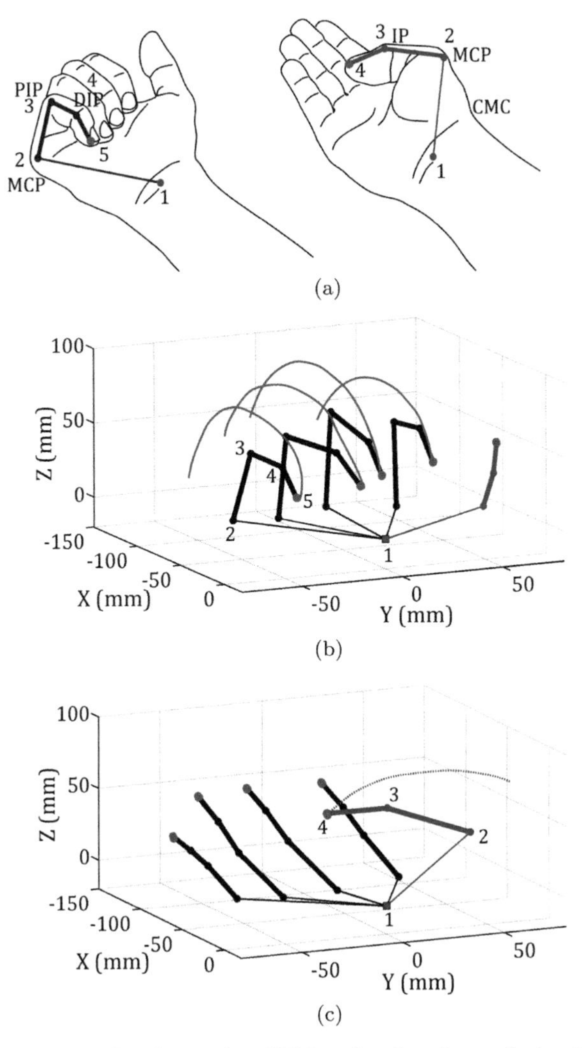

Figure 5. (a) Illustration showing the numbered EM trackers location on the hand. (b) The measured trajectories for the index, middle, ring and small fingers while the thumb remains extended. (c) The measured trajectory of the thumb while performing an opposition motion while all the rest of the fingers remain extended. Location numbered as 1 indicates the reference EM tracker at the wrist (reprinted from Ref. [26]).

3.3. *Matching actuator ROM with hand*

To compare the range of motion of the multi-segment actuators with the thumb and finger, EM tracking sensors were placed along the bottom face of the soft actuators for the index finger and thumb. The actuators were pressurized until they matched the maximum of the range of motion of each biological finger (345 kPa). These experiments were repeated five times and their average is presented in

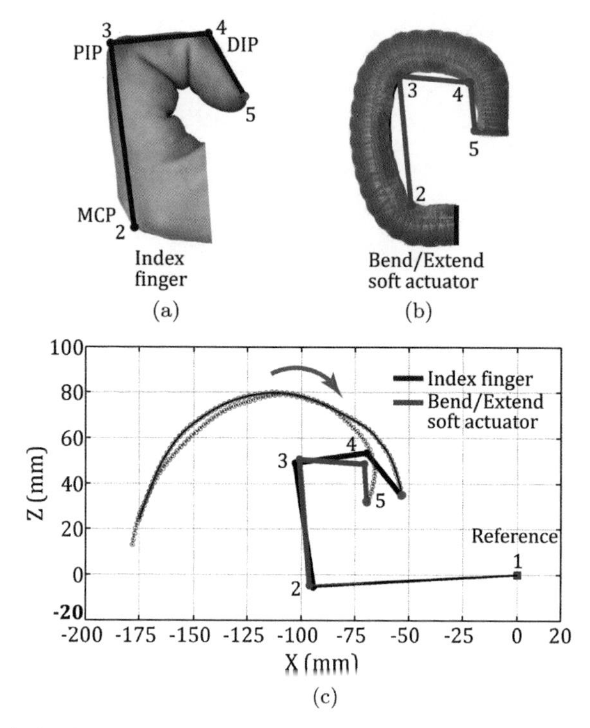

Figure 6. (a) The index finger in a flexed position and the numbered EM tracking sensor locations. (b) The pressurized state (at 345 kPa (50 psi)) of the multi-segment soft actuator designed for the index finger. The numbers represent the EM tracking sensors location. (c) Comparison between index linger motion and soft actuator as measured by EM sensors (reprinted from Ref. [26]).

Figs. 6(b)–6(c) and 7(b)–7(c). for the index finger experiment, the trajectory of the distal end (labeled number 5 in Fig. 6(c)) of the soft actuator and the biological finger follow similar paths while transitioning from fully extended to flexed. The thumb actuator operated at a lower input pressure of 275 kPa (40 psi) due to the twisting segment and produced a trajectory that matched the biological thumb (Fig. 7(c)). It should be noted that both actuator types are capable of producing motions that exceed those measured in the biomechanics studies by bending, twisting, and extending more at higher fluidic pressures. However, we found that when the actuators were integrated into the glove and constrained by the hand anatomy, they could be pressurized up to 400 kPa ($\sim$60 psi) and provide comfortable forces to the wearer.

3.4. *Integrating actuators into a glove*

The soft wearable robotic glove features an open palm concept with a modular actuator attachment method (Fig. 8(a)).[34] The actuators are housed in lightweight spandex knit with a pocket for the finger at one end and a hook pad at the other

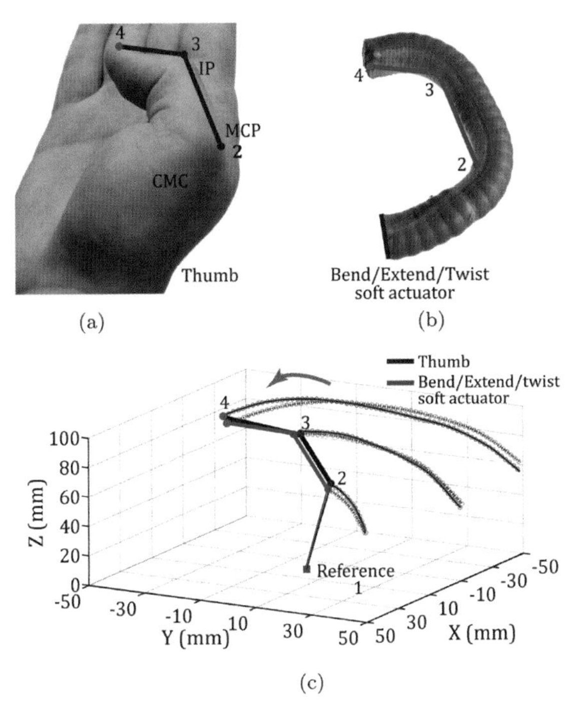

Figure 7. (a) The flexed opposition state of thumb and the numbered EM tracking sensor locations. (b) The pressurized state (at 275 kPa (40 psi)) of the multi-segment bending, extending and twisting soft actuator designed for the thumb. The numbers represent the location of the EM tracking sensors. (c) Comparison between thumb motion and soft actuators as measured by EM sensors (reprinted from Ref. [26]).

for securing to the wrist strap (Fig. 8(b)). The spandex was chosen as a method to comfortably attach the actuator to the finger without significantly impeding the range of motion of the actuator. The wrist strap serves as a ground for the soft actuators and also supports the wrist. Based on preliminary studies of individuals with impaired hands, we found a strong correlation between weak hand strength and weak wrist strength. While it is not the focus of this work, supporting wrist motion in addition to hand motion is an unmet need that has been expressed by several participants. The actuators anchor to the wrist strap via hook and loop straps rather than being permanently sewn to the wrist strap. This allows the actuators to be adjusted to a position that will hold the hand in the extended position. In this design, the pressurized actuators apply force to flex the fingers, and upon depressurization, the soft actuators behave as elastic return springs to return the fingers to the extended hand state — active flexion and passive extension (Fig. 9). Further, the hook and loop straps provide modular approach to insert and/or remove actuators that fail or are not needed. For example, depending on the impairment, the glove could be easily adjusted to support fewer than five fingers.

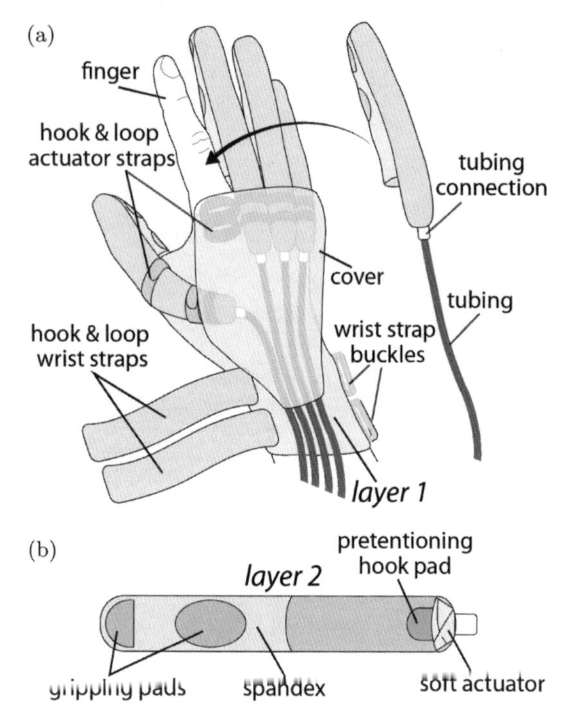

Figure 8. Schematic of the soft robotic glove outlining the textile components that couple the soft actuators to the user's hand (reprinted from Ref. [27]).

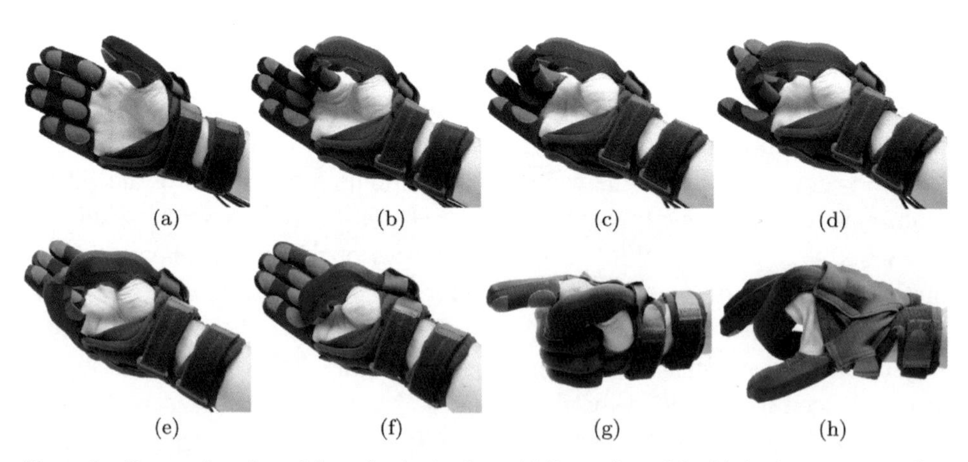

Figure 9. Range of motion of the soft robotic glove. (a) Pretension of the fabric sleeves surrounding the fiber-reinforced actuators offers full hand extension. (b)–(f) Executing the Kapandji[35] test with the soft robotic glove for thumb range of motion. (g) Finger flexion with index finger straight, (h) Index finger flexion (reprinted from Ref. [27]).

3.5. *System description*

Given the physical limitations of our intended user, we minimize the resulting distal mass of the glove by supplying power from a control unit via lightweight tubing. The prototype control box (Fig. 10) houses (a) the power components, including a lithium polymer (Li-Po) battery of 5Ah, and a wall mount power supply; (b) the electronics, including voltage regulators, PWM signal controllers for the valves, and a microcontroller (Arduino Yun, Arduino) with two embedded processors — one that facilitates wireless transmission of data regarding the glove state, and the other that computes the glove control algorithms, and (c) the hydraulics, which include fluidic pressure sensors (150PGAA5, Honeywell, Morristown, NJ) for the regulation of pressure within each finger actuator, solenoid valves (M series, Gems Sensors & Controls, Plainville, CT), a miniature diaphragm hydraulic pump (LTC series, Parker Hannifin Corp.) and a water reservoir. The onboard battery is capable of providing continuous operation for approximately 3 hours, and the voltmeter displays inform when recharging is required. The mechanical action switches on the box lid enable manual control of the glove's individual finger actuators, and a red, emergency stop button can shut down all glove functionality in the event of malfunction. Quick disconnect tube connectors located at the side of the box facilitate glove switching procedures.

3.6. *Control*

Selecting a suitable control interface is one of the most challenging aspects of developing an assistive hand device. Each user presents a different set of limitations such that no one control solution can satisfy all users. In this work, we present some of our preliminary works using surface mount EMG sensors as a method to trigger the glove to open and close. This control solution aims to work in line with the

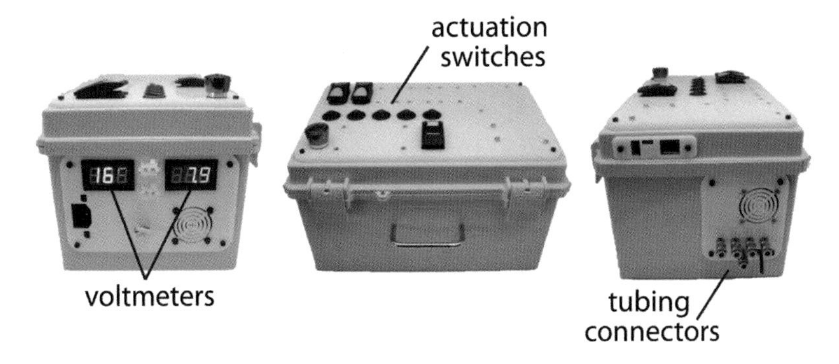

Figure 10. Views of the soft robotic glove control box (adapted from Ref. [27]).

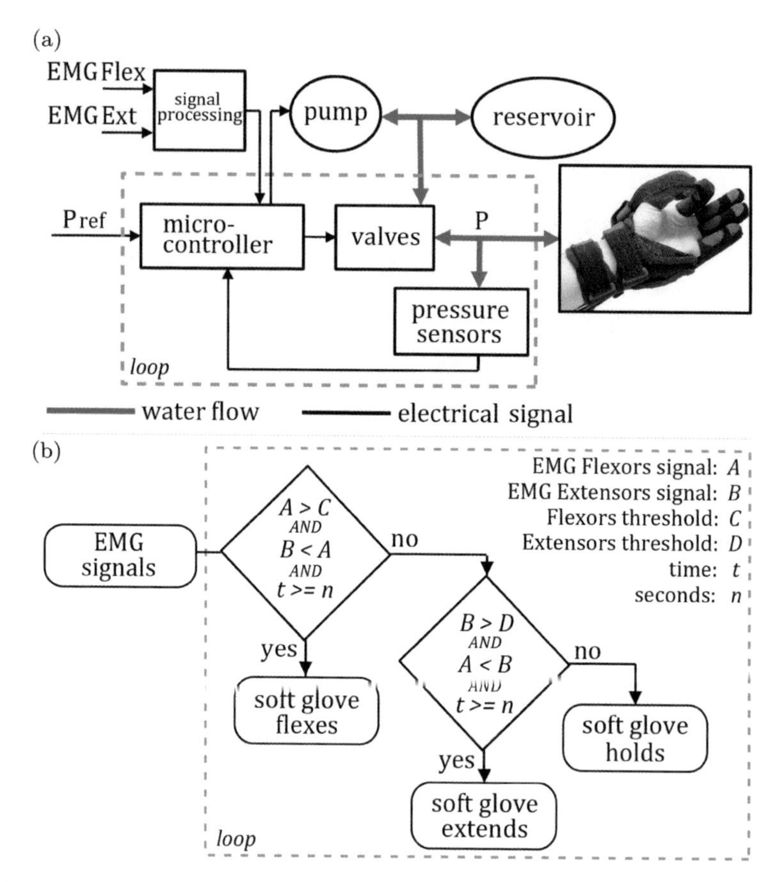

Figure 11. (a) The control scheme for the soft robotic glove. The processed sEMG signals are measured from FDS and EDC muscles and sent to the microcontroller, which regulates the pressurization level of the soft actuators and (b) flowchart of the EMG logic used to detect user intent. The state of the two sEMG signals is compared to three predefined conditions that result in the glove flexing, extending, or holding its form (reprinted from Ref. [33]).

user's biomechanics where signals from the muscles responsible for hand opening and closing are used to control the glove. The implemented control scheme for the soft robotic glove is shown in Fig. 11(a), where surface electromyography (sEMG) sensors readings are captured from two muscle groups on the forearm, amplified, filtered, and quantified. The processed information from the signals is sent to a microcontroller where it progresses through a series of conditions (EMG logic) that are responsible for the activation and deactivation of a low-level controller. In turn, the low-level controller uses pulse width modulation (PWM) to command the opening and closing of the valves and pump based on pressure measurements within the fluidic lines of the actuators.

3.7. *sEMG logic*

Hand flexion and extension can be detected by measuring the electrical activity of two muscle groups on the forearm with sEMG sensors: one electrode placed at the Flexor Digitorum Superficialis (FDS) muscle to measure gross finger flexion, and the other at the Extensor Digitorum Communis (EDC) to detect gross finger extension. The electrical signals of these two muscles are monitored and signal gains along with threshold parameters can be adjusted to initiate triggering events with minimal muscle contraction effort.

The open-loop sEMG logic hierarchy (see example flowchart in Fig. 11(b)) can control the soft robotic glove by continuously monitoring and comparing the state of the two muscle signals (FDS and EDC) to three predefined conditions: "flex", "extend", and "hold". The parameters of these conditions are set and adjusted based on initial assessments relating to the user's pathology and residual muscle activity. The "flex" condition is satisfied when the processed signal from the FDS muscle crosses over a flexor threshold for a pre-specified minimum amount of time (i.e. time-over-threshold statement), while at the same time, the EDC muscle signal is less than the FDS signal. Once this condition is met, the soft actuators are pressurized to close the glove. To trigger the glove to open or "extend", the EDC muscle signal must cross over an extensor threshold for a pre-specified duration, while at the same time exceed the magnitude of the FDS muscle signal. When this condition is met, the actuators will depressurize and passively return the fingers to the extended position. Finally, if neither the "flex" nor "extend" conditions are met, the "hold" condition is activated to maintain the fluidic pressure within the soft actuators. Any of the three glove states — flex, extend, and hold — have the ability to remain active for as long as the corresponding condition of the sEMG logic hierarchy remains true. The time-over-threshold statement within the conditions is designed to prevent involuntary muscle contractions from triggering glove assist commands.

4. Preliminary Human Subjects Testing

The soft robotic glove with EMG controls was evaluated in a preliminary user study with a healthy participant and a participant with muscular dystrophy. For the participant studies, two sEMG sensors (Myomo Inc., Boston, MA) were mounted on the forearm on the FDS and EDC muscle groups for each participant. The study was approved by the Harvard Medical School Institutional Review Board.

4.1. *Healthy participant*

4.1.1. *Grasping muscle effort*

An experiment with a healthy participant was conducted to examine the strength and stability of the glove's grip without the influence of any biological muscle effort. For this experiment, two, double differential sEMG electrode sensors (Trigno Wireless System — Delsys, Boston, MA) were placed on top of the FDS and EDC muscles to record the user's muscle activity in three sub-experiments (note this experiment is not considering glove control) (Fig. 12(a)). The first was a baseline test that measured maximum muscle effort of voluntary muscle contractions (VMC) during hand flexion and extension. The second sub-experiment required the user to perform an isometric muscle contraction to grasp, lift and hold, and then put down and release a 75 mm diameter, 500 g tin can. The user then repeated the second sub-experiment with the glove on and allowed the glove to perform the grasping motion. In all experiments, the position of the sEMG sensors on the forearm remained unchanged so that readings could be easily compared across trials.

Due to the inherent variability of EMG signals, during post-processing, the collected raw signals were full-wave rectified, filtered with a 4th order low-pass Butterworth filter with cut-off frequency of 10 Hz, and normalized against the baseline VMC. This follows the signal conditioning process suggested by the International Society of Electrophysiology and Kinesiology (ISEK) guidelines that enables physiological interpretation of EMG data.[36] For all sub-experiments, electrical muscle data were collected with a sampling rate of 2000 Hz. In Fig. 12(b), the graph on top shows the unprocessed and processed muscle activation signals of FDS muscle for the baseline test along with the normalized muscle effort (Fig. 12(b) lower graph). Figures 12(c) and 12(d) display the sEMG signals from grasping the tin can with and without assistance from the soft robotic glove, respectively. The normalized muscle effort for grasping the tin can unassisted was measured to be 12.7% of the VMC. In contrast, the normalized muscle effort with glove assistance was found to be close to zero and within the noise levels of the EMG sensor. This experiment demonstrated that the glove can grasp and hold an object while requiring minimal to no muscle effort.

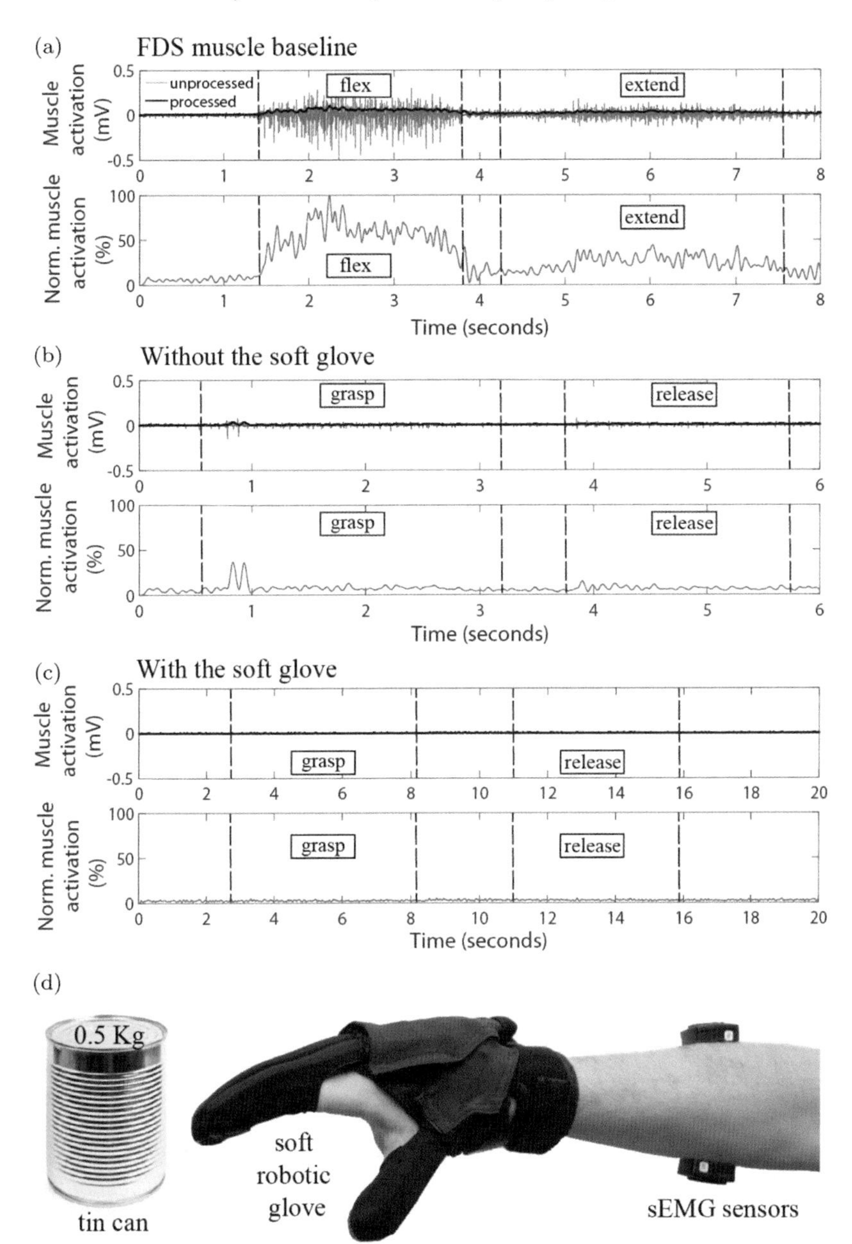

Figure 12. The unprocessed, processed, and normalized muscle activation (EMG) signals for FDS: (a) the placement of the wireless Delsys sEMG sensors on the forearm, (b) baseline test without assistance from the soft robotic glove, (c) grasping and releasing of a tin can without assistance from the soft robotic glove, and (d) grasping and releasing of a tin can with assistance from the soft robotic glove (reprinted from Ref. [33]).

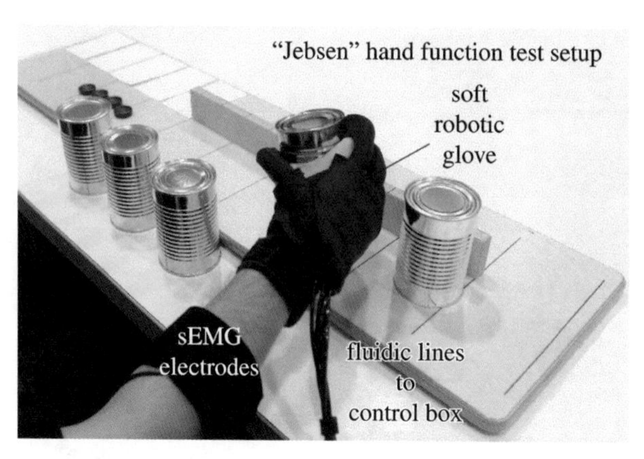

Figure 13. User performing the standardized Jebsen hand function test wearing the robotic glove that is controlled through sEMG signals read from the fingers' flexor and extensor muscles on the forearm (reprinted from Ref. [33]).

4.1.2. *Glove control*

The glove with EMG control was tested on a healthy subject to evaluate the robustness of the control logic for simple activities. Following the EMG logic discussed in Sec. 3.7, the user was able to control the state of the glove with only the activation signals from the two muscle groups. In a timed experiment, the participant was tasked with completing several of the subtests in the Jebsen hand function test (Fig. 13), namely, lifting five large, light objects (50 g tin can), lifting five large, heavy objects (500 g tin can), stacking four 1-1/4″ diameter checkers, and simulated page turning of five 3″ × 5″ index cards.[37] The participant completed the tasks in 29, 39, 26, and 44 seconds, respectively. While these times are approximately an order of magnitude slower than reported normative data for healthy individuals with no assistance, for individuals with hand impairment, the added support from the soft robotic glove could mean the difference between completing a task and not.

4.1.3. *Glove pressure distribution*

To further understand the influence of the glove on the hand's biomechanics, a simple force distribution experiment was performed. The setup comprised a 100 mm diameter acrylic tube wrapped with an ultra-thin pressure sensitive sensor film (Tekscan 5250, Tekscan Inc., Boston, MA) (Fig. 14(a)). At the start of the experiment, the participant wearing the glove relaxed all hand muscles to minimize the influence of biological hand strength. The glove was then pressurized to 413 kPa.

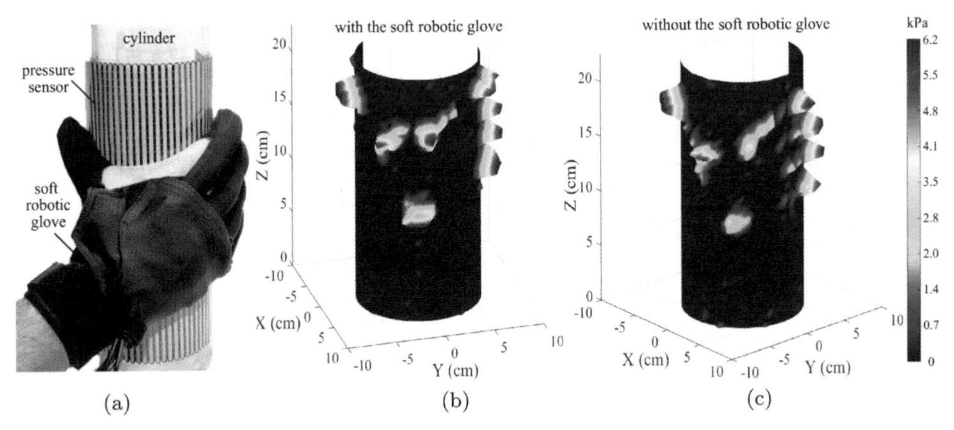

Figure 14. (a) Setup for obtaining contact pressure distribution, (b) pressure distribution on cylinder when all actuators of the soft robotic glove are pressurized, and (c) pressure distribution while the individual grasps the cylinder using his hand without the soft robotic glove (reprinted from Ref. [33]).

Figure 14(b) shows the resulting pressure distribution when all soft actuators of the glove were pressurized, and the user was not contributing to the grasp with their physical strength. The total contact force generated by the glove was 14.15 N, which was calculated by integrating the volume under the pressure distribution surface. For comparison, Fig. 14(c), presents the pressure map when the participant grasped the cylinder without the glove with a similar amount of force (approximately 14.4 N). The data from the maps show that the pressure distribution obtained using the soft robotic glove is qualitatively similar to the distribution obtained using a functional hand.

4.2. *Hand impaired participant*

A preliminary evaluation of the system was performed on a participant with muscular dystrophy. The participant demonstrated some proximal arm strength (i.e. able to lift arms), but had extremely weak hand strength with little to no spasticity or contractures. In a preliminary evaluation of the participant's sEMG signal strength, both FDS and EDC muscles were found to be sufficient (i.e. large enough amplitude) for the user to operate the soft robotic glove with the sEMG control logic described in Sec. 3.7. Figure 15(a) shows still photographs of the three glove states that include grasping, holding, and releasing a wooden block using the soft robotic glove with sEMG control. Figure 15(b) shows data collected for the two sEMG signals alongside their corresponding thresholds. The three glove conditions — flex, hold, extend — are shown in the same graph.

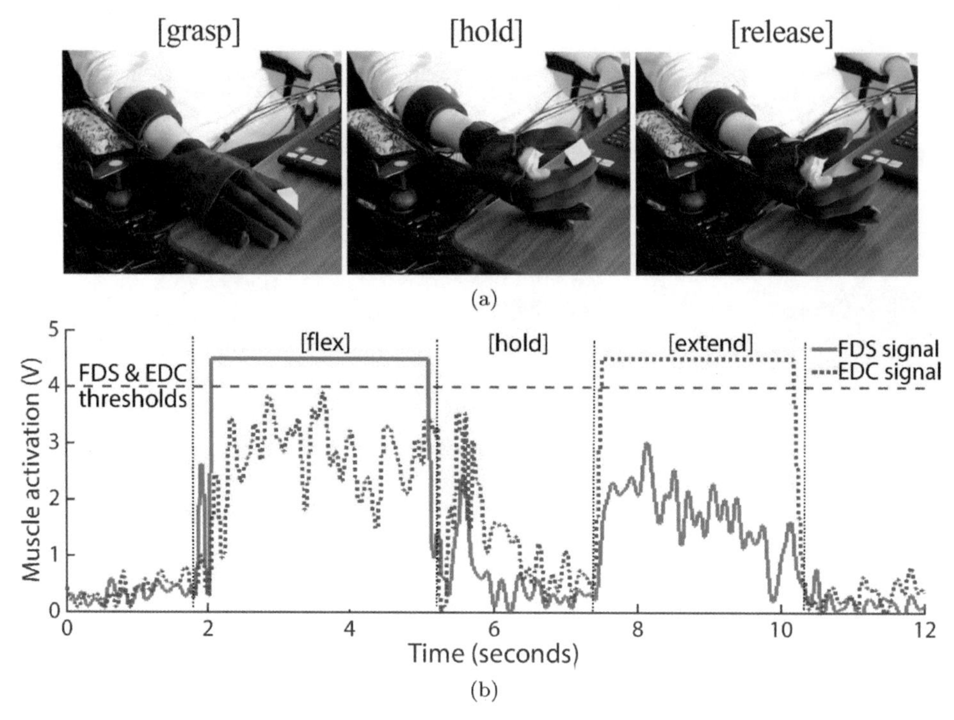

Figure 15. (a) Video stills showing a hand impaired participant grasping, holding, and releasing a wooden block using sEMG control logic with a soft robotic glove. (b) Conditioned sEMG signals and their thresholds. The graph shows how the flexor muscle triggers pressurization of the glove where flexor signal (FDS) is above the threshold and extensor muscle signal is smaller than the flexor muscle signal (left). The middle portion represents the hold condition where both muscle signals are below their thresholds. The last portion (right) illustrates how the extensor muscle can depressurize the glove and extend the hand by making the extensor signal (EDC) exceed the threshold for a short duration while keeping the flexor muscle signal less than the extensor muscle signal. Note that the saturation level for the EMG signal is 4.5 V (reprinted from Ref. [33]).

5. Discussion and Conclusion

In this chapter, a soft robotic glove is presented which is intended to combine assistance with ADL for individuals with hand disabilities. Hydraulically actuated multi-segment soft actuators were designed and fabricated using elastomers with fiber reinforcements. The soft actuators demonstrated the ability to replicate the finger and thumb motions suitable for many typical grasping motions. Furthermore, the actuators were mounted to the dorsal side of the hand, providing an open palm interface so as to not impede object interaction.

We have shown that the actuation, control, and power for such systems can be packaged in a control box that could be mounted on a wheelchair. With continued optimization, these components could also be reduced to the form factor of a waist belt suitable for ambulatory patients.

Our preliminary human subjects testing on healthy individuals demonstrated that the soft robotic glove is capable of applying sufficient force to assist with typical activities of daily living. However, its current form may not be suitable for patients with significant hand stiffness or spasticity or those who require assistance with hand extension as this is currently provided passively. Thus, the glove in its current form is most likely suitable for patients with muscular dystrophy, incomplete SCI or ALS where the hand is still flaccid. Going forward, we plan to refine the design of the actuators and will seek to reduce their form factor and increase the force-generating capacity. This will make the glove more suitable for a wider variety of individuals with upper extremity impairments. Additionally, the robustness and life cycle of the multi-segment soft actuators will be investigated during fatigue tests.

The soft wearable system presented here has the potential to provide increased freedom and independence for individuals with functional grasp pathologies and reduce care costs. For example, as an assistive device, it can facilitate grasping in ADLs such as eating and grooming, and making therapy part of a daily home program. The concept of combined rehabilitation and physical assistance necessitates wearable robotic systems which can be worn at home for extended periods to provide assistance with ADLs. Such devices could also incorporate sensors that measure the state of the user's limb and estimate the activities that they are performing. This information can be relayed to a therapist for remote monitoring and provides the opportunity for applying continuous rehabilitation tailored to the user's capabilities and lifestyle. Such an approach to rehabilitation also promises to increase motivation. Assistance with ADLs will increase compliance with exercise regimens, and quantified performance metrics will communicate progress to the user. Furthermore, combining therapy and assistive functionality into a wearable system promises to reduce costs and improve outcomes. Present occupational and physical therapy is inherently expensive and such a system suitable for home use can increase the dose of therapy for patients and increase the impact and productivity of therapists.

Acknowledgments

Kevin C. Galloway and Panagiotis Polygerinos have contributed equally to this chapter. This work is partially supported by the National Science Foundation (Grant Nos.: 1317744, 1454472), DARPA (Award No.: W911NF-11-1-0094), and the Wyss Institute for Biologically Inspired Engineering and the School of Engineering and Applied Sciences at Harvard University. We would like to thank Zheng Wang, Siddharth Sanan, Maxwell Herman, Kathleen O'Donnell, and Zivthan Dubrovsky for their advice and contributions.

References

1. M. H. P. Janssen, *et al.* (2014). Erratum to: Patterns of decline in upper limb function of boys and men with DMD: an international survey, *Journal of Neurology* 261(7):1289–1290.
2. R. P. Erhardt. (1994). Developmental hand dysfunction: theory, assessment, and treatment 2nd edn. *Therapy Skill Builders* 235.
3. J. Liepert, *et al.* (2000). Treatment-induced cortical reorganization after stroke in humans, *Stroke* 31(6):1210–1216.
4. H. Krebs, *et al.* (1998). Robot-aided neurorehabilitation, *IEEE Transactions on Rehabilitation Engineering* 6(1):75–87.
5. P. Heo, *et al.* (2012). Current hand exoskeleton technologies for rehabilitation and assistive engineering, *International Journal of Precision Engineering and Manufacturing* 13(5):807–824.
6. P. Maciejasz, *et al.* (2014). A survey on robotic devices for upper limb rehabilitation, *Journal of NeuroEngineering and Rehabilitation* 11(1):3.
7. P. M. Aubin, H. Sallum, C. Walsh, L. Stirling and A. Correia. (2013). A pediatric robotic thumb exoskeleton for at-home rehabilitation: The Isolated Orthosis for Thumb Actuation (IOTA), *2013 IEEE 13th International Conference on Rehabilitation Robotics (ICORR)*, Seattle, WA, pp. 1–6.
8. A. Chiri, *et al.* (2012). Mechatronic design and characterization of the index finger module of a hand exoskeleton for post-stroke rehabilitation. Mechatronics, *IEEE/ASME Transactions* 17(5):884–894.
9. L. Dovat, *et al.* (2008). HandCARE: a cable-actuated rehabilitation system to train hand function after stroke. *IEEE Transactions on Neural Systems and Rehabilitation Engineering* 16(6):582–591.
10. S. B. Godfrey, *et al.* (2013). A synergy-driven approach to a myoelectric hand, in *IEEE International Conference on Rehabilitation Robotics* (*ICORR*) 1–6.
11. Y. Hong Kai, *et al.* (2015). A soft exoskeleton for hand assistive and rehabilitation application using pneumatic actuators with variable stiffness, in *IEEE International Conference on Robotics and Automation (ICRA)* 4967–4972.
12. I. Hyunki, *et al.* (2015). Exo-Glove: A wearable robot for the hand with a soft tendon routing system, *Robotics & Automation Magazine*, IEEE, 22(1):97–105.
13. Y. Kadowaki, *et al.* (2011). Development of soft power-assist glove and control based on human intent, *Journal of Robotic Mechatronics* 23(2):281.
14. K. Tadano, *et al.* (2010). Development of grip amplified glove using bi-articular mechanism with pneumatic artificial rubber muscle, *IEEE International Conference on Robotics and Automation (ICRA)* 2363–2368.
15. P. Polygerinos, S. Lyne, Z. Wang, B. Mosadegh, G. Whitesides and C. Walsh (2013). Towards a Soft Pneumatic Glove for Hand Rehabilitation, in *Proc. Inter. Conf. on Intelligent Robots and Systems*, Tokyo, pp. 1512–1517.
16. F. Vanoglio, *et al.* (2013). Evaluation of the effectiveness of Gloreha (Hand Rehabilitation Glove) on hemiplegic patients. Pilot study, *XIII Congress of Italian Society of Neurorehabilitation* 18–20.
17. I. Gaiser, *et al.* editor (2012). Compliant robotics and automation with flexible fluidic actuators and inflatable structures, *Smart Actuation and Sensing Systems — Recent Advances and Future Challenges* Ed. D. G. Berselli. 2012, INTECH. 22.
18. G. K. Klute, J. M. Czerniecki and B. Hannaford. (1999). McKibben artificial muscles: pneumatic actuators with biomechanical intelligence, *1999 IEEE/ASME International Conference on Advanced Intelligent Mechatronics (Cat. No. 99TH8399)*, Atlanta, GA, USA, pp. 221–226.
19. K. Suzumori. (1996). Elastic materials producing compliant robots, *Robotics and Autonomous Systems* 18(1–2):135–140.

20. J. Bishop-Moser and S. Kota. (2015). Design and modeling of generalized fiber-reinforced pneumatic soft actuators, in *IEEE Transactions on Robotics* 31(3):536–545.
21. J. Bishop-Moser, *et al.* (2012). Design of soft robotic actuators using fluid-filled fiber-reinforced elastomeric enclosures in parallel combinations, *2012 IEEE/RSI International Conference on Intelligent Robots and Systems*, Vilamoura, pp. 4264–4269.
22. F. Connolly, *et al.* (2015). Mechanical Programming of Soft Actuators by Varying Fiber Angle, *Soft Robotics* 2(1):26–32.
23. P. Maeder-York, *et al.* (2014). Biologically Inspired Soft Robot for Thumb Rehabilitation, *Journal of Medical Devices* 8(2):020933–020933.
24. K. C. Galloway, P. Polygerinos, C. J. Walsh and R. J. Wood. (2013). Mechanically programmable bend radius for fiber-reinforced soft actuators. *2013 16th International Conference on Advanced Robotics (ICAR)*, Montevideo, pp. 1–6.
25. P. Polygerinos, Wang, Z., Overvelde J. T. B., Galloway, K. C., Wood, R. J., Bertoldi, K., Walsh, C. J. (2015). Modeling of Soft Fiber-reinforced Bending Actuators, *IEEE Transactions on Robotics* 31(3):778–789.
26. D. Sasaki, *et al.* (2004). Wearable power assist device for hand grasping using pneumatic artificial rubber muscle, *13th International Workshop on Robot and Human Interactive Communication*, IEEE 655–660.
27. P. Polygerinos, Z. Wang, K. C. Galloway, R. J. Wood and C. J. Walsh (2015). Soft robotic glove for combined assistance and at-home rehabilitation, *Robotics and Autonomous Systems (RAS) Special Issue on Wearable Robotics* 73:135–143.
28. P. Polygerinos, Galloway, K., Savage, E. A., Herman, M., O'Donnell, K., Walsh, C. (2015). Soft Robotic Glove for Hand Rehabilitation and Task Specific Training, *Proc. Inter. Conf. on Robotics and Automation*, Seattle, Washington, USA.
29. R. Loureiro and W. Harwin. (2007). Reach & Grasp Therapy: Design and Control of a 9-DOF Robotic Neuro-rehabilitation System. *Proceedings of the IEEE 10th International Conference on Rehabilitation Robotics (ICORR)* 757–763.
30. P. Seidenberg and A. Beutler. (2008). *The Sports Medicine Resource Manual*. Elsevier.
31. I. N. Gaiser, *et al.* (2009). The FLUIDHAND III: A Multifunctional Prosthetic Hand. *Journal of Prosthetics and Orthotics* 21(2):91–96.
32. V. Mathiowetz, *et al.* (1985). Grip and pinch strength: normative data for adults. *Archives of Physical and Medical Rehabilitation* 66(2):69–74.
33. K. Matheus and A. M. Dollar. (2010). Benchmarking grasping and manipulation: Properties of the Objects of Daily Living, *2010 IEEE/RSJ International Conference on Intelligent Robots and Systems* 5020–5027.
34. P. Polygerinos, K. C. Galloway, S. Sanan, M. Herman and C. J. Walsh. (2015). EMG controlled soft robotic glove for assistance during activities of daily living, *2015 IEEE International Conference on Rehabilitation Robotics* (*ICORR*), Singapore, pp. 55–60.
35. A. Kapandji, (1986). Cotation clinique de l'opposition et de la contre-opposition du pouce. 5(1):67–73.
36. R. Merletti, (1999). Standards for Reporting EMG data. *Journal of Electromyography and Kinesiology* 9(1):III–IV.
37. R. Jebsen, *et al.* (1969). Journal of Electromyography and Kinesiology, *Archives of Physical Medical Rehabiliation* 50(6):311–319.

Chapter 7

REHABILITATION ROBOTICS: WEARABLE SYSTEMS

Changsoo Han

Hanyang University, Department of Robot Engineering, Engineering Building V, 55, Hanyangdaehak-ro, Sangnok-gu, Ansan-si, Gyeonggi-do, Republic of Korea

Since the wearable system is intended to be worn and manipulated by humans, the system provides intuitive motions that supplement and enhance the limited, insufficient, lost or absent human physical functions. With more advances in autonomous robotic technology, the wearable system has been well applied in the rehabilitation area, and it is about to open a new era where many disabled people can function as able ones. Several wearable systems are presented in this chapter. The types of the system include upper body wearable system, lower limb wearable system, ankle rehabilitation system, treadmill gait training system, physical assistive system and soft robotic system. The purpose of this chapter is to present the state-of-the-art wearable systems of rehabilitation, so as to provide a potentiality that the readers can utilize this knowledge and may even apply it for further development.

1. Upper Body Wearable System

1.1. *ARMin*

ARMin is an upper limb wearable robot to assist, enhance, evaluate, and document neurological and orthopedic rehabilitation. For people with upper limb paralysis, it is possible to consider therapies where intelligent assistance from a robot is able to provide varying degrees of compensatory movements for the affected limb. The devices provide a varying degree of assistance to patient's active movements with no assistance to full assistance where the patient behaves passively.

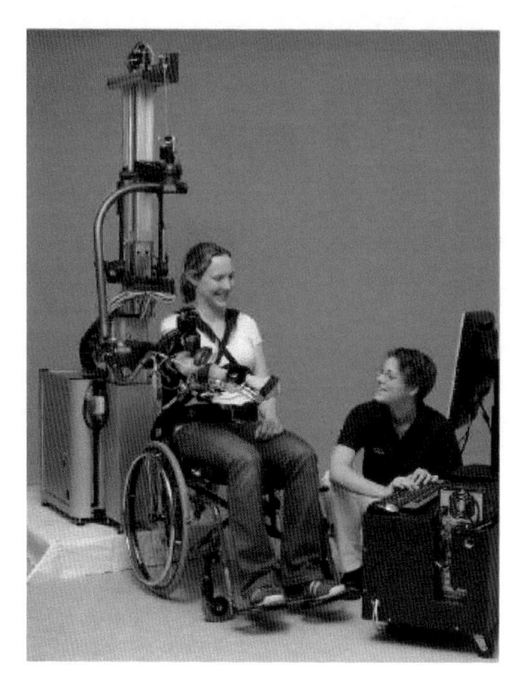

Figure 1. ARMin-II.[3]

The second version of ARMin and ARMin-II is shown in Fig. 1. The patient sits in a wheelchair beneath the robot. Her torso is attached to the wheelchair with straps and bands. The end-effector-based mechanics enable actuation of two degrees of freedom of the shoulder joint, namely, arm elevation (flexion–extension in the sagittal plane, abduction–adduction in the frontal plane) using a vertically oriented linear drive actuator and arm horizontal flexion–extension using an ordinary rotary actuator. The exoskeletal mechanics actuate the upper arm internal–external rotation, elbow flexion–extension, forearm pronation–supination, and wrist flexion–extension.[3] Due to the limited functional importance of the wrist ulnar–radial deviation, this joint is constrained in a neutral position in order to reduce the complexity of the device. Fingers are not obstructed by the mechanics of the forearm exoskeleton.

ARMin III shown in Fig. 2 is the third version of the ARMin series. It is equipped with six motors moving the shoulder joint in 3-DOF, the elbow joint, lower-arm pronation supination and wrist flexion–extension.[4] The mechanics are symmetric and the robot can be used for the right or the left arm. Advanced control algorithms allow controlling not only the position of the device but also the interacting force between the robot and the patient.

Along with the hardware improvements, ARMin utilizes a game therapy mode. In the game therapy mode, a game-like scenario is presented to the patient.

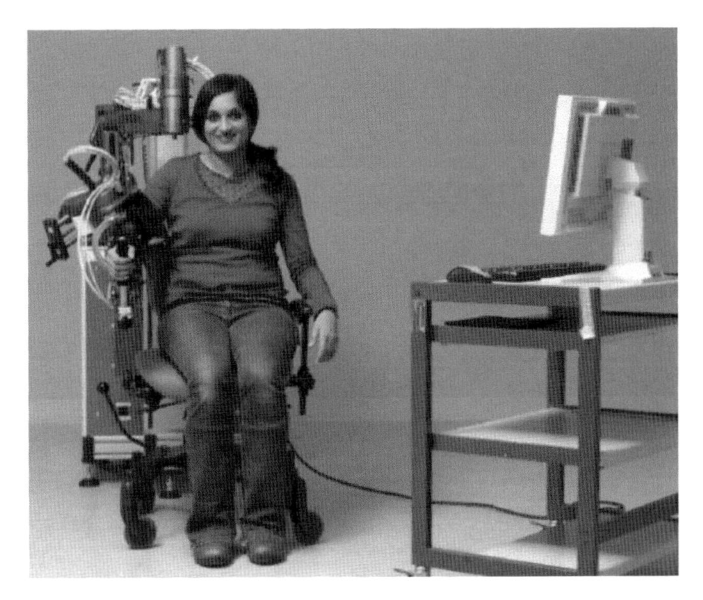

Figure 2. ARMin-III.[4]

The patient tries to fulfill the task while he is supported by the robot. The device detects how much the patient contributes to the movement and delivers support as much as needed.

The ARMin series is now provided by a company called Hocoma, which is the global market leader for the development, manufacturing, and marketing of robotic and sensor-based devices for functional movement therapy. The Swiss-based medical technology company made ARMEO THERAPY CONCEPT(ArmeoPower, ArmeoSpring, ArmeoBoom) with ARMin exoskeleton rehabilitation robot. This ARMEO series provides rehabilitation training for people with upper limb paralysis and scientific results show that robotic training with the ARMEO reduced motor impairment faster and more effectively than the conventional therapy after stroke.

1.2. *Kiguchi robot*

Kazuo Kiguchi research team has been developing exoskeleton robots in order to assist the motion of physically weak persons such as elderly persons or handicapped persons.

In 2003, they developed an exoskeletal robot to assist the motion of a shoulder. The exoskeletal robot consists of a frame, two main links, an arm holder, two DC motor drive wires, wire tension sensors, and the mechanism of the moving center of rotation (CR) of the shoulder joint.[5] The exoskeleton robot worn by a human subject is supposed to assist the subject's shoulder joint motion by manipulating the subject's upper arm with the arm holder.

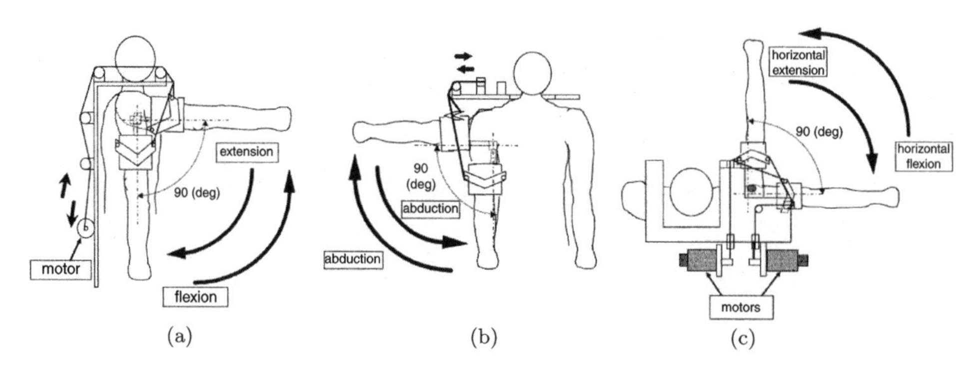

Figure 3. Assisted shoulder joint motion.[5]

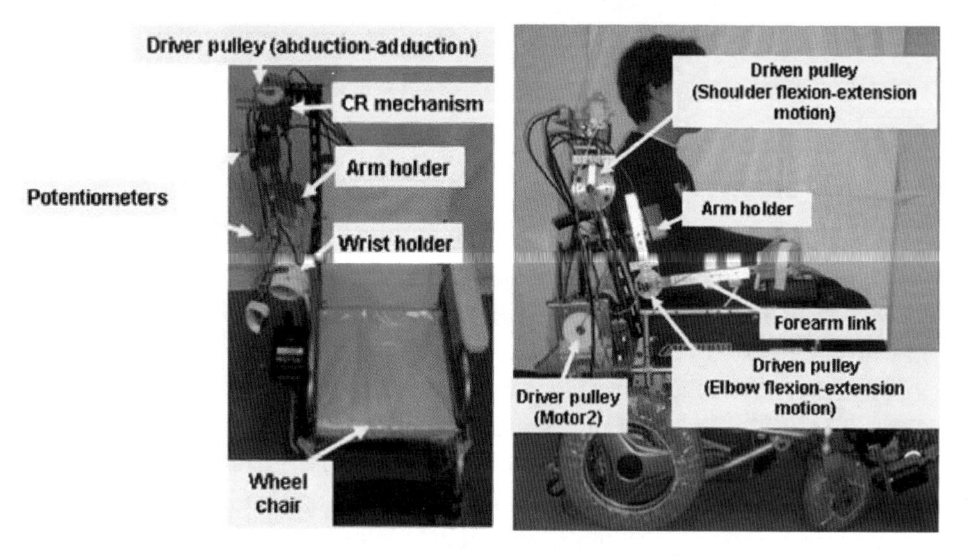

Figure 4. Assisted shoulder joint motion.[6]

The robot in Fig. 3 uses EMG signals that describe the muscle activity level. By adjusting the amount of force generated by the shoulder muscles based on the EMG signals, the shoulder motion can be moderately controlled.

The upper limb exoskeleton robot system, shown in Fig. 4, has been developed to assist rehabilitation and daily activities of physically weak persons. The redesigned exoskeleton robot mainly consists of a shoulder motion support part, an elbow motion support part, a wrist force sensor, and a mobile wheelchair.[6]

In 2010, they used task-oriented perception-assist, which is described in Fig. 5. In order to identify the tool used by the user in the task, they used the stereo camera. After the tool was identified, the task carried out by the user was estimated based on the identified tool. Then the suitable motion for the candidate's estimated task can be predicted by the exoskeleton robot.[7]

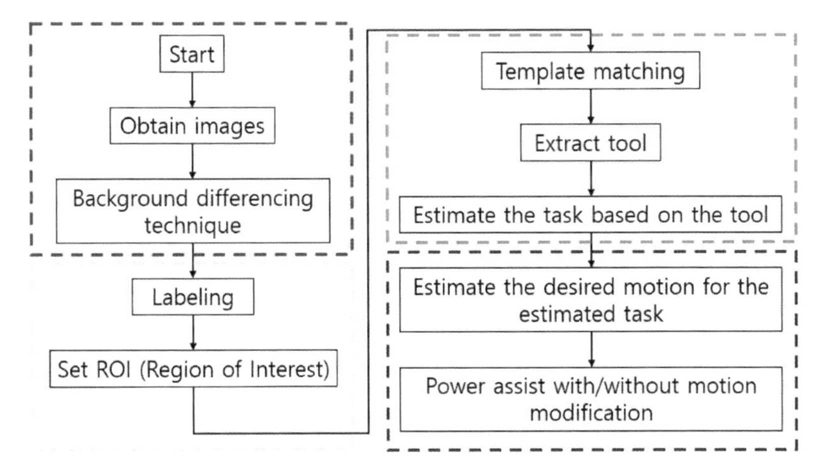

Figure 5. Flowchart of task-oriented perception-assist.[7]

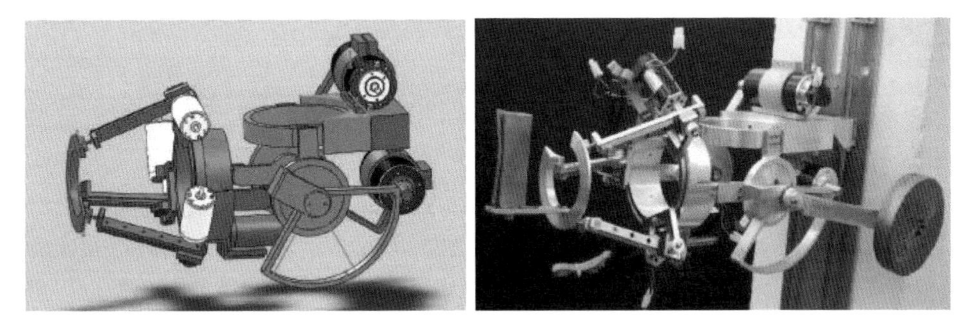

Figure 6. MAHI Exo-2 Elbow, forearm wrist exoskeleton for stroke and spinal cord injury (SCI) rehabilitation.[8]

1.3. *MAHI EXO*

The MAHI (Mechatronics and Haptic Interfaces) Lab focuses on the design, manufacture, and evaluation of mechatronic or robotic systems to model, rehabilitate, enhance or augment the human sensorimotor control system.[9] The basic kinematic structure of the 5-DOF MAHI exoskeleton is depicted in Fig. 6. The exoskeleton comprises a revolute joint at the elbow, a revolute joint for forearm rotation, and a 3-RPS(revolute-prismatic-spherical) serial in parallel wrist. MAHI EXO-1 has a frameless and brushless DC motor with encoder and is used to drive the forearm joint. In the new design of MAHI EXO-2, a high torque DC motor with cable drive mechanism is implemented.

In comparison with other rehabilitation robots, MAHI EXO-2 poses several advantages. First, the parallel design of the wrist provides increased rigidity and torque output, decreased inertia and isometric force distribution throughout the workspace, as compared to a serial configuration. Also, the alignment of the biomechanical axes of joint rotation with the controlled DOF of the RiceWrist makes it possible to constrain the movement of desired joints.[8]

1.4. *Intelliarm*

Biodynamics Lab at the Rehabilitation Institute of Chicago studied the neurological impairments and sports-related injuries, and developed state-of-the-art rehabilitation robotics. Arm impairments in stroke survivors involve the shoulder, elbow, and wrist simultaneously with abnormal coupling between the joints and the muscles acting at each joint. The intelligent rehabilitation robot controls the shoulder, elbow, and wrist individually and allows natural trunk and scapular motions. It has unique capacities for diagnosis, multi-joint stretching, voluntary movement training, and outcome evaluation.

Intelliarm has four active DOFs and two passive DOFs at the shoulder, 2-DOFs at the elbow, 1-DOF at the wrist, and 1-DOF at the finger. Intelliarm designs the hand part with four-bar linkage for hand grasping motion (see Fig. 7).

1.5. *Carex*

Sunil Kumar Agrawal and Ying Mao in the Robotics and Rehabilitation Lab (ROAR LAB) are focused on developing new and innovative technologies to improve the quality of care and patient outcomes.

CAREX is a light-weight exoskeleton designs for the upper arm, in which rigid links of the exoskeleton are replaced by lightweight cuffs attached to the moving limb segments of the human arm. Cables, driven by motors, are routed through these cuffs to move the limb segment. Because of this structure, it is nearly an order of magnitude lighter than the conventional exoskeletons. This upper arm exoskeleton that is mounted on a 5-DOF arm is shown in Fig. 8. The 5-DOFs of the anthropomorphic arm consist of three at the shoulder joint, flexion, and extension at the elbow joint, and pronation and supination of the forearm.[13,15]

CAREX makes it possible to allow agile arm motions with the weight of the exoskeleton at merely 1.55 kg.

1.6. *WREX*

The Wilmington Robotic Exoskeleton (WREX) is a powered, gravity-balanced upper limb orthosis for children with muscular weakness present in conditions such as muscular dystrophy and spinal muscular atrophy (see Fig. 9). The WREX has

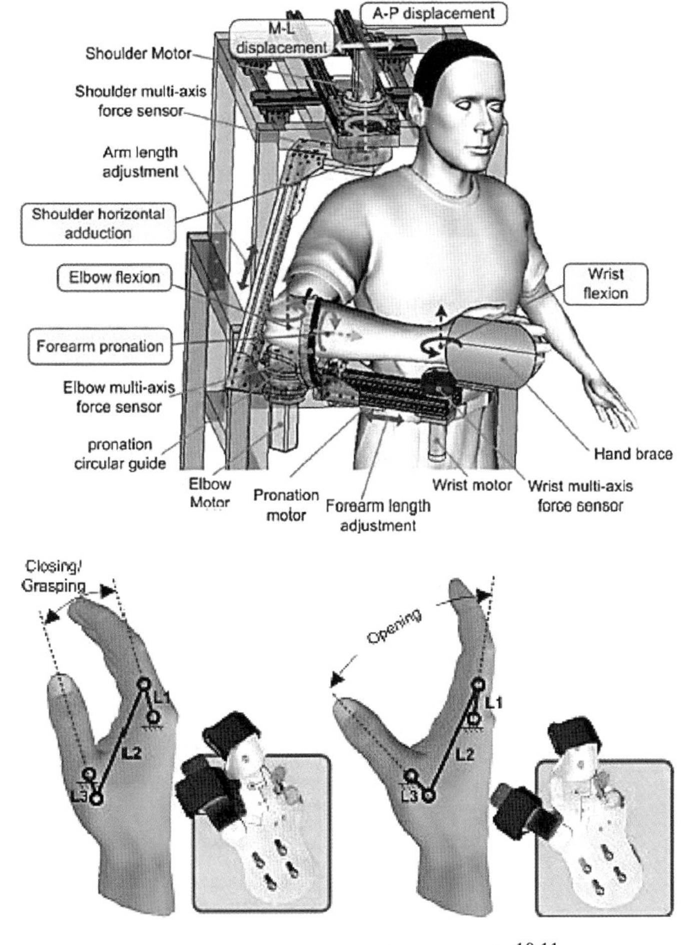

Figure 7. Intelliarm and finger module.[10,11]

4-DOF to allow full range of motion and is assisted by gravity-balancing elastic bands. In addition, the WREX is powered at the shoulder and elbow joint against gravity, to provide user-directed assistance similar to power steering. A force sensor at the forearm picks up the user's intention, which is sent to the motors to provide assistance. The WREX can be attached to a wheelchair or to a body jacket.

1.7. *HEXAR UR/KR series*

HEXAR, which stands for Hanyang EXoskeletal Assistive Robot, is a start-up business company in CnR-LAB at Hanyang University. The CnR-LAB started the research on the human–robot cooperation system in 2006. Then in 2011, HEXAR, the venture company, appeared as a spin-off of the exoskeleton technology. The company develops wearable robots for industry/military use and for elderly and

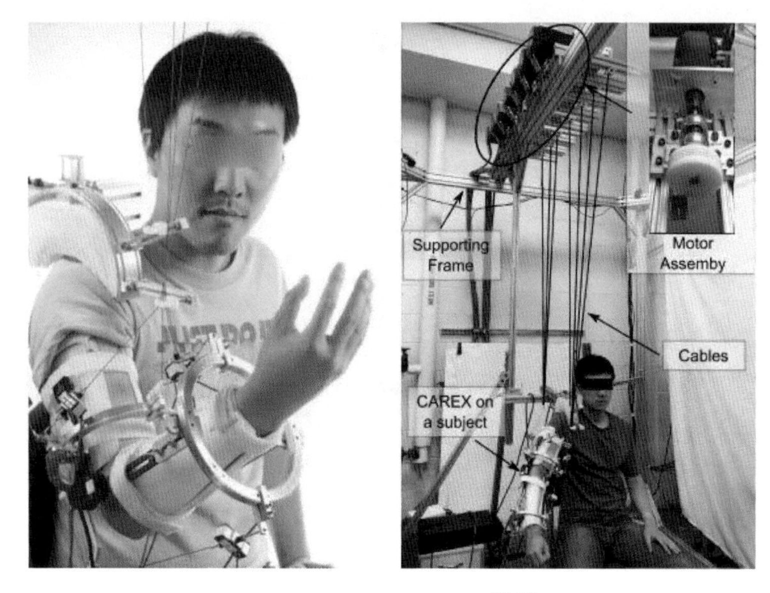

Figure 8. CAREX robot.[13,14]

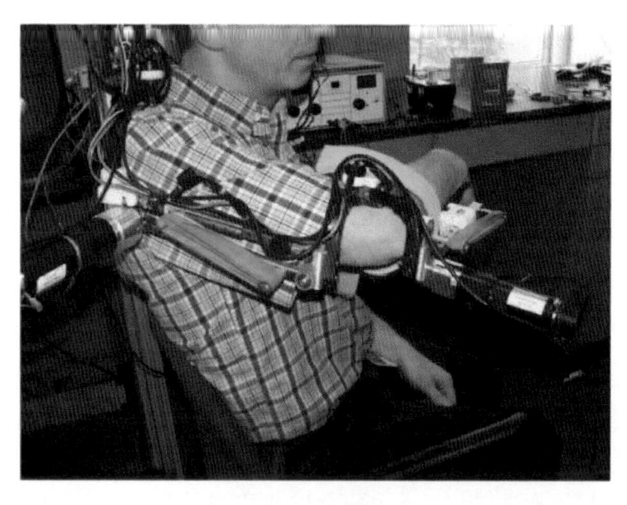

Figure 9. WREX.[14]

disabled people. The area of development on the robots for elderly/disabled people includes continuous passive motion (CPM) system, continuous active motion (CAM) system, overground gait training exoskeleton for hemiplegic and paraplegic patients.

Knee-CPM, KR-20, was the first application of the rehabilitation of the musculoskeletal system (see Fig. 10). The development of the robot for shoulder and elbow joints came after KR-20. In particular, the shoulder CPM is organized

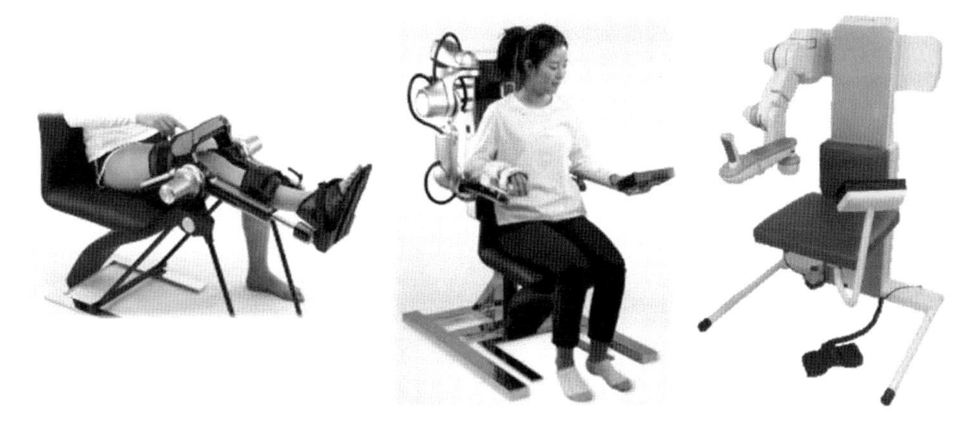

Figure 10. Hexar KR-20, UR-10, UR-20.

with multiple joints for the user's maneuverable convenience and it is designed to easily change the pose and right/left configuration. A clinical study of rehabilitation of knee joint using KR-20 was conducted for 105 patients.[16] The study showed that after using KR-20, the range of motion of knee joint and lower limb muscular power of patients improved as well as other statistically significant results on the timed-up-and-go test and short physical performance battery test.

For the gait rehabilitation, a lower limb powered exoskeleton is developed to provide the rehabilitative training for both hemiplegic and paraplegic patients by applying different algorithms of corresponding patient's condition.

Currently, the researches such as on upper limb muscular power assisting robot, and a robot for the rehabilitation of upper limb neural network are in progress.[17–19]

2. Lower Limb Wearable System

2.1. *Ekso*

Ekso is a lower limb wearable robot for patients with complete SCI, developed by Ekso Bionics (see Fig. 11).[22] It allows the paraplegic patient to sit, stand up and walk over the ground. Since the official announcement on the development of eLEGs in 2009, which was the earlier version of Ekso, Ekso Bionics has been continuously improving its robot hardware and software. The company has also been conducting clinical tests to verify the robot's feasibility and safety.

Dr. Homayoon Kazerooni is the key developer at Ekso. Back in 1990s, Dr. Homayoon Kazerooni, who was a professor in Mechanical Engineering Department at the University of California, Berkeley, was developing a powered exoskeleton that could allow a wearer to carry heavy equipments without feeling the load weight.[23] The efforts of Kazerooni and his team led to the development of

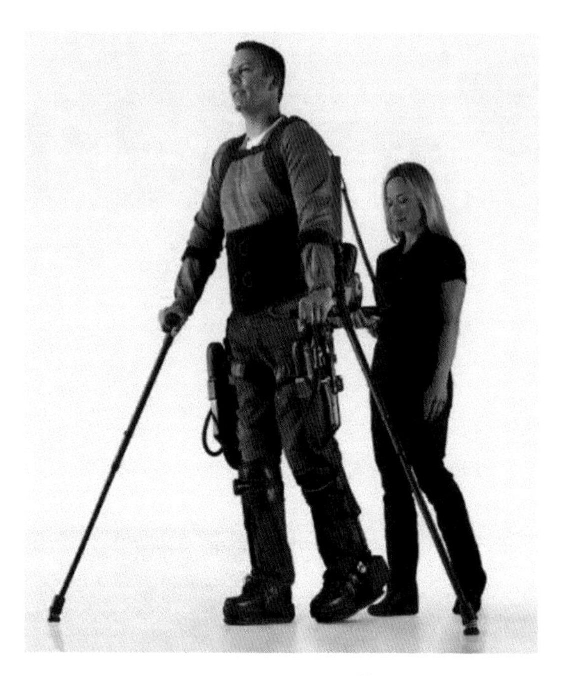

Figure 11. Ekso.[20]

the powered exoskeleton called Berkeley Lower Extremity Exoskeleton (BLEEX), the first functional load-carrying and energetically autonomous exoskeleton.[24] The development of BLEEX later led to HULC in 2008 which stands for Human Universal Load Carrier.

The development of Ekso was initiated by Berkeley ExoWorks, founded in 2005, by Homayoon Kazerooni, Russ Angold, and Nathan Harding.[25] The founders originally belonged to the Berkeley Robotics and Human Engineering Laboratory at the University of California. After the formation of the campany, ExoWorks developed ExoHiker and ExoClimber, exoskeletons that could allow users to carry heavy objects while the users are in motion.

In 2007, the company changed its name from Berkeley ExoWorks to Berkeley Bionics. The company licensed HULC™ to the Lockheed Martin Corporation in 2009 for further research and development for military use. In 2010, the company developed eLEGs (see Fig. 12). This exoskeleton was the father of Ekso that could allow the paraplegic patients to stand up from the wheel chair and walk. With one more change of company name from Berkeley Bionics to Ekso Bionics in 2011, it finally developed Ekso in 2012, the first commercialized robotic exoskeleton for use in rehabilitation and medical facilities.

Ekso weighs about 20 kg and can speed up to 3.2 km/h. Its battery lasts 6 hours. The pilot requirements include 220 pounds of weight, height between 5 ft 2 in and

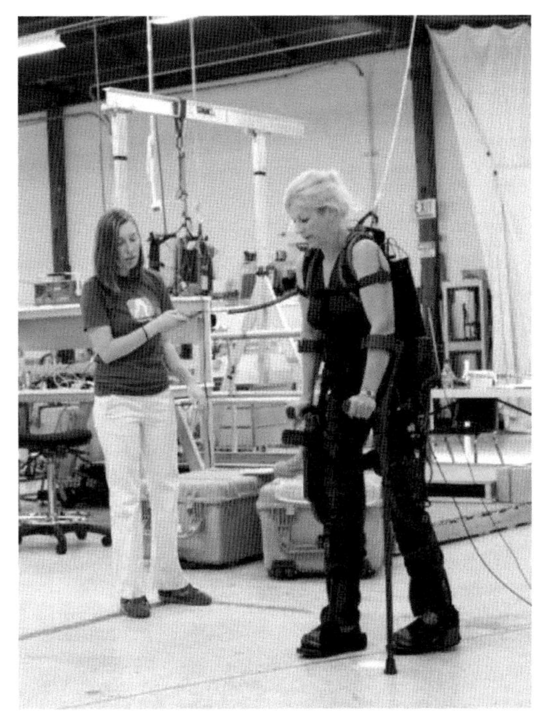

Figure 12. eLEGs.[21]

6 ft 4, an enough upper body strength to transfer themselves from a wheelchair to a chair. With ground reaction force sensors on the crutches, the robot can figure out its walking state automatically, such as swing-phase and standing, and it provides appropriate motion to the user. One study showed that this automatic system provides better ambulation and reduces human effort while operating the robot.[26]

In the medical area, the Ekso has been tested for the rehabilitation of individuals with SCI.[27–29] One study was based on the research conducted at the Santa Clara Valley Medical Center in San Jose, CA, USA.[27] The purpose of this study was to evaluate the feasibility and safety of Ekso to aid ambulation in individuals with SCI. To do so, eight individuals with complete T1 SCI or below underwent 6 weekly sessions with graduated time and less assistance in the Ekso device. During the sessions, parameters such as blood pressure, pain level, or spasticity to quantify the feasibility and safety were measured. The result showed that no major skin effects, minimal pain reports, no known fractures, swelling, or other adverse events occurred. Level of assistance ranged from dependent to moderately independent, the average set up time was 18.13 minutes, and the loss of balance and falls were infrequent. The study concluded that bionic exoskeletons such as Ekso were safe and could enhance the mobility of the patients having disorders in lower extremity functions.

2.2. *Rewalk*

Rewalk (Fig. 13) is a commercial bionic powered exoskeleton walking robot that enables paraplegic patients to sit up, walk, and ascend/descend stairs. It is by far the only exoskeleton that received U.S. Food and Drug Administration clearance.[31] Rewalk Bionics, Inc. (originally Argo Medical Technologies) is the company that has developed the robot. Rewalk has two computer-controlled bilateral hip and knee joint motors with on-board computerized control system and contains rechargeable batteries to allow the users to use Rewalk for an extended period of time.[32] To perceive the human intention, Rewalk uses two kinds of sensors. One is a ground force sensor. The other is a tilt sensor that senses the gravitational shift of the user.[33] Currently, Rewalk is used in several medical areas including Rewalk Robotics's own training centers.

Dr. Amit Goffer developed Rewalk. It is not clear when the development of Rewalk began. However, the exoskeleton revealed its technology on the media. The first showcase was a prototype Rewalk on the American TV series Glee. Then on 8 May 2012, a paralyzed athlete Claire Lomas finished the London Marathon while wearing Rewalk.[34] She was recorded to be the first person to complete the marathon using a bionic suit. Today, a number of medical centers are importing Rewalk as a gait training device for the paraplegic patients.

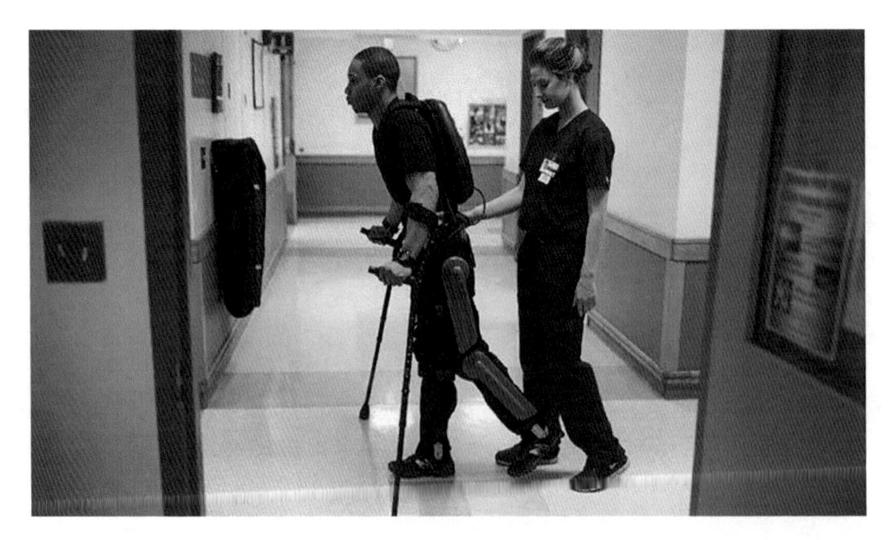

Figure 13. Rewalk.[30]

With more advances in development and marketing, Rewalk Robotics provides two types of Rewalk, Rewalk Rehabilitation and Rewalk Personal 6.0.[35] Although the technology has grown to be suitable in practical use, the cost of Rewalk is still an obstacle when an individual tries to buy such a device. The cost of Rewalk is estimated to be $69,500 and health insurance in the U.S. does not cover the robot.[36] Thus, it requires some financial challenges if someone wants to operate Rewalk at his or her home.

The Rewalk system contains rechargeable batteries and on-board Windows-operated computer.[37] The Rewalk system weighs about 46 pounds (21 kg) and its battery is designed to last a full day of intermittent walking. However, if the user walks continuously, the system will last for about three to four hours.

A wrist device that has physical buttons allows the user to choose one of the three modes of exoskeleton: standing, sitting, and walking. Once the button is pushed, the wrist device sends a signal to the control system and the system engages proper motions. In the walking mode, the user does not have to trigger each step since the robot uses tilt sensors to detect the center of gravity of the user and initiate preset walking pattern.

The Rewalk has a unique feature that no other exoskeleton possesses.[33] It is a wearable airbag. This airbag is intended to be engaged when either the user alerts or the robot senses a fall. Accelerometers with control units are equipped in the backpack.

Rewalk has been adopted in the medical area for the rehabilitation of paraplegic patients. Although the Rewalk has gained US FDA clearance for medical use, it seems the scientific data to support the validity of utilization of such powered exoskeleton is not sufficiently proved. Therefore, like other lower limb exoskeletons such as HAL and Ekso, the Rewalk has been on clinical tests to evaluate the feasibility and safety of the device. So far, it is reported that the use of Rewalk is not risky in the controlled environment, and any adverse events occur infrequently. Still, more data concerning the effectiveness of using exoskeleton for the rehabilitation of paraplegic patients is required. Once it is clearly found that the use of exoskeleton triggers the restoration of damaged nerve systems, all the paraplegic patients may wear the powered exoskeleton in the future. An interested reader should refer to Refs. [38–41] for more information about the clinical data of Rewalk.

2.3. *HAL*

HAL (Hybrid Assistive Limb) is a powered robotic suit that assists physical human strength. It has been developed by Tsukuba University and Cyberdyne, Inc. in Japan (see Fig. 14).[43] The robot senses user's intention through electromyography (EMG)

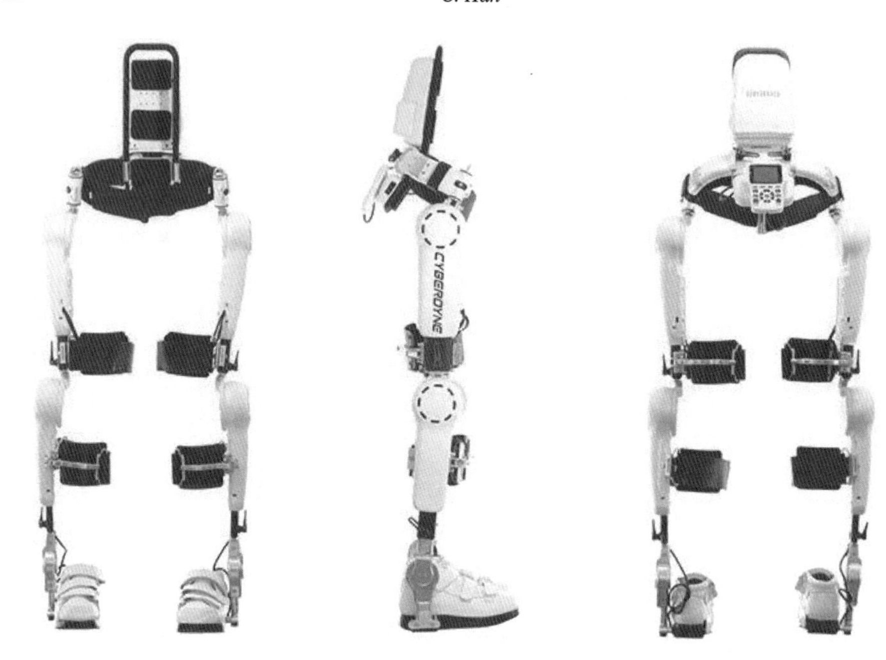

Figure 14. Hybrid Assistive Limb (HAL)[42]

sensors and floor reaction force (FRF) sensors, and it moves its robotic limb based on the information gathered from the sensors. Dr. Sankai, Professor of the Graduate School of Systems and Information Engineering in the University of Tsukuba, is the main developer of HAL™, and he is also the President of Cyberdyne, Inc.

In the late 1990s, Dr. Sankai and his research team started the development of the HAL series. At that time, HAL was the acronym for "Hybrid Assistive Leg". HAL-1 had two hip joints and two knee joints, and the joints used the DC motor and ball screw to generate the necessary torque.[44] The robot used myoelectricity for the estimation of an operator's intention. It was the first stage of HAL series, hence it was only for research purpose and not for practical use.

After HAL-1, HAL-3 was developed toward a more suitable system to be used in actual daily life (see Fig. 15).[45,46] Unlike HAL-1, all the actuators of HAL-3 consisted of DC servo motor with a harmonic drive to assist torques at each joint. In addition, the robot used not only the EMG signals but also the floor reaction force (FRF) sensors to acquire the human intention.[47] HAL-3, with the control method called Cybernic Autonomous Control, successfully enhanced a healthy person's walking, stair-climbing, standing up from a sitting posture and cycling, synchronizing with his/her body condition.[48]

With more advances in their research, Dr. Sankai and his team developed HAL-5 in 2005 which was a full-body exoskeleton for the arms, legs, and torso.

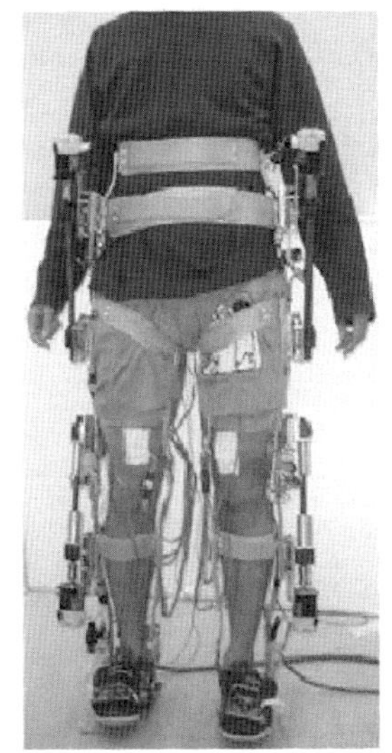

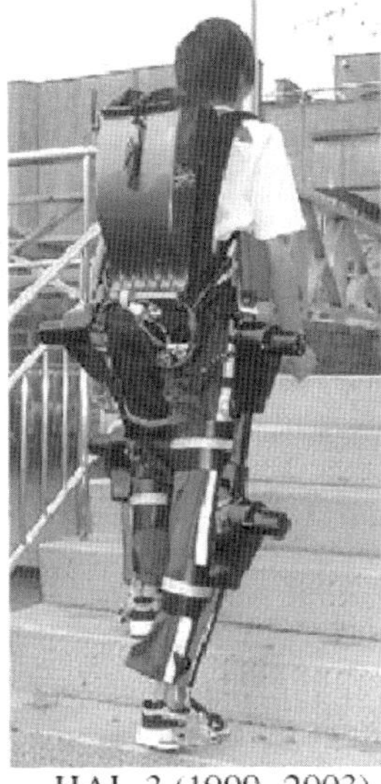

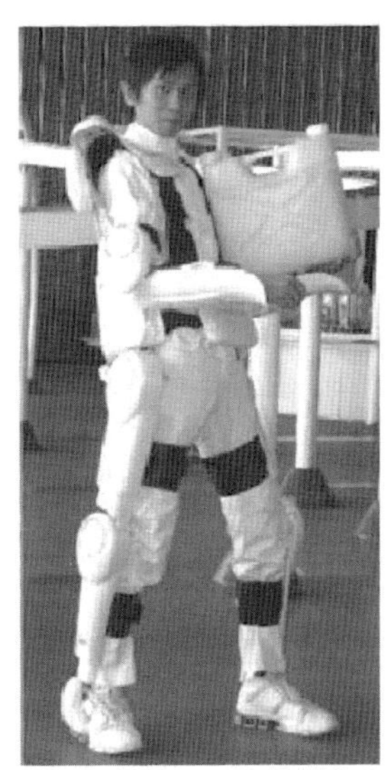

HAL-1 Type-B (1996–1999) HAL-3 (1999–2003) HAL-5 Type-B (2005–)

Figure 15. HAL series HAL-1, HAL-3, and HAL-5.[49]

It could hold and lift heavy objects up to 70 kg.[49] The robot was more compact and lasted for a longer period of time than the previous versions.

Since 2008, HAL™ has been marketed by Cyberdyne, Inc. At first, the company let people to use HAL™ through rental service in Japan. With the gains of several qualified certificates, HAL is now available in Japan and Europe for medical purposes.

The HAL-5 (Fig. 15) specifications include 15 kg for lower body type, battery life for approximately 2 h 40 min under continuous operation, daily activities assist function (standing up from a chair, walking, climbing up and down stairs), heavy load-carrying ability up to 70 kg, and hybrid control system (Cybernic Voluntary Control and Cybernic Autonomous Control). Today, a more advanced version of HAL exists, although the specification of HAL for medical use is not clearly unveiled yet.

These days, HAL is being applied in the medical area for the rehabilitation of paraplegic patients. In August 2013, the suit received an EC certificate, permitting its use for medical purposes in Europe. Since then, multiple clinical tests have been conducted both in Japan and Europe. These tests are mostly aiming for the evaluation of feasibility and safety of the robot when the robot is being worn by the disabled people.

For further information on HAL, please see Refs. [50–56] regarding the clinical testing of such robots (see Fig. 16). An interested reader can look for further information about how HAL is being utilized in the medical area.

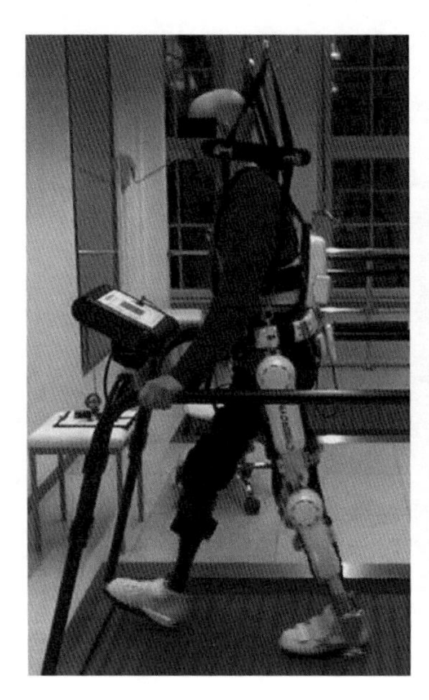
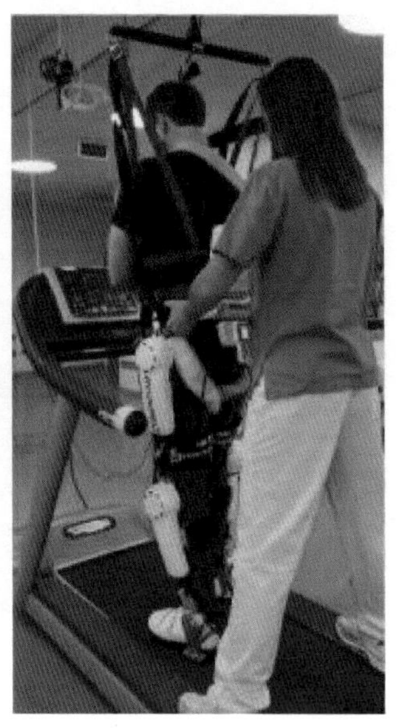

Figure 16. HAL on the treadmill for gait training.[55,56]

3. Ankle Rehabilitation System

3.1. *Anklebot*

In 2007, Anklebot was developed at Massachusetts Institute of Technology (MIT) for the rehabilitation of the ankle following a stroke, and was commercialized by Interactive Motion Technologies.[57] The robot supports the posture for rehabilitation therapy; walking on the treadmill and seated. In 2011, MIT developed the child version of the Anklebot (see Fig. 17).

The company conducted the clinical test to determine the feasibility of using the Anklebot as a gait training tool by increasing the contribution of the paretic ankle in the walking function.[58]

A pioneer of the Anklebot's class, MIT-MANUS, a robotic upper limb manipulandum for shoulder and elbow training, was developed in 1991. Along with the success of MIT-MANUS, the robot has motivated the development of new modules designed for the rehabilitation of the wrist, of the hand, and of the ankle.[59]

The Anklebot weighs about 3.6 kg and provides actuation in two of the ankle's 3-DOF. It allows 25° of dorsiflexion (DF), 45° of plantarflexion (PF), 25° of inversion, 20° of eversion, and 15° of internal or external rotation.[57]

A 6-week clinical study utilized the Anklebot modules three times per week for one hour therapy sessions. An equal number of chronic stroke survivors and

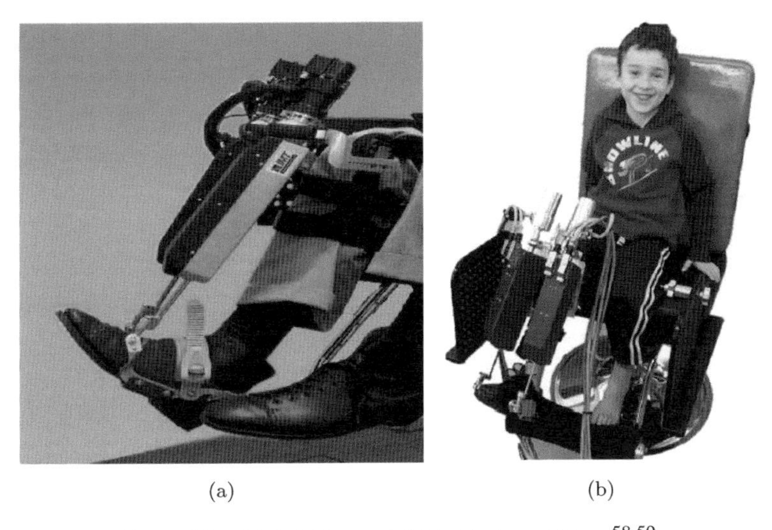

Figure 17. (a) Anklebot and (b) Pediatric Anklebot.[58,59]

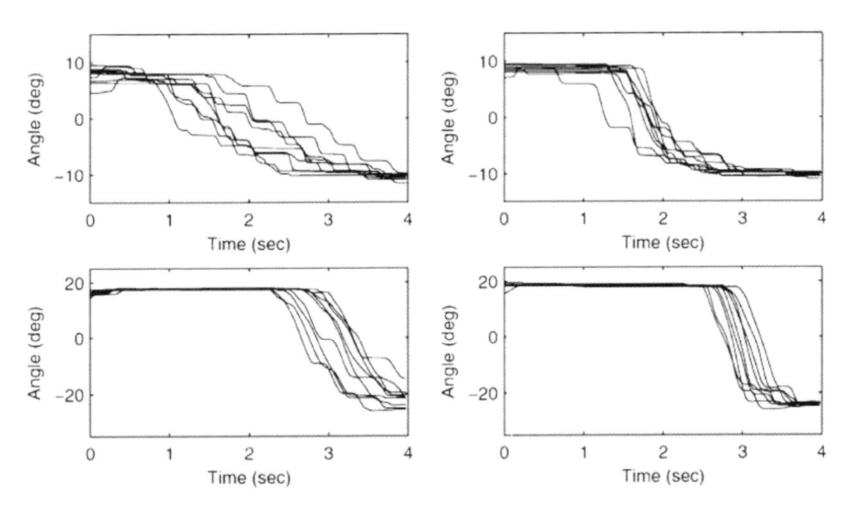

Figure 18. Exemplar point-to-point unassisted movements made by a typical (upper) stroke and (lower) healthy subject before (left) and after training (right).[57]

healthy subjects participated. Both groups were given to perform the training that consisted of playing the racer video game in certain DF/PF of ankle motion. The result of the study is shown in Fig. 18. The left side shows the ankle motion of subjects before the training and the right side shows the ankle motion subjects after the training. The upper and lower figures are cases of chronic stroke survivors and healthy people, respectively. It showed that after training the trajectory of DF/PF motion of chronic stroke survivors became more condensed into the similar patterns, meaning that the motion got more stable. As a result, subjects after chronic stroke showed improved control of the impaired ankle, smoother movement and quicker response. The study concluded that the ankle was used on a seated position. The clinical outcome consistent with all subjects was that on average they showed a 20% improvement in the walking speed.[49]

3.2. *Arizona state univ. AAFO (active ankle foot orthosis)*

Dr. Thomas Sugar at the Arizona State University has developed the ankle rehabilitation devices that assist stroke patients during gait.[60] He began to develop the Robotic Gait Trainer (RGT) and the Powered Ankle Foot Orthosis (PAFO) (see Fig. 19). Both models were used in clinical tests to collect qualitative data from patients and verify the effects of robotic gait therapy.[61,62]

In 2005, Dr. Sugar developed the RGT which is a walking device on a treadmill. The device is a tripod mechanism consisting of a flat plate and two bi-directional actuators[63] and it is capable of moving the foot about the ankle joint in dorsiflexion and plantarflexion as well as inversion and eversion. In 2007, he made a different type of model which is called the Powered Ankle Foot Orthosis. It consists of a powered orthosis using a robotic tendon that uses a motor to correctly position a tuned spring in the gait pattern. This device supports motion with a single degree of freedom, ankle rotation in the sagittal plane.[64]

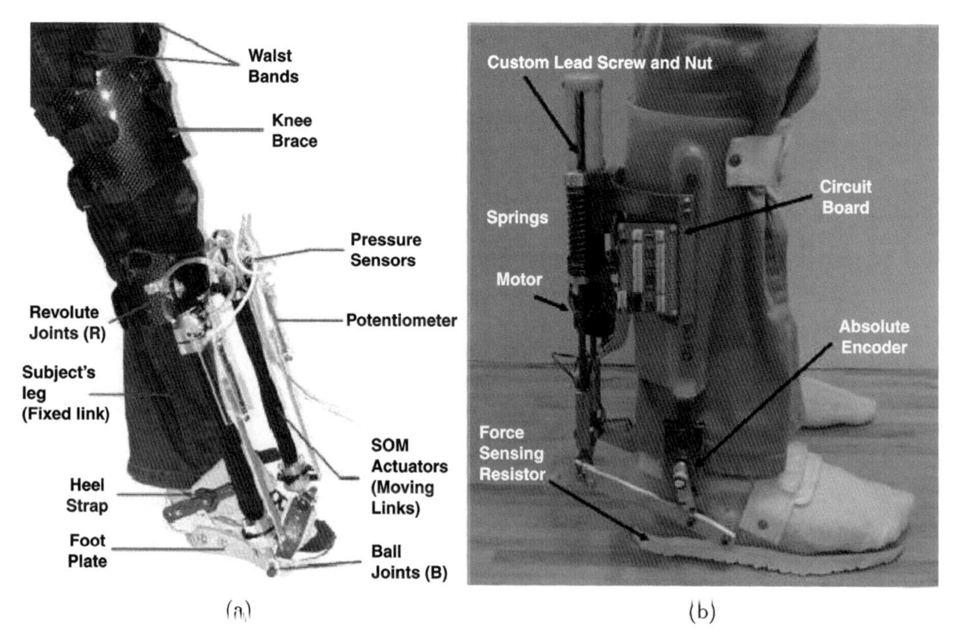

Figure 19. (a) Robotic gait trainer (RGT) and (b) Powered ankle foot orthosis (Photo courtesy of Arizona State University).[61,64]

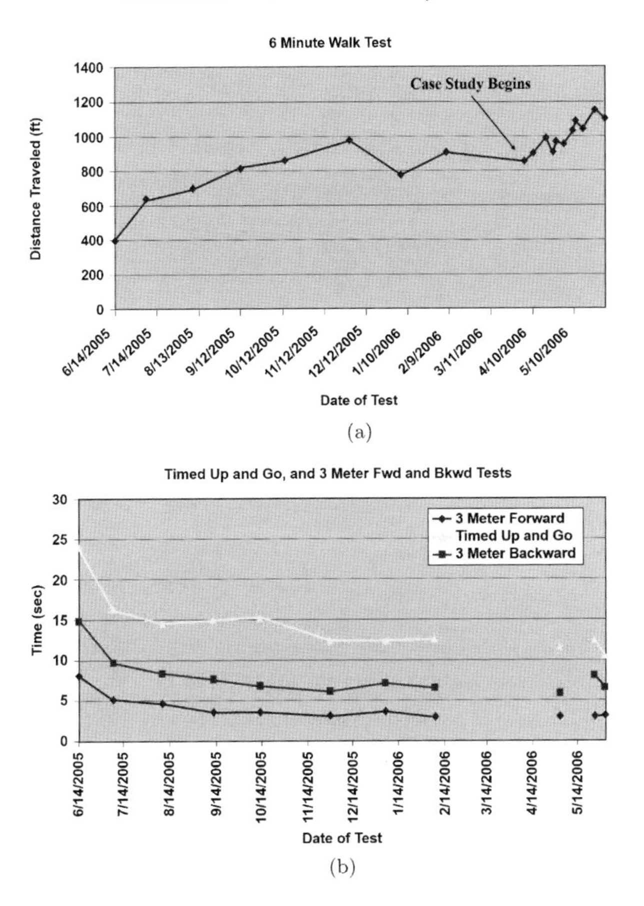

Figure 20. (a) 6 Minute Walk Test and (b) Timed Up and Go, and 3 Meter Fwd and Bkwd Tests.[61]

The RGT was tested to determine the usability for ankle rehabilitation. The study was performed at the Southwest Advanced Neurological Rehabilitation Center.[61] This study was conducted twice per week for 8 weeks on a 22 year old female stroke survivor. The patient would walk on the treadmill in five-minute intervals. The patient's performance was measured by "six minute walk" test and "timed-get-up-and-go" test. The result of the test is shown in Fig. 20. Based on this result, it can be seen that the RGT therapy was beneficial for the stroke survivor.

4. Treadmill Gait Training

4.1. *Lokomat*

Lokomat is a treadmill-utilized robotic system for gait rehabilitation of hemiplegic and paraplegic patients. Since Professor Gery Colombo proposed the idea in 1995, research has been conducted, and now a company called Hocoma leads this study.

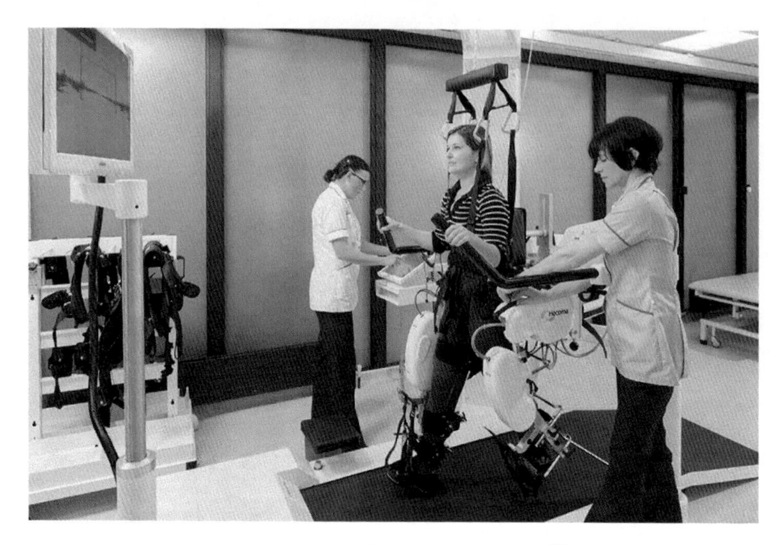

Figure 21. LokomatPro(Hocoma).[65]

Lokomat (Fig. 21) is a combination of exoskeleton robot and treadmill system. The system helps the rehabilitation training of the patients by providing and controlling a preset gait pattern for the user to follow the correct motion.[66] Using four linear actuators with force sensors mounted on, the system can control the motion of hip and knee joints. In addition, it utilizes a four-bar linkage to both express vertical motion and prevents the collapse of lateral balancing.[67] Hocoma developed the LokomatPro in 2005 with Pediatric Orthoses included, and Free D in 2014 that aids the left/right body weight movements.[68]

4.2. *Walkbot*

In Korea, a robotic system called Walkbot (Fig. 22), which is similar to Lokomat, has been developed by P&S Mechanics. Like Lokomat, Walkbot is robotic rehabilitation system that is a combination of treadmill and exoskeleton robot. The system helps the rehabilitation of paraplegic patients.[69] Unlike Lokomat, however, Walkbot uses powered actuator on the ankle joint, and provides a motion linked with EMG and FES. Moreover, there exists a pressure sensor below the sole to detect the contact between the robot and the ground. The system is designed to adjust its length of lower limb frame.

5. Walking Assist for Activities of Daily Living

5.1. *Walking assist device*

Honda in Japan found the basic research center in Saitama in Japan and started a research on the exoskeleton robot. In late 2008, the company showed a walking

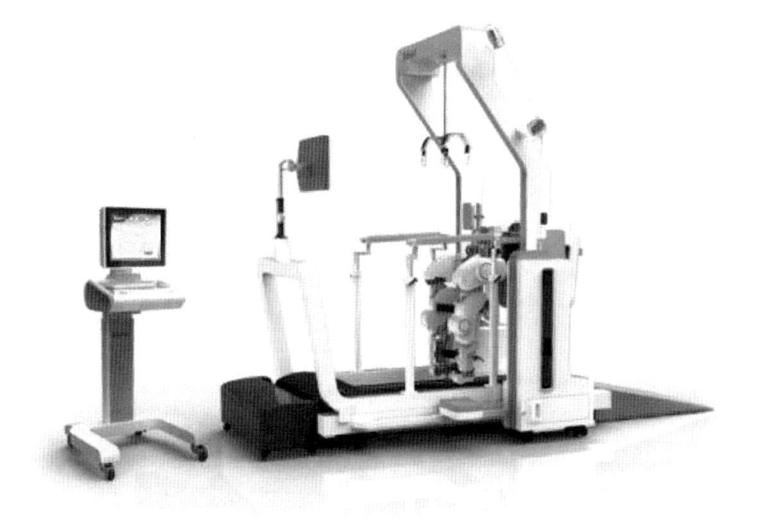

Figure 22. Walkbot (P&S Mechanics).[71]

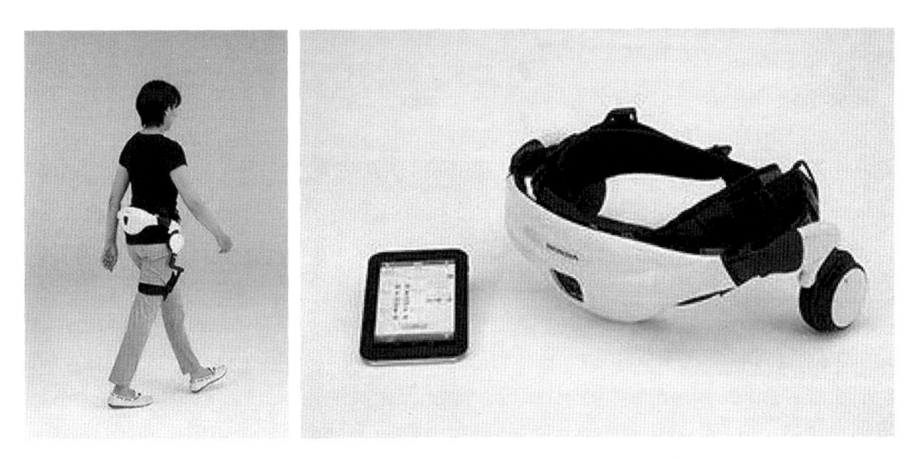

Figure 23. Walking Assist Device (Honda).[72]

assistance robot (see Fig. 23).[73] In 2009, the company published a report about the effectiveness of the robot by applying it on elderly people for 5 months.[74] The robot presented in the report used two motors to maintain the cadence and gait frequency at an adequate level so that the user could experience an easier and better ambulation. After the application of the robot for 5 months, it was found that the gait speed increased due to the effects of exercising while wearing the robot, and the heart rate decreased. The robot weighs 2.7 kg and has a lithium-ion battery that lasts for an hour and actuators that can exert 4 Nm, the maximum torque.[75]

6. Soft Robotic System

6.1. *SNU-Exo-Glove*

In South Korea, the BioRobotics Laboratory at Seoul National University has been developing soft biologically inspired mechanisms and robots with the goal of developing innovative ways of creating motion without rigid joints and links. They are extending interest to soft wearable robots that require biologically inspired design to create effective ways of assisting the movement of people with disability.

The goal of the robot is to develop a compact and wearable assistive device for the people who have paralysis of the hand. The main drawback of exoskeletons with rigid frames is that they do not have simple and compact assistive devices. One of the alternatives to overcome this limitation is to have wearable robots without rigid frames and driven by tendons. The rigid frames of conventional exoskeletons have the functions of weight bearing and power transmission. A wearable frame without rigidity is based on the concept of replacing the role of a rigid frame structure with the user's skeletal structure. The tendons of the robot act as the tendons of the human body, which pulls the skeletal structures (see Fig. 24).[77]

Based on the structure of the human hand, the EXO-Glove has two tendons for each finger and the thumb, several types of straps that together form the pulley, and supporting structures that form the origin of the muscles. These components are designed to transmit normal forces to the body. To generate an appropriate finger trajectory for different users, the tendon path of the routing system can be adjusted by changing the length and position of the fabric straps.[78]

The Exo-Glove (Fig. 25) is most suitable for people incapable of closing or opening their hands but able to use other joints of the upper limb including wrist, elbow, and shoulder joints. The Exo-Glove can also be used by people with medium to low level finger spasticity, as long as all finger joints exhibit the same degree of spasticity. This robot is especially used for occupational therapy rehabilitation.[77]

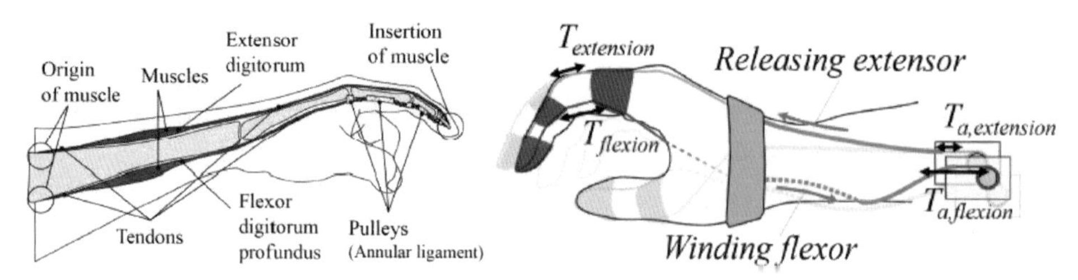

Figure 24. The human finger works via tendons, muscles, and pulleys acting on the skeleton and while the tendon moves toward the joint, the tension applied to the joint is greater than the tension at the actuator.[77]

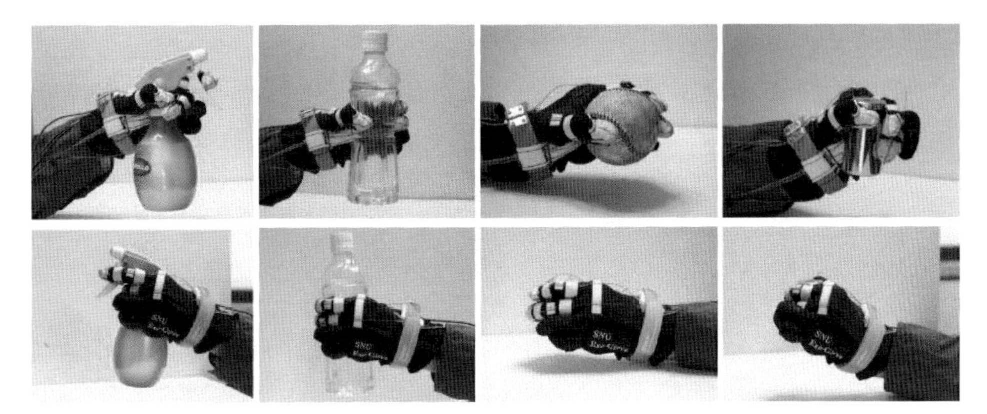

Figure 25. Various grasping motions achieved by a tetraplegic subject using the Exo-Glove. The simple human–robot interface and underactuation mechanisms made it easy for the subject to grasp the objects.[77]

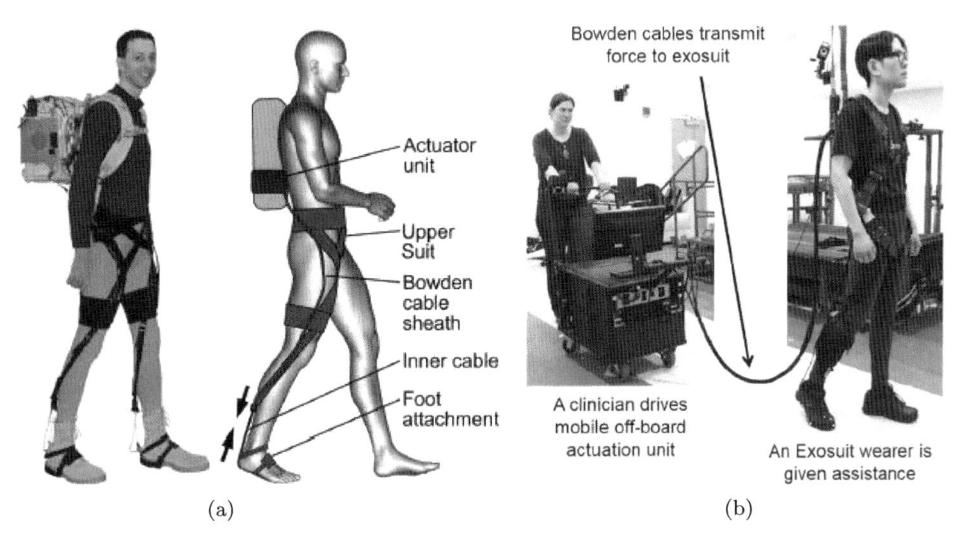

Figure 26. (a) Exosuit system and (b) Overground walking wearing an exosuit actuated by a mobile off-board actuation unit (Photo courtesy of Harvard University).[80]

6.2. *Soft Exosuit*

Conor J. Walsh at Harvard University developed the soft cable-driven exosuit. This device's feature is that it can generate forces passively due to the body's motion, similar to the body's ligament and tendon. This exosuit was tested with five healthy subjects that showed a minimal effect on gait kinematics and an average best-case metabolic reduction of 6.4%.[79] The study concluded that a soft exosuit (Fig. 26) could improve patient's gait symmetry and paretic limb progression.[80] Clinical trials for stroke survivors were also attempted during the study.

References

1. M. Mihelj, T. Nef and R. Riener. (2006). ARMin-toward a six DoF upper limb rehabilitation robot. In Biomedical Robotics and Biomechatronics, *The First IEEE/RAS-EMBS International Conference on BioRob* 1154–1159.
2. T. Nef, M. Mihelj, G. Colombo and R. Riener. (2006). ARMin-robot for rehabilitation of the upper extremities, in *Proceedings IEEE International Conference on Robotics and Automation, ICRA* 3152–3157.
3. T. Nef, M. Mihelj, G. Kiefer, C. Perndl, R. Müller and R. Riener. (2007). ARMin-Exoskeleton for arm therapy in stroke patients, in *IEEE 10th International Conference on Rehabilitation Robotics, ICORR* 68–74.
4. T. Nef, M. Guidali, V. Klamroth-Marganska and R. Riener. (2009). ARMin-exoskeleton robot for stroke rehabilitation. In *World Congress on Medical Physics and Biomedical Engineering* September 7–12, 2009, Munich, Germany 127–130. Springer: Berlin Heidelberg.
5. K. Kiguchi, K. Iwami, M. Yasuda, K. Watanabe and T. Fukuda. (2003). An exoskeletal robot for human shoulder joint motion assist. Mechatronics, *IEEE/ASME Transactions on Mechatronics* 8(1):125–135.
6. K. Kiguchi, M. H. Rahman, M. Sasaki and K. Teramoto. (2008). Development of a 3 DOF mobile exoskeleton robot for human upper-limb motion assist, *Robotics and Autonomous Systems* 56(8), 678–691.
7. K. Kiguchi, Y. Kose and Y. Hayashi. (2010). Task-oriented perception-assist for an upper-limb powerassist exoskeleton robot, in *World Automation Congress (WAC)* 2010:1–6.
8. A. U. Pehlivan, O. Celik and M. K. Malley. (2011). Mechanical design of a distal arm exoskeleton for stroke and spinal cord injury rehabilitation, in *IEEE International Conference on ICORR* 1–5.
9. Mechatronics and Haptic Interfaces Lab, (2015). http://mahilab.rice.edu
10. Y. Ren, H. S. Park and L. Q. Zhang Sr. (2009). Developing a whole-arm exoskeleton robot with hand opening and closing mechanism for upper limb stroke rehabilitation, in *IEEE International Conference on ICORR* 761–765.
11. Rehabilitation Institute of Chicago, (2015). http://smnorthwestern.edu/.
12. D. Ragonesi, S. K. Agrawal, W. Sample and T. Rahman. (2013). Quantifying anti-gravity torques for the design of a powered exoskeleton. Neural systems and rehabilitation engineering, *IEEE Transactions on Neural Systems and Rehabilitation Engineering* 21(2):283–288.
13. Y. Mao and S. K. Agrawal. (2012). Design of a cable-driven arm exoskeleton (CAREX) for neural rehabilitation. *IEEE Transactions on Robotics* 28(4):922–931.
14. ROAR LAB, (2015). http://roar/me.columbia.edu/projects/wex/
15. S. K. Agrawal, V. N. Dubey, J. J. Gangloff, E. Brackbill, Y. Mao and V. Sangwan. (2009). Design and optimization of a cable driven upper arm exoskeleton, *Journal of Medical Devices* 3(3):031004.
16. Kim, Mi Jung, Dong Hun Lee, Taikon Kim, Seongho Jang, Hee-Sang Kim, Jinmann Chon, Seung Don Yoo *et al.* (2014). Lower extremity exercise of knee osteoarthritis patients using portable assistive robot (HEXAR-KR40P), *International Journal of Precision Engineering and Manufacturing* 15(12):2617–2622.
17. Kim, Wooram, Dongbock Lee, Deokwon Yun, Younghoon Ji, Minsung Kang, Jungsoo Han, and Changsoo Han. (2015). Neurorehabilitation robot system for neurological patients using H-infinity impedance controller, in *IEEE International Conference on ICORR*, 876–881.
18. Khan, M. Adnan Deok-won Yun, Jung-Soo Han, Kyoosik Shin, and Chang-Soo Han. (2014). Upper extremity assist exoskeleton robot, in *The 23rd IEEE International Symposium on RO-MAN*, 892–898.

19. Abdul Manan Khan, Deok-won Yun, Mian Ashfaq Ali, Jungsoo Han, Kyoosik Shin and Changsoo Han. (2015). Adaptive impedance control for upper limb assist exoskeleton, in *International Conference on Robotics and Automation*, 4359–4366.
20. Ekso Bionics, (2015). http://intl.eksobionics.com/ekso
21. Berkeley Robotics and Human Engineering Laboratory (2015). http://intl.eksobionics.com/ekso
22. Wikipedia, the free encyclopedia (2015). https://en.wikipedia.org/wiki/Ekso_Bionics
23. H. Kazerooni. (1996). The human power amplifier technology at the University of California, Berkeley, *Robotics and Autonomous Systems* 19(2):179–187.
24. H. Kazerooni, J. L. Racine, L. Huang and R. Steger. (2005). On the control of the berkeley lower extremity exoskeleton (BLEEX), in *Proceedings of the IEEE International Conference on ICRA*, 4353–4360.
25. Ekso Bionics, (2015). http://intl.eksobionics.com/ourstory
26. K. A. Strausser and H. Kazerooni. (2011). The development and testing of a human machine interface for a mobile medical exoskeleton, in *International Conference on IEEE/RSJ*, 4911–4916.
27. S. A. Kolakowsky-Hayner, J. Crew, S. Moran and A. Shah. (2013). Safety and feasibility of using the EksoTM bionic exoskeleton to aid ambulation after spinal cord injury. *Journal of Spine* S4.
28. J. Kressler, C. K. Thomas, E. C. Field-Fote, J. Sanchez, E. Widerstrøm-Noga, D. C. Cilien and M. S. Nash. (2014). Understanding therapeutic benefits of overground bionic ambulation: exploratory case series in persons with chronic, complete spinal cord injury, *Archives of Physical Medicine and Rehabilitation* 95(10):1878–1887.
29. Y. Gerasimenko, R. Gorodnichev, T. Moshonkina, D. Sayenko, P. Gad and V. R. Edgerton. (2015). Transcutaneous electrical spinal-cord stimulation in humans, *Annals of Physical and Rehabilitation Medicine* 58(4):225–231.
30. Technology Vista, (2015). http://www.technologyvista.in/pin/the-rewalk-6-0-robotic-exoskeleton-soon-to-make-wheelchairs-an-obsolete-thing/
31. U.S. Food and Drug Administration, (2015). http://www.fda.gov/NewsEvents/Newsroom/PressAnnouncements/ucm402970.htm.
32. A. Esquenazi. (2013). New bipedal locomotion options for individuals with thoracic level motor complete spinal cord injury, *Journal of Spinal Research Found* 8(1):26–28.
33. A Goffer. (2013). Enhanced Safety of Gait in Powered Exoskeletons, Conference on Dynamic Walking 2014.
34. The Telegraph, (2012). http://www.telegraph.co.uk/sport/othersports/athletics/london-marathon/marathon/9252424/Paralysed-Claire-Lomas-finishes-London-Marathon.html
35. Rewalk Robotics, (2015). http://rewalk.com/about-products-2
36. Strange, Adario (2014). FDA Approves First Robotic Exoskeleton for Paralyzed Users. Mashable. Retrieved 30 July 2014.
37. A. Esquenazi and A. Packel. (2012). Robotic-assisted gait training and restoration, *American Journal of Physical Medicine and Rehabilitation* 91(11):S217–S231.
38. G. Zeilig, H. Weingarden, M. Zwecker, I. Dudkiewicz, A. Bloch and A. Esquenazi. (2012). Safety and tolerance of the ReWalk™ exoskeleton suit for ambulation by people with complete spinal cord injury: A pilot study, *Journal of Spinal Cord Medicine* 35(2):96–101.
39. A. Esquenazi, M. Talaty, A. Packel and M. Saulino. (2012). The ReWalk powered exoskeleton to restore ambulatory function to individuals with thoracic-level motor-complete spinal cord injury, *American Journal of Physical Medicine and Rehabilitation* 91(11):911–921.
40. M. Talaty, A. Esquenazi and J. E. Briceno. (2013). Differentiating ability in users of the ReWalk TM powered exoskeleton: An analysis of walking kinematics, in *IEEE International Conference on ICORR* 1–5.

41. Hollie Samantha Forbes White, Stephen Hayes and Matthew White (2014). The Effect of Using a Powered Exoskeleton Training Programme on Joint Range of Motion on Spinal Injured Individuals: A Pilot Study, *International Journal of Physical Therapy and Rehabilitation* 1:102.
42. Cyberdyne INC, (2015). http://www.cyberdyne.jp/english/products/LowerLimb_medical.html
43. (2015) https://en.wikipedia.org/wiki/HAL_(robot)
44. K. Kasaoka and Y. Sankai. (2001). Predictive control estimating operator's intention for stepping-up motion by exo-skeleton type power assist system HAL. In Intelligent Robots and Systems, *Proceedings International Conference on IEEE/RSJ* 3:1578–1583.
45. H. Toda, T. Kobayakawa, Y. Sankai. (2006). A multi-link system control strategy based biological movement, *Advanced Robotics* 20(6):661–679.
46. H. Toda and Y. Sankai. (2006). Three-dimensional link dynamics simulator base on N-single-particle movement, *Advanced Robotics* 19(9):977–993.
47. H. Kawamoto and Y. Sankai. (2005). Power assist method based on phase sequence and muscle force condition for HAL, *Advanced Robotics* 19(7):717–734.
48. H. Imai, M. Nozawa, Y. Kawamura and Y. Sankai, (2002). Human motion oriented control method for humanoid robot, in *Proc. Int. Workshop on Robot and Human Interactive Communication*, Berlin, 221–226.
49. Y. Sankai. (2011). HAL: Hybrid assistive limb based on cybernics. In Robotics Research 25–34. Springer: Berlin Heidelberg.
50. S. Maeshima, A. Osawa, D. Nishio, Y. Hirano, K. Takeda, H. Kigawa and Y. Sankai. (2011). Efficacy of a hybrid assistive limb in post-stroke hemiplegic patients: a preliminary report. *BMC Neurology*, 11(1):116.
51. H. Sakakima, K. Ijiri, F. Matsuda, H. Tominaga, T. Biwa, K. Yone and Y. Sankai. (2013). A newly developed robot suit hybrid assistive limb facilitated walking rehabilitation after spinal surgery for thoracic ossification of the posterior longitudinal ligament: a case report, *Case Reports in Orthopedics*.
52. S. Kubota, Y. Nakata, K. Eguchi, H. Kawamoto, K. Kamibayashi, M. Sakane and N. Ochiai. (2013). Feasibility of rehabilitation training with a newly developed wearable robot for patients with limited mobility, *Archives of Physical Medicine and Rehabilitation* 94(6):1080–1087.
53. H. Kawamoto, K. Kamibayashi, Y. Nakata, K. Yamawaki, R. Ariyasu, Y. Sankai and N. Ochiai. (2013). Pilot study of locomotion improvement using hybrid assistive limb in chronic stroke patients, *BMC Neurology* 13(1):141.
54. O. Cruciger, T. A. Schildhauer, R. C. Meindl, M. Tegenthoff, P. Schwenkreis, M. Citak and M. Aach. (2014). Impact of locomotion training with a neurologic controlled hybrid assistive limb (HAL) exoskeleton on neuropathic pain and health related quality of life (HRQoL) in chronic SCI: a case study*, *Disability and Rehabilitation: Assistive Technology* 1–6.
55. A. Nilsson, K. S. Vreede, V. Häglund, H. Kawamoto, Y. Sankai and J. Borg. (2014). Gait training early after stroke with a new exoskeleton — the hybrid assistive limb: a study of safety and feasibility, *Journal of Neuroengineering and Rehabilitation* 11(1):92.
56. M. Aach, O. Cruciger, M. Sczesny-Kaiser, O. Höffken, R. C. Meindl, M. Tegenthoff and T. A. Schildhauer. (2014). Voluntary driven exoskeleton as a new tool for rehabilitation in chronic spinal cord injury: a pilot study, *Spine Journal* 14(12):2847–2853.
57. Interactive Motion Technologies. (2015). http://interactive-motion.com/healthcarereform/inmotion-anklebot/
58. A. Roy, H. I. Krebs, J. E. Barton, R. F. Macko and L. W. Forrester. (2013). Anklebot-assisted locomotor training after stroke: A novel deficit-adjusted control approach, in *IEEE International Conference on ICRA* 2175–2182.
59. H. Krebs, S. Rossi, S. J. Kim, P. K. Artemiadis, D. Williams, E. Castelli and P. Cappa. (2011). Pediatric anklebot, in *IEEE International Conference on ICORR* 1–5.
60. Arizona State University. (2015). https://webapp4.asu.edu/directory/ person/227786?pa=true

61. J. Ward, S. Balasubramanian, T. Sugar and J. He. (2007). Robotic gait trainer reliability and stroke patient case study. In Rehabilitation Robotics, *IEEE 10th International Conference on ICORR* 554–561.
62. J. Ward, T. Sugar, J. Standeven and J. R. Engsberg. (2010). Stroke survivor gait adaptation and performance after training on a powered ankle foot orthosis. In Robotics and Automation, *IEEE International Conference on ICRA* 211–216.
63. K. Bharadwaj, T. G. Sugar, J. B. Koeneman and E. J. Koeneman. (2005). Design of a robotic gait trainer using spring over muscle actuators for ankle stroke rehabilitation, *Journal of Biomechanical Engineering* 127(6):1009–1013.
64. J. Ward, T. Sugar, J. Standeven and J. R. Engsberg. (2010). Stroke survivor gait adaptation and performance after training on a powered ankle foot orthosis. In Robotics and Automation, *IEEE International Conference on ICRA* 211–216.
65. Hocoma, (2015). https://www.hocoma.com/world/en/partners/clinical-partners/
66. G. Colombo, M. Wirz, and V. Dietz. (2001). Driven gait orthosis for improvement of locomotor training in paraplegic patients, *Spinal Cord* 39(5):252–255.
67. Jezernik, Sašo, *et al.* (2003). Robotic orthosis lokomat: a rehabilitation and research tool, Neuromodulation, *Technology at the Neural Interface* 6(2):108–115.
68. Hocoma. (2015). http://www.hocoma.com/world/en/about-us/company/history
69. P & S Mechanics. (2015). http://www.walkbot.co.kr/xe/kor_main
70. J.-H. Jung, *et al.* (2009). Validity and feasibility of intelligent Walkbot system. *Electronics Letters* 45(20):1016–1017.
71. P & S Mechanics. (2015). http://www.walkbot.co.kr/eng/page2_21.html
72. Honda Motor Co., Ltd. (2015). http://world.honda.com/news/2015/p150721eng.html
73. Bogue, Robert. Exoskeletons and robotic prosthetics: a review of recent developments. *Indus Trail Robot: An International Journal* 36(5):421–427.
74. K. Yasuhara, *et al.* (2009). Walking assist device with stride management system. *Honda R&D Technical Review* 21(2):54–62.
75. http://world.honda.com/news/2015/p150721eng.html
76. H. In and K. J. Cho. (2013). Analysis of the forces on the finger joints by a joint-less wearable robotic hand, SNU Exo-Glove. In Converging Clinical and Engineering Research on Neurorehabilitation. Springer: Berlin Heidelberg, pp. 93–97.
77. H. In, B. B. Kang, M. Sin and K. J. Cho. (2015). Exo-glove: A soft wearable robot for the hand with a soft tendon routing system. *IEEE Robotics and Automation Magazine* 22(1): 97–105.
78. U. Jeong, H. K. In and K. J. Cho. (2013). Implementation of various control algorithms for hand rehabilitation exercise using wearable robotic hand, *Intelligent Service Robotics* 6(4):181–189.
79. A. T. Asbeck, S. M. De Rossi, K. G. Holt and C. J. Walsh. (2015). A biologically inspired soft exosuit for walking assistance. *International Journal of Robotics Research* 0278364914562476.
80. J. Bae, S. M. M. De Rossi, K. O'Donnell, K. L. Hendron, L. N. Awad, T. R. Teles Dos Santos and C. J. Walsh. (2015). A soft exosuit for patients with stroke: Feasibility study with a mobile off-board actuation unit. *IEEE International Conference on Rehabilitation Robotics ICORR* 131–138.

Chapter 8

A REVIEW OF HOME-BASED ROBOTIC REHABILITATION

Aliakbar Alamdari*, Seungkook Jun†, Daniel Ramsey‡, and Venkat Krovi§

**Harmac Medical Products, Inc.*
†*Orbital ATK*
‡*D'Youville College, Department of Health Professions Education, NY, USA*
§*Clemson University, International Center for Automotive Research, SC, USA*

The Smart Health paradigm has opened up immense possibilities for designing modern cyber–physical/robotic systems for implementing data-, information- and knowledge-driven execution of healthcare decision making processes.

Human movement arises from a complex dynamic interplay of the neuromusculoskeletal system with the environment. From the rehabilitation perspective, a therapist seeks to better understand these bi-directional power interactions (motion and forces) with the ultimate intent of customizing and modulating ensuing patient behaviors. Advances in quantitative sensing, computational analysis, data-driven decision-making and flexible-modulation of human behaviors through data-capture devices and wearable robotic systems have served to further this approach. However, logistics constraints (infrastructure requirements, cost, trained personnel) limit the scope of deployment to best outpatient clinic settings.

In recent times, many exemplary cyber–physical/robotic frameworks for home-based progressive rehabilitation have emerged. Immense flexibility ensues from a service-deployment perspective which need no longer be confined to the inpatient clinic. Numerous studies have shown that the most effective therapeutic results are from transferring rehabilitation process from clinic setting to patient's home. The scheduling logistics are significantly simplified (for the specialized equipment and personnel at the clinic) while patients are now afforded enhanced access in a self-directed manner.

We will first survey existing clinic-based rehabilitation frameworks for upper limb motor rehabilitation (for stroke patients) and lower limb rehabilitation (for osteoarthritic (OA) patients). Subsequently, we examine several commercial-off-the-shelf (COTS) technologies and examine the viability of their adaptation to support in-home therapeutic frameworks. We will evaluate these frameworks for both patient and provider benefits, including ease-of-use by all parties; modulating the intensity, duration and consistency of therapy; and logistics of monitoring and deployment for home-based use.

1. Introduction

The Smart Health paradigm has opened up immense possibilities for designing cyber–physical systems with integrated sensing and analysis for data-driven healthcare decision-making. Clinical motor-rehabilitation has traditionally tended to entail labor-intensive approaches with limited quantitative methods and numerous logistics deployment challenges. We believe such labor-intensive rehabilitation procedures offer a fertile application field for robotics and automation technologies, which can be easily applicable to home-based rehabilitation systems. To give greater clarity, we will examine this in the context of upper limb motor rehabilitation for stroke patients, and lower limb rehabilitation for OA patients.

1.1. *Societal needs*

Several neurological disorders including stroke, spinal cord injury (SCI), cerebellar disorders, and neuromuscular diseases exhibit themselves via generation of abnormal patterns of lower and upper limb motions.

Stroke is one of the principal causes of disability worldwide. Stroke affects over 800,000 people annually in the US, leaving 75% of those afflicted with some form of disabilities that reduce their quality of life.[1] The principal consequence is the reduction of functional performance (of both lower and upper extremities) which limits independence of the affected subjects. Recovery strategies depend on the duration, strength and specificity of training.[2] Studies have shown that short-term and goal-oriented robotic rehabilitation on individuals with chronic motor impairment after a stroke significantly improve motor abilities at the end of the therapy.[3] Repetitive practices of daily activities are thought to help stroke survivors due to neurological remapping and brain plasticity, thereby increasing motor capabilities. Thus, these key issues have encouraged many researchers to develop rehabilitative devices for affected patients. These treatment processes commence immediately after discharge from hospital with constant medical care.

Osteoarthritis is a progressive degenerative disease that afflicts a large and growing number of Americans,[4] and is predicted to become the fourth leading cause of disability as the population ages and with steadily increasing obesity rates. OA-induced pain and knee instability limit function and slow or interrupt locomotion.[5] An estimated 24–37% of arthritic adults in the US report reduced capacity for "normal daily activity", which predisposes them to further health decline associated with inactivity. Thus, with earlier onset, increasing patient populations, and chronic and prolonged course, the costly treatments make OA an important public health issue.[5,6] According to Hootman *et al.*,[7] by 2030, it is estimated that the prevalence of clinically-diagnosed arthritis will afflict nearly 67 million US adults (25% of the projected total adult population). By 2015, the number of knee replacements and joint realignment surgery (osteotomy) performed is expected to reach 1.3 million at a cost of $49 billion.[8] Both these procedures are expensive, with variable success rates, require long recoveries, and carry the risk of surgical morbidity.[9]

1.2. *Challenges*

Numerous studies have noted that the systematic deployment of rehabilitation regimen (of adequate intensity, duration, and consistency) can help restore motor functionalities in such patients. However, significant challenges exist for realization of these rehabilitation systems.

Immense variability exists across a population, which is based on gender and age, and this is compounded by individual differences stemming from the level of conditioning and the degree of disease severity and/or therapy. Hence, there is great interest in carefully personalizing entire rehabilitation programs, both in terms of user-device ergonomics and regimen parameters, to enhance patient outcomes. However, a sound understanding of the interplay between such design and control strategies of articulated bracing for realizing desired dynamic interaction patterns is lacking among persons with neuromusculoskeletal deficits. Moreover, such a rehabilitation process tends to be labor-intensive, relying on inpatient diagnostic and therapeutic procedures that are administered by a clinician working with a single patient at a time. As the number of patients increases, limited availability of rehabilitation centers with specialized equipment/personnel support offer serious constraints, which is particularly acute for persons who reside in rural or remote locations.

To address these shortcomings, we undertook a visual-sensing/dynamical-systems perspective, building upon the following features: (i) Robotics therapy allows for more complex therapies like constraint-induced therapy that guides patients through intensive, repetitive functional movement; (ii) home-based deployment to empower access and overcome the traditional logistics constraints that limited the duration intensity and regularity of exercise performances; and (iii) computer-enhanced therapy which leverages ubiquitous computational power and responsiveness that allows for immersive experiences, quantitative automated, and transparent assessment of patient performance.

The remainder of this chapter is organized as follows: Sec. 2 focuses on a review of the different trends in rehabilitation therapy, including current clinical motor-rehabilitation devices, home-based rehabilitation therapy, computerized exercise systems, and enhanced computerized exercise systems for home-based rehabilitation. The current challenges of using cyber–physical-systems at home for rehabilitation purposes include motion capture using Kinect, static measurement using the Wii balance board, human motion analysis, and user-specific customization for appropriate design which are presented in Sec. 3. Section 4 describes various Quantitative Progressive Exercise Rehabilitation Regimens, whereas Sec. 5 presents an implementation example of a cyber–physical system. Finally, Sec. 6 highlights the concluding remarks.

2. State of the Art in Rehabilitation Therapy

Conventional rehabilitation therapy has traditionally relied on quantitative motion capture with subsequent computational analysis to help with diagnosis and treatment of various movement disorders. While surgical as well as more conservative (non-operative) interventions are available to mediate pain and improve function and quality of life for chronic cases, a structured exercise regimen may also alleviate and slow disease progression. However, given the immense variability across a population based on gender and age, this is compounded by individual differences stemming from the level of conditioning and the degree of disease severity and/or therapy. Hence, there is great interest in carefully personalizing rehabilitation programs in terms of exercise-regimen parameters to enhance patient outcomes. Here, we therefore examine a continuum of approaches currently available, ranging from clinic-based rehabilitation with robotic devices to computerized at-home exercise systems for rehabilitation.

2.1. *Clinic-based robotic therapy*

Traditionally, lower and upper limb motor therapies are performed manually that perhaps require multiple physiotherapists. The inconsistency from one session to the next has motivated researchers to develop robotic devices to provide consistent motion. These robotic assistive devices have been widely used for motor function therapy and rehabilitation of individuals with neurological impairments. Robotic devices enable longer and more frequent utilization in the clinic. Recent therapeutic modalities, such as constraint-induced therapy, have been shown to significantly restore function faster using intensive, supervised training.[10,11] It must be noted that labor-intensive neuro-rehabilitation can be greatly aided by robot-assisted therapy devices ("rehabilitators") that physically interact with patients in order to assist in movement therapy.[12–15] Such robotic devices augment the therapist by guiding the patient through intensive, repetitive practice of functional movement, with several studies documenting their successes.[16–18]

Task-oriented repetitive movements reportedly improve muscle strength and movement coordination among patients with neurological impairments. Robotic and automation technologies have been used to assist, enhance, evaluate, and document rehabilitation. Here, we therefore focus on two broad categories of robotic rehabilitation therapy that are utilized in the clinic: lower limb and upper limb rehabilitation devices.

2.1.1. *Clinic-based lower limb rehabilitation therapy*

Classic gait rehabilitation can be classified under two sub-categories: neurophysiological and motor learning. In the neurophysiological rehabilitation approach described by Bobath,[19] the patient is the passive recipient of the physiotherapist's direct corrective and assistive movements whereas in motor learning, as described by Perfetti,[20] the emphasis is on active patient participation. Although these two distinct approaches are used for hemiparetic gait rehabilitation, each method is customized for each specific condition and patient. Yet, States *et al.*[21] have shown that there are no benefits with these methods, but that body weight supported treadmill training is more effective. Classic gait rehabilitation methods alone are reportedly unable to restore a normal walking pattern in many stroke patients.[22] Robotic rehabilitation devices potentially offer many advantages for gait rehabilitation including: (i) reduction of physical assistance and therapy cost, (ii) data acquisition, measurement and assessment, and (iii) repeatability.[23] When robotic devices have been included into gait rehabilitation, the evidence suggests improved endurance, lower limb balance, functional balance, gait symmetry, double stance support, and stride length.[24,25] To date, numerous assistive orthosis systems for gait rehabilitation have been deployed, including treadmill gait trainers, overground gait trainers, and stationary gait and ankle trainers for the neurologically impaired. These systems implement unique mechanical structures, designs, actuators, methods, control schemes and rehabilitation strategies, as well as various procedures to ensure the reliability and robustness of the systems when compared to others.

Lokomat is one of the best examples of a gait orthosis that can be used for lower limb disabilities.[26,27] As shown in Fig. 1(a), it consists of three main parts: body weight support, a treadmill, and a powered leg orthosis. Control algorithms improve performance, such as position, adaptability, impedance controllers, etc.[26] The electromechanical exoskeleton employs a zero-impedance control mode or path control thereby allowing patients to freely move their limbs while walking. Shown

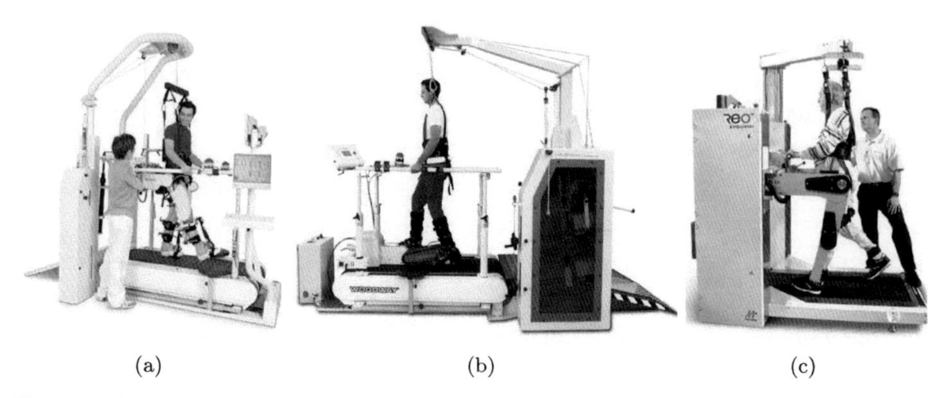

(a) (b) (c)

Figure 1. Examples of clinic-based robotic therapy devices for lower limb extremities: (a) Lokomat,[26] (b) LOKOhelp,[28] and (c) ReoAmbulator.[28]

in Fig. 1(b), the LokoHelp treadmill gait trainer incorporates an electromechanical foot-powered orthosis that mediates a gait motion during the training session. The control device moves the patients' foot trajectory with a fixed step length of 400 mm.[28] The ReoAmbulator shown in Fig. 1(c) has been used for rehabilitation therapies. The robotic arms attach to the thigh and ankle of the patient's leg, and a stepping pattern is performed using the implemented control scheme and strategy.[28]

2.1.2. *Clinic-based upper limb rehabilitation therapy*

Among the earliest robotic upper limb rehabilitation systems is the MIT-Manus. As shown in Fig. 2(a), the MIT MANUS is a planar, two-revolute-joint robot which assists acute stroke patients in sliding their arms across a tabletop. Developed to influence the recovery process, subjects perform a series of movement tasks such as moving targets and tracing figures, and receive mechanical assistance from the robot if needed. Functional motor recovery was evident in two sets of trials, 3 years apart, in which significant improvements in motor recovery were reported for the treatment groups.[29]

Exoskeletons for force feedback and gravity support exoskeletons have shown significant improvements in clinical measures of stroke patients.[30] The ARM Guide shown in Fig. 2(b) is active-assistive robotic device that serves as a therapeutic and diagnostic tool for evaluation of several key motor impairments, including abnormal tone, coordination, and weakness. As a therapeutic tool, the device provides a means to implement and evaluate active assistive therapy for the arm.

Force feedback devices quantify the performance of a patient for measuring improvement. The Rutgers Master II haptic depicted in Fig. 2(c) serves as an

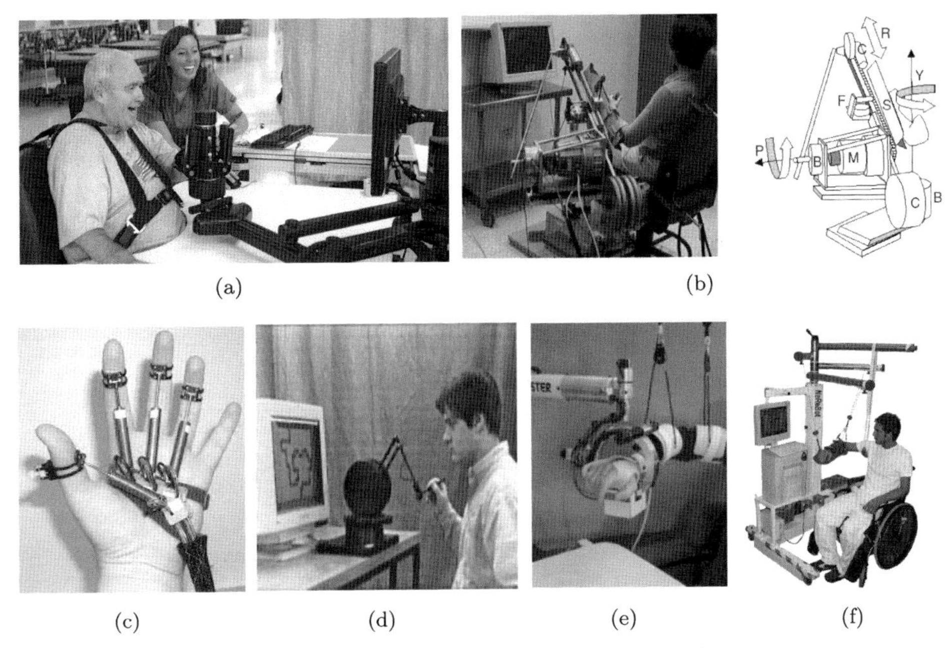

Figure 2. Examples of clinic-based robotic therapy devices for upper limb extremities: (a) MIT-Manus,[29] (b) ARM guide,[34] (c) Rutgers Master II,[35] (d) Phantom-based therapy,[31] (e) Haptic master,[33] and (f) NeRebot.[36]

instrumented interface to sample hand position and provides suitable resistive forces. The enhanced system includes an input device (cyber glove) and immersive virtual environment (VE)-based exercise protocols from hand movement studies. Another force feedback phantom therapy developed by Bardorfer *et al.*[31,32] utilizes a haptic interface as a kinematic measuring device for providing tactile feedback to the patient (see Fig. 2(d)).

The Haptic master in Fig. 2(e) is a 3-DOF robot that interfaces with a haptic display. Used for rehabilitating stroke patients,[33] the Haptic master is part rehabilitation device for training arm movements by attaching the patients' wrist to the end-effector of the robot. Two ropes of a weight-lifting system support the arm against gravity and interactive support for patient movements is enabled by admittance control strategies.

The NeReBot (NEuroREhabilitation roBOT) is a 3-DOF wire-driven robot that is also used for post-stroke upper limb rehabilitation. Three wires independently driven by three electric motors (Fig. 2(f)) are connected to the patient's upper limb by means of a splint and are supported by a transportable frame located above the patient. By controlling the wire length, rehabilitation treatment can be delivered over a wide working space.

2.1.3. *Translating from the clinic- to home-based rehabilitation*

Despite their demonstrated effectiveness, the significant logistic constrains (infrastructure, cost, and trained personnel) often limit deployments to at least outpatient clinic settings. In contrast, most home-based rehabilitation employ relatively simple passive devices, if at all.

Thus, it is in the final stages of translating these advances to the home-based rehabilitation setting that things have slowed, principally due to the lack of easily available specialized equipment that is affordable by each patient. For example, the recommended home-based exercises for OA patients, who are (mildly) affected by the disease, are principally unassisted exercise prescriptions. However, the lack of structured exercise and monitoring of performance (by therapist or machine) can lessen the achievable benefits as they may not appropriately stress the affected limbs/joints/muscles.

2.2. *Traditional home-based rehabilitation*

While inpatient therapy remains the preferred means for rehabilitation (in terms of recovery times), home-based programs have gained importance and relevance due to the considerable flexibility afforded in tailoring the scheduling, intensity and duration of the rehabilitation regimen.

2.2.1. *Self-directed rehabilitation exercises at home*

Recent evidence highlights the benefits of home-based rehabilitation as a viable approach to provide treatment for patients.[37] Figure 3 depicts various self-directed

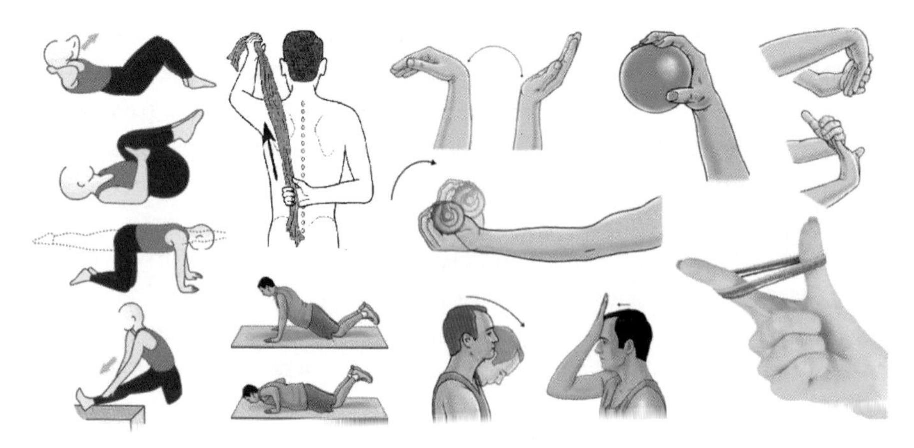

Figure 3. Self-directed exercises at home for rehabilitation including wrist stretch, wrist flexion–extension, grip strengthening, push-up, single knee to chest stretch, double knee to chest, isometric neck extension, etc.

Table 1. Highlights of comparative studies of between home-based and day hospital/outpatient therapies.

Author	Intervention	Period	Sample	Main Results
Anderson *et al.*[38,39]	Hospital versus home-based rehabilitation (RCT)	6 months	86	No difference in outcomes, lower costs in rehabilitation.
Byford *et al.*[40]	Short-term family placement scheme	3 months	120	Increased functional outcome, decreased cost
Gladman *et al.*[41]	Domiciliary versus hospital based rehabilitation	6 months	327	No difference in outcomes, cost in domiciliary service
Hui *et al.*[42]	Day hospital versus conventional care (RCT)	6 months	120	No difference in functional outcomes, no difference in cost
Young and Forster[43]	Home physiotherapy versus day hospital	8 weeks	95	No difference in functional outcomes, decreased cost in home physiotherapy

exercises and over-the-counter devices for home-based rehabilitation. Flexible intensity and duration of the rehabilitation regimen, and comparable outcomes with hospital functional gains are the benefits of home-based rehabilitation. However, the lack of a structured and monitored exercise program may reduce achievable benefits, and specialized exercise machines are limited.

Numerous studies have shown that a program of continuing self-directed exercises for home-bound patients, and supervised once a week by therapists, was as effective as outpatient day hospital therapy (and definitely more resource efficient). Table 1 highlights some comparative studies between home-based and day hospital/outpatient therapy, and supports the assumption that home-based rehabilitation may be more economical with comparable outcomes in terms of functional gains.

2.2.2. *Self-rehabilitation with devices at home*

For lower limb rehabilitation, the MOTOmed is shown in Fig. 4(b) and its cycling device with Functional Electrical Simulation (FES) is illustrated in Fig. 4(c). Rhythmic arm cycling was shown to increase upper limb performance and reduce arm spasticity.[44] To date, there are several commercially available training devices for stroke patients which are affordable for home-based rehabilitation. In Fig. 4(a),

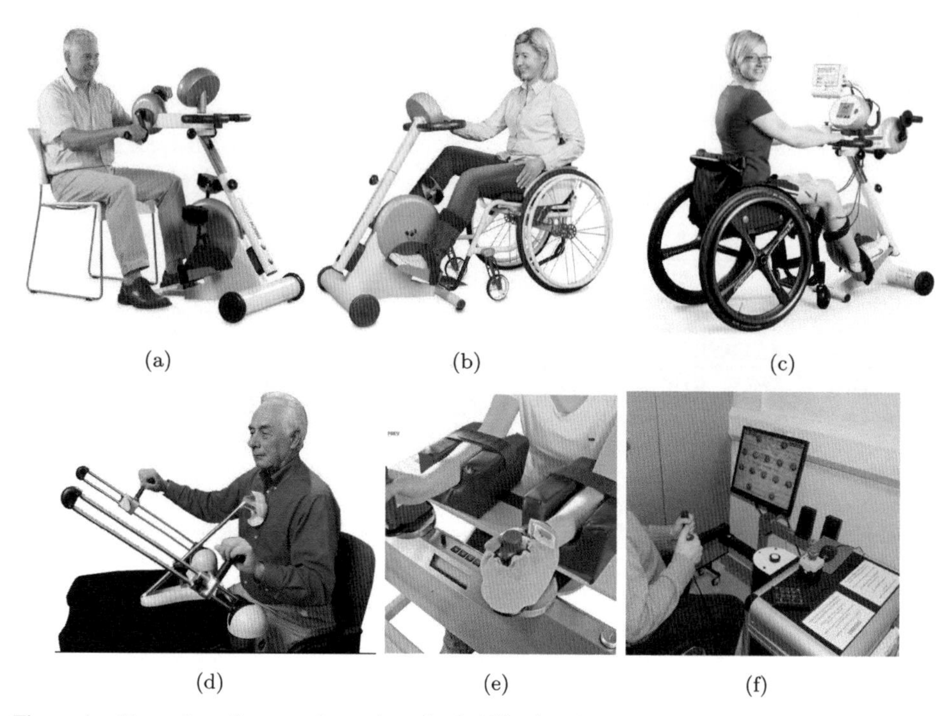

Figure 4. Examples of current home-based rehabilitation devices at home: (a) MOTOmed viva2 offers a number of preassigned therapy programs for upper limbs from which the user can select a suitable training flow, (b) MOTOmed by Reck (courtesy of eurorehab.com), (c) The MOTOmed lower limb cycling device with Functional Electrical Simulation (FES), (d) Tailwind/BATRAC for bimanual rehabilitation, (e) Bi-Manu-Track, and (f) Home-based Computer Assisted Arm Rehabilitation (hCAAR).

the affordable MOTOmed arm cycling training device is customizable and can be used passively, or with motor-assist, or active resist.

Self-rehabilitation using bi-manual rehabilitation is very well suited for home-based stroke therapy since much of the required force could be provided by the person's sound limb with minimal or no external assistance required from a caregiver or motor.[45] These devices rely solely on the patients' impaired arm to generate motion, but do not provide assistive forces. Recent research has shown that bimanual therapies target the brain stem pathways.[46] The study by Whitall *et al.*[47] (developers of the BATRAC as shown in Fig. 4(d)) reported significant improvement in the affected arm, with as little as one hour of training per week over several weeks. Improvements from 12% to 26% on two different motor improvement scales were evident with patients independently moving their hands along the linear slide with in-phase or out-of-phase motions.

Another passive bi-manual device, the Bi-Manu-Track, enables patients to perform forearm pro- and -supination and exercises to train wrist flexion and extension, as shown in Fig. 4(e). The entire effort to move the handles, including friction, is controlled by the sound limb. Because the Bi-Manu-Track addresses specifically both sides of the human musculoskeletal system, lost movements are reanimated with the assistance of the healthy arm.[48] The home-based Computer Assisted Arm Rehabilitation (hCAAR) robot (see Fig. 4(f)) comprises a joystick that is controlled by the weak upper limb to perform tasks shown on a computer monitor. The device assists movements depending on user ability, and statistically significant improvements have been reported.[49]

As discussed, although several home devices for upper limb rehabilitation are commercially available, complications related to balance and stability during standing or walking preclude the ready availability of home devices for lower limb rehabilitation.

2.3. *Recent advances in computer-enhanced home-based rehabilitation systems*

In recent years, advances in miniaturization of processors/sensors/actuators have created a new generation of smart embedded products that offer significant and cost-effective functionality and performance. For example, numerous commercial-off-the-shelf (COTS) computer-interface devices e.g. Kinect, the Wii balance board and Novint Falcon, are intended primarily for gaming applications. These not only sense a person's motions but they also register forces during such motions. Similar to the existing robotic therapy, these devices may serve as interfaces that stimulate human movement profiles, as well as create customizable patterns of active/passive motion and force assists respective to the user motions. Additional benefits come from their ability to quantitatively monitor (record/replay) the patient's performance and most importantly to post-process (analyze/compare) this data against various normal cohorts. Thus, it is believed that there is a class of problems where low-cost commercial-off-the-shelf (COTS) devices, coupled with rehabilitation therapy protocols, open up the possibility of widespread deployment as truly inexpensive home-based trainers.

Several research groups have been motivated to create the framework, algorithms, and augmentative hardware and software to facilitate interactive performance as well as an online method for control/tasking/updating of a rehabilitation regimen.

2.3.1. *Home-based upper limb rehabilitation*

In recent years, by leveraging, the power of the internet real-time video transmission has come to supplement audio and data transmission for telerehabilitation applications.[50] In a representative scenario, the clinic-based telerehabilitation

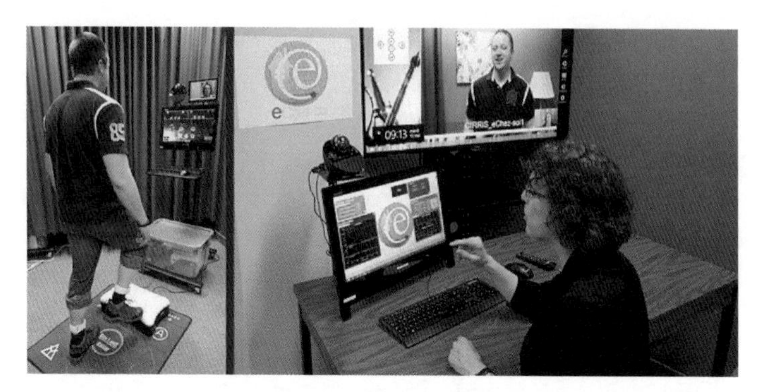

Figure 5. Delivering in-home telerehabilitation services.[52]

specialist observes the remote-clients tasks, and subsequently instructs/coach the home-based team (see Fig. 5). Real-time video teleconferencing provides a visual and explicit exchange of information during this process with significant consumer (both patient and therapist) acceptance. However, multiple camera views may be necessary for the therapist to recognize patients' activity patterns, thereby increasing the infrastructure (cameras, network-bandwidth) requirements of such a telecounseling approach. To date, quantitative assessment has been difficult owing to inexpensive videoconferencing systems, which are unable to leverage the quantitative computational infrastructure to assist the assessment.

Early home-based, computer-enhanced rehabilitation prototypes focused on telerehabilitation, such as home-based telerehabilitation. The Training-Wilmington Robotic Exoskeleton (T-WREX), developed at the University of California-Irvine,[51] was designed for adults with significant arm weakness resulting from stroke, and provided intense movement training without continuous supervision of a therapist. In a 5-DOF passive anti-gravity orthosis and computer workstation, the orthosis relieved the weight of the arm using elastic bands attached around its frame.

However, devices tend to be specialized/custom-built which limit ubiquitous access. As a result, researchers have begun to examine the use of truly low-cost, mass-produced COTS force-feedback devices (commonly for gaming applications) for rehabilitation therapy applications. A modified COTS force-feedback joystick (Microsoft Sidewinder) with an arm support was coupled to a target tracking scenario to serve as an exercise protocol and implemented as a downloadable web-based, Java applet game. While emphasis was on examining the use of artificial assistive forces (generated via the force feedback joystick) on mediating arm movements, the quantitative measurement capabilities to facilitate diagnosis were not explored.

The feasibility of patients undertaking therapy at home was further evaluated to facilitate training duration without financially burdening the client's caregivers

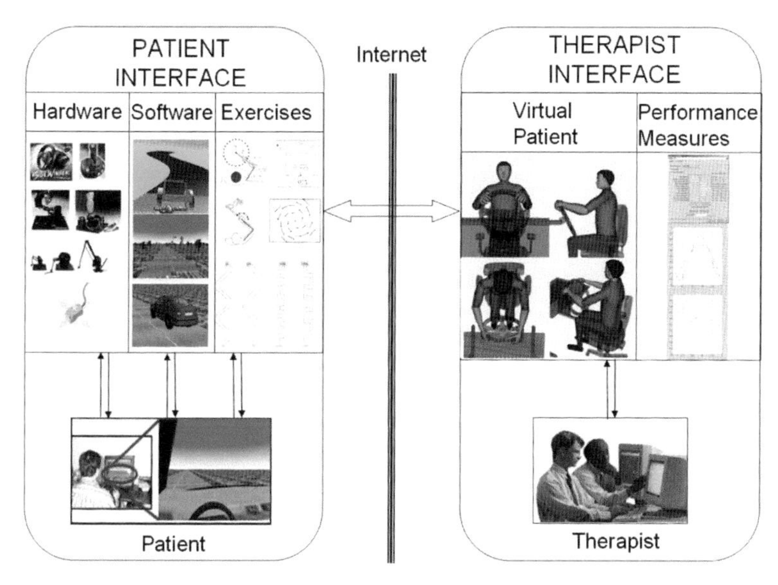

Figure 6. Haptic Virtual Driving Environment (hVDE) for individualized interactive telerehabilitation.

or impacting their ability to participate in other activities. A PS3 gaming console was transformed into a rehabilitation station by integrating a sensing glove, a customized therapy-oriented games.[53–55]

At the University at Buffalo, a haptic telerehabilitation framework (shown in Fig. 6) was developed for home-based rehabilitation of patients with upper limb dysfunction.[56] A COTS haptic force-feedback driving wheel interfaced with a PC to create a haptic Virtual Driving Environment (hVDE). Coupling this framework with movement protocols structured as driving exercises along paths of varying complexity was key to the creation of an inexpensive, immersive, and individualized personal-movement trainer.

Many research groups are therefore beginning to consider augmenting video information with collected quantitative physiological information.[57] Such approaches have been intended principally for cardiac, respiratory and diabetes management, they have not been explored in the telerehabilitation context.

2.3.2. *Home-based lower limb rehabilitation*

We focus on the conservative, and more technically and economically feasible intervention by developing intelligent mechanical OA braces designed to not only passively constraint motion but also to redirect and reuse energy at various stages of the gait cycle. The OA brace is actively adjustable and articulated, incorporating external in-parallel elastic tendons, which modulate the transfer of stored spring energy to limb-segment potential energy at appropriate intervals

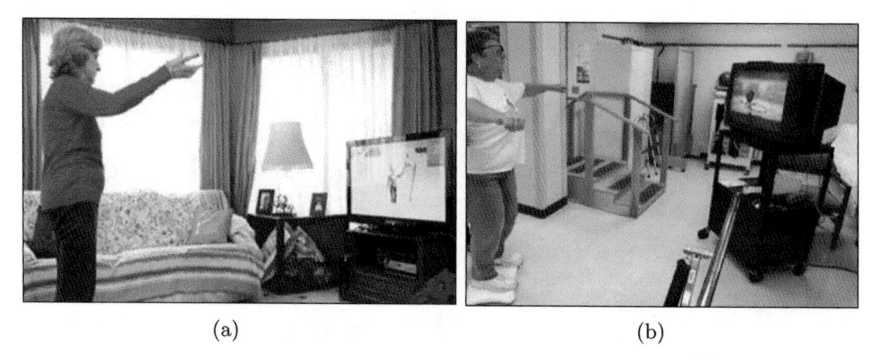

(a) (b)

Figure 7. Examples of home-based rehabilitation system by using (a) Kinect[26] and (b) Wii Balance Board.[28]

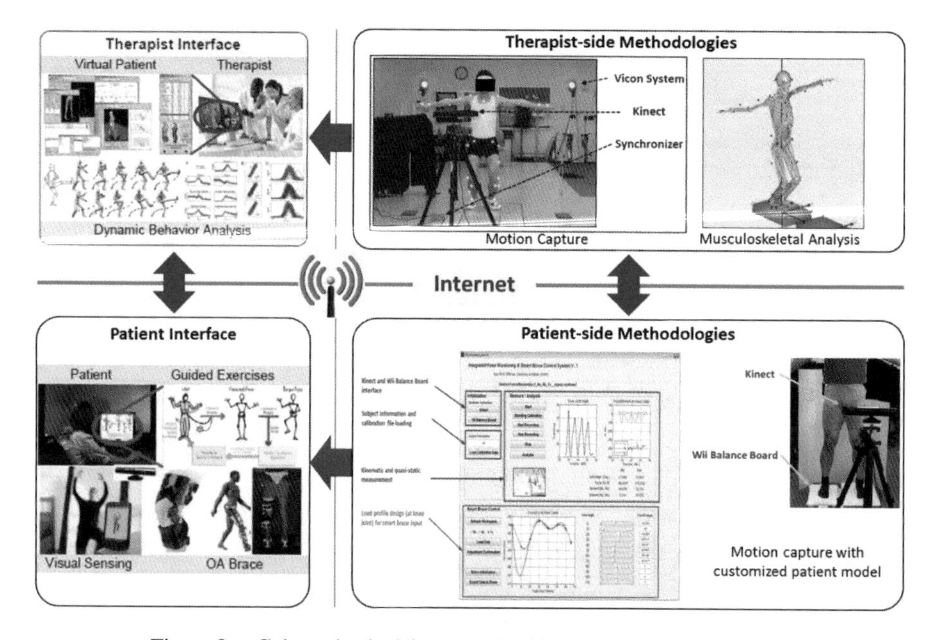

Figure 8. Cyber–physical framework of home-based rehabilitation.

of the gait cycle. Therefore, this low-cost, home-based hardware coupled with a customizable regimen of motion-based limb movement therapy (Fig. 7) has tremendous potential to make telerehabilitation services a viable option. A validated framework is necessary to facilitate both the quantitative diagnostic monitoring and individualized motor rehabilitation of limb dysfunction.

The overall cyber–physical framework consists of (i) Patient Interface (ultimately intended to be home-based) and (ii) Therapist Interface (intended to be at a remote central hospital location) that are connected through the Internet (Fig. 8).

The emphasis on modularity and bi-directional parametric coupling in all aspects of development of this framework is intended to facilitate "plug-in-play" functionality and to achieve distributed implementation on different computational platforms. As illustrated in the physical (left) module of Fig. 8, a knee OA patient at home interacts with a patient interface using the home-based COTS devices (Kinect sensor, Wii Balance Board) and OA brace, which serves as a manipulandum to quantitatively capture the patient motion, activity characteristics, and deploy customized exercises. By leveraging internet-based networking, such a patient interface could then be connected with a therapist interface at a knee OA rehabilitation center. The remote rehabilitation therapist would then be able to monitor this patient's sensorimotor performance.

3. Current Challenges in Home-based Computerized Exercise Systems (CES)

Biomechanical assessment of human movement typically involves acquiring kinematic (movement) and kinetic (force) measures of normative and aberrant mechanics with emphasis on comparing compensatory musculoskeletal adaptations with rehabilitative strategies to restore normal function. In what follows, we will discuss some of the challenges entailed and the advances being made to support home-based CES.

- **3D Motion Analysis:** A motion capture system is used to acquire 3D kinematic information about human movement by tracking reflective surface markers placed over segments, thereby providing a quantitative assessment of the movement pattern.
- **Force Platforms:** Force platforms are used to measure the ground reaction forces during various activities and the data is often combined with kinematic measures acquired from motion analysis using link segment modeling to calculate joint moments and joint reaction forces.
- **Electromyography:** The electrical activity skeletal muscle can be monitored simultaneously during the movement performance using electrodes affixed over the muscle, and the relative amount and sequencing of muscle activity can be monitored simultaneously.
- **Data Post-processing and Analysis:** Proprietary 3D analysis software is needed to acquire and quantify 3D biomechanics modeling, analysis, and reporting functions.

The digital revolution has prompted the development of new COTS low-cost computer-interface-devices for capturing patient performance. The Microsoft Kinect camera is a motion sensing device that reconstructs 3D full-body images from depth and color video information under any ambient light condition. Kinect's

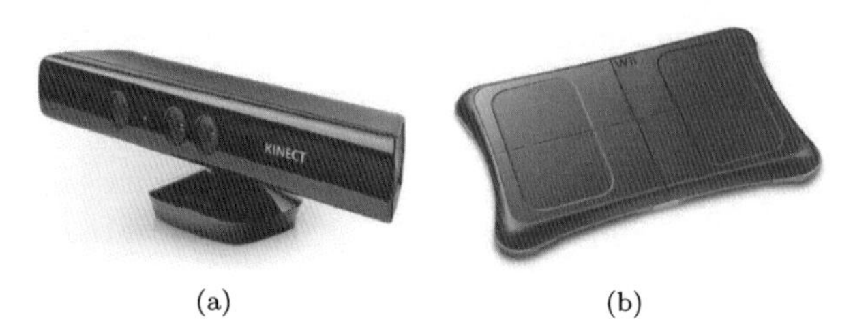

(a) (b)

Figure 9. (a) Kinect by Microsoft and (b) Wii Balance Board by Nintendo.

depth camera uses infrared projection to detect the distance of objects from it. This depth image makes it easy for proprietary software to detect the "skeleton" of the person in front of it. Various software development kits and libraries track the skeleton figure and process the kinematic data of the person recorded from the camera.

3.1. *Human exercise measurement*

Human motion- and force-capture systems have played a significant role in a variety of product-design, biomechanics and ergonomics settings for over a quarter-century. Translating these advances to home-based rehabilitation is where momentum has slowed principally due to affordable measurement systems. Thus, we believe there is a class of pathologies where low-cost COTS devices, coupled with rehabilitation therapy protocols, open up the possibility of widespread deployment as a truly inexpensive home-based treatment modality.

3.1.1. *Limitations of Kinect and Wii Balance Board*

The Kinect/Wii-based system (Fig. 9) offers an opportunity to track human motion in real-time at a fraction of the cost of conventionally-equipped gait labs. Together with computational human modeling and analysis tools, this offers an opportunity to potentially gain insight into functional performance of humans outside the restrictive gait or biomechanics labs. However, multiple factors need to be considered in supporting the deployment of such a framework. There exist significant differences in the capabilities and ease-of-use between the clinic-based and home-based tools, necessitating a careful evaluation. The Kinect system streams color image, depth image data and can recognize and track human motion up to 30 Hz in the frontal plane. The Kinect can recognize up to six human objects in the field of view but only two objects can be tracked in detail. Kinect's skeletal tracking recognizes users facing the sensor and tracks persons within 0.8 to 4.0 m from the camera, suggesting a practical range of 1.2–3.5 m. Evidence suggests that Kinect depends critically on the person's location within the workspace.[58] As shown in Fig. 10,

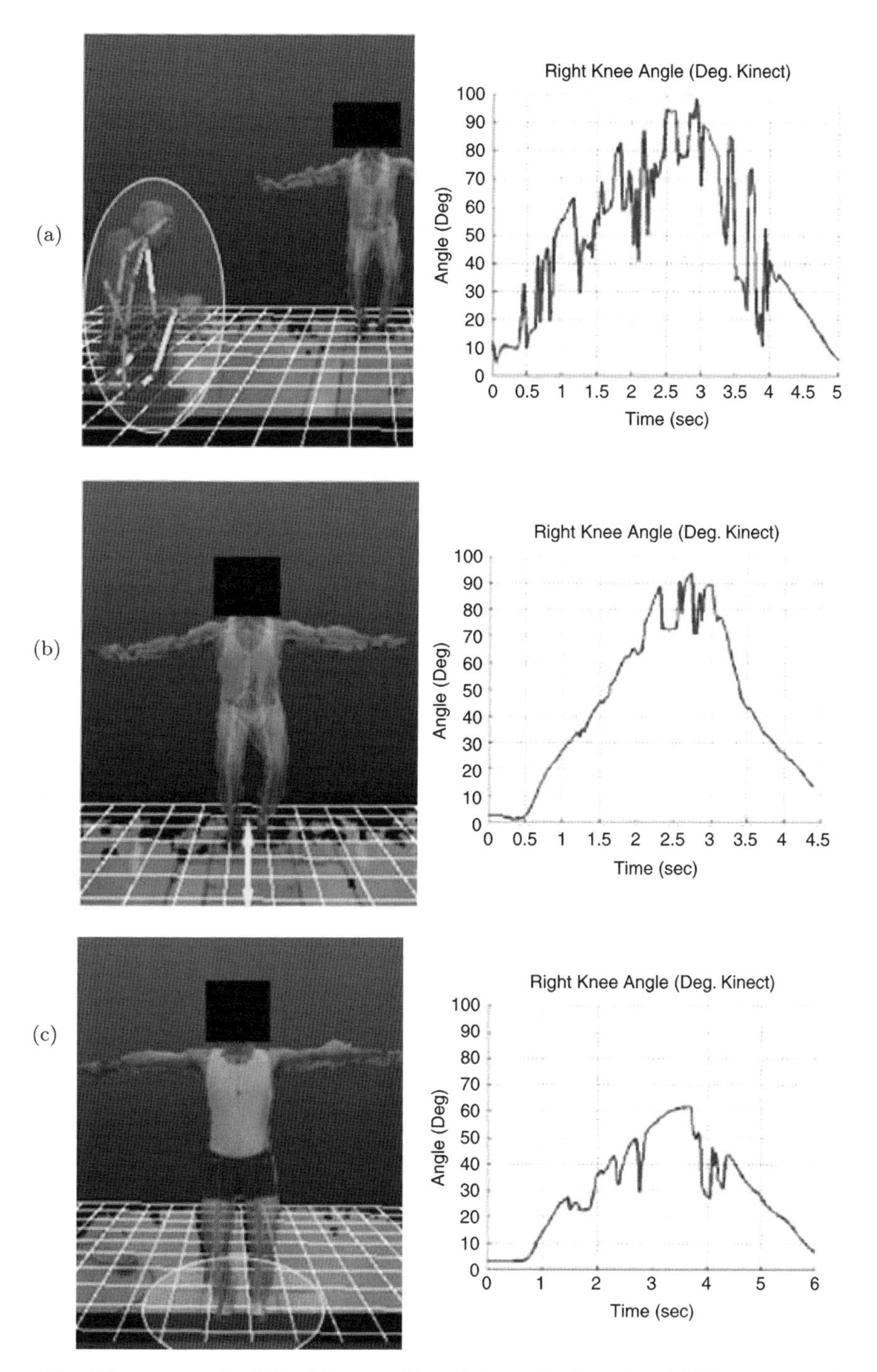

Figure 10. Kinect system's skeletal frame and knee joint angle data when (a) Kinect system detects the second subject, (b) and (c) part of body is not in the workspace, and (d) subject is located in ideal position.[58]

(d)

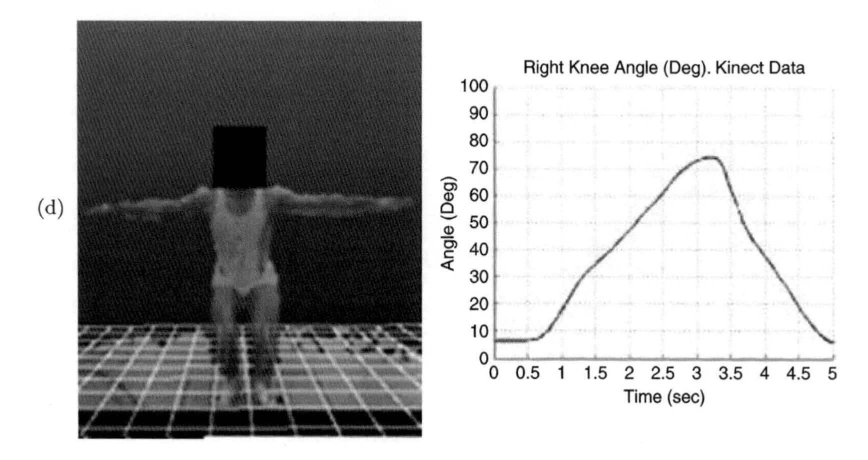

Figure 10. *(Continued)*

the appearance of a second person or object diminishes the ability to track the primary subject. Thus, although it is able to simultaneously track multiple human subjects: (i) recordings were restricted to one subject at a time and (ii) all body segments were visible within the workspace. Figure 10(a) illustrates the effect of a second subject, (b) and (c) depict the relationship between subject's position in the workspace and Kinect performance, while (d) illustrates the ideal subject location for motion capture and corresponding inferred knee joint angles. For more information about the limitation of Kinect, see Ref. [58].

The Nintendo Wii Balance Board (WBB) as shown in Fig. 9(b) is similar to a force platform although it is intended primarily as a gaming device that measures the center of gravity and weight of the subject. Although developed for entertainment, it has the potential to be an inexpensive and readily accessible vertical force measuring device that can be used for home-based rehabilitation. The accuracy and repeatability of individual WBB weight sensors reportedly have an accuracy of ± 0.61 kg and repeatability error of ± 0.52 kg,[59] but they are different in resolution, accuracy and degree of freedom compared to force plates.

3.2. *Human motion analysis*

Clinicians who treat human movement pathologies not only assess movement but also simultaneous neuromuscular function both before and after treatment interventions. However, synthesizing detailed descriptors of the elements of the neuromusculoskeletal system with measurements of movement to create an integrated understanding of normal movement, and establishing a scientific basis for correcting abnormal movement remain major challenges. Using experiments alone to understand movement dynamics has two fundamental limitations. First, important variables, including the forces generated by the muscles, are not generally measurable. Second, it is difficult to establish cause–effect relationships in complex dynamic systems from experimental data alone.[60]

Dynamic simulation of movement that integrates anthropometric, anatomic and physiologic elements of the neuromusculoskeletal system combined with multi-joint mechanics provides such a framework. Muscle-driven dynamic simulations complement experimental approaches by providing estimates of muscle and joint forces, which are difficult to measure experimentally. Simulations may also identify cause–effect relationships allowing for "what if?" studies to be performed where for example, the excitation pattern of a muscle can be altered and the resulting motion can be observed.

Proprietary 3D analysis software is needed to acquire and quantify 3D biomechanics modeling, analysis, and reporting functions. The AnyBody (AnyBody Technology Inc.)[61] modeling system is a computational framework for simulating the human musculoskeletal performance, used to estimate individual muscle force, joint force and moment, metabolism, elastic energy and antagonistic muscle actions. An alternative is OpenSim, a free open-source platform for modeling, simulating, and analyzing the neuromusculoskeletal system. OpenSim,[62] developed and maintained on Simtk.org, provides a platform on which a library of simulations are being tested, analyzed, and improved by the biomechanics community through multi-institutional collaboration. Visual3D (Visual 3D, C-Motion Inc.) is another commercial analysis tool for biomechanical modeling and analysis, which is used to measure and quantify movement as collected by a 3D motion capture systems.

3.3. *Appropriate design*

For modeling, analyzing and understanding of human–robot interaction, the musculoskeletal model of the human body as well as multi-body dynamics of exoskeleton need to be integrated and modeled. Therefore, the model is able to estimate the muscle activities in cooperative motions and enables the design analysis and optimization of robotic exoskeleton.

Exoskeletons, designed to augment human performance, comprise an articulated mechanical structure, with actuators, or visco-elastic components, sensors and control elements. They are also intended to improve rehabilitation for people with disabilities caused by strokes,[63] muscle disease, SCIs,[64] etc. The state of the art for lower limb exoskeletons presented by Dollar and Herr[63] showed that having knowledge of the biomechanics of walking is important to build an exoskeleton that can interact with the user with minimal chances of harm. For training patients undergoing rehabilitation with an exoskeleton, physical human–robot interaction is a major concern for safe and comfortable usage. For example, the PACER[65,66] is a cable-driven end-effector-based exoskeleton that directly integrates with the human arm for safe human–robot interaction. Another articulated cable-driven exoskeleton for the lower limbs is the ROPES[64,67] that interfaces with the lower limbs. The comprehensive design and analysis of ROPES in assisting with lower-extremity rehabilitation and analyzing its performance have been examined by Alamdari.[68]

Compared to exoskeletons, braces employ simpler and less complex designs and focus primarily on passive structural equilibration of the externally applied loads. A new class of "semi-active" (adjustable passive spring-magnetic fluid/dampers) or "active" (powered actuators) braces for rehabilitation has spawned development (see Fig. 11). Intelligent mechanical braces equipped with electronic sensors, i.e. gyroscopes and tri-axial accelerometers, detect respective rotations and accelerations and actively modulate knee motion. Potentiometers measure joint angles, foot switches are used to identify stance and swing during the gait cycle, and dampers control the knee during the loading response phase of gait. Similar to existing robotic devices, such apparatuses serve as interfaces to stimulate movement, as well as to create customizable patterns of active/passive motion and force assists to user motions.

Traditionally, the design of exoskeletons (from choice of configuration to selection of parameters) as well as the process of fitting the exoskeleton (to the individual user/patient) has largely depended on intuition and/or practical experience of the designer/physiotherapist. However, improper exoskeleton design and/or incorrect fitting may cause buildup of significant residual forces/torques (both at the joint and fixation site). Performance can be further compromised by the innate complexity of human motions and need to accommodate the immense individual variability (in terms of patient-anthropometric, motion-envelopes and musculoskeletal-strength).

Recent research on exoskeletons design has examined ways of improving flexibility, wearability as well as reducing the overall weight. Very few exoskeletal systems, however, have succeeded in satisfying all these criteria due to the complexities engaged in human joint motions and loading. Some robotic exoskeletons are shown in Fig. 12.

Our initial brace design was configured with an adjustable passive torque-assist, focusing on knee flexion–extension, to assist with squatting.[58] In future designs, addressing multiple degrees of freedom is critical for real-world deployment of smart knee-braces, and currently remains an active research endeavor.

3.3.1. *User-specific customization*

There is considerable variation of performance, function and disability across individuals in a population and hence rehabilitative devices and services have to

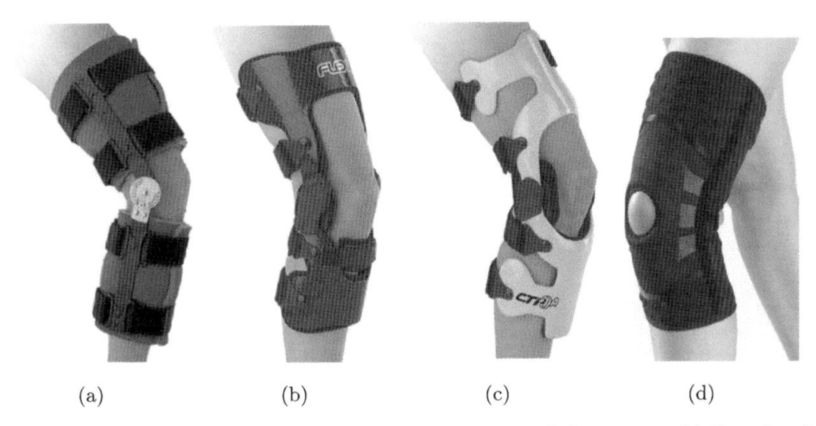

(a) (b) (c) (d)

Figure 11. (a) Rehabilitation knee braces by Ossur courtesy of Ossur.com, (b) Functional knee brace: Unilateral and bilateral hinged upright functional knee braces by Ossur, (c) off-the-shelf and custom medial offloader knee brace by Ossur, and (d) patellofemoral braces MxSpider knee by Ossur.

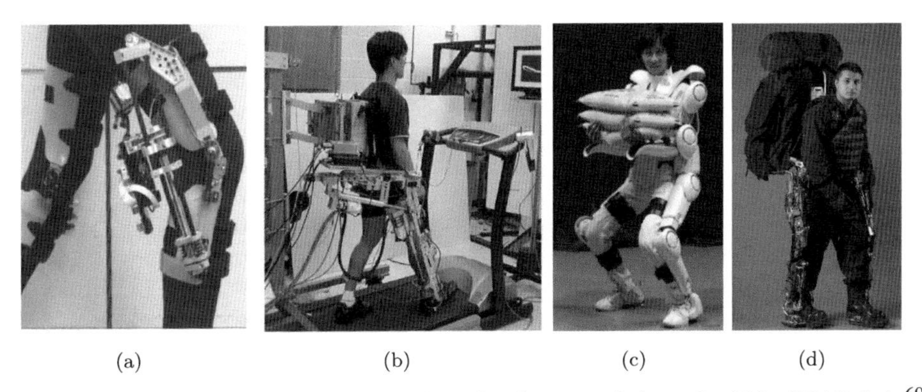

(a) (b) (c) (d)

Figure 12. Robotic exoskeletons (a) Quasi-passive knee exoskeleton by Yale GRAB Lab,[69] (b) active leg exoskeleton (ALEX)[70] (c) HAL-5 exoskeleton,[71] and (d) University of California at Berkeley BLEEX exoskeleton.[72]

be one-of-a-kind and subject specific.[73] However, traditional user-customization models have had limited success. On the one hand, categorizing individuals into one of the many "stock sizes" (on the basis of limited physiological measurements) and using "off-the-rack" products (with a few adjustable features) results in poor fit and diminished performance.

On the other hand, adopting a "tailor-made" approach for enhanced user-customization comes with the significant expense for skilled manual labor and an iterative fitting process. In light of this, new paradigms for rapid development of inexpensive, high quality rehabilitation aids customized to the specific needs of the individual patients have emerged over the past decade.[74] As such, implementing an automated process of deriving user-specified and iterative design refinement

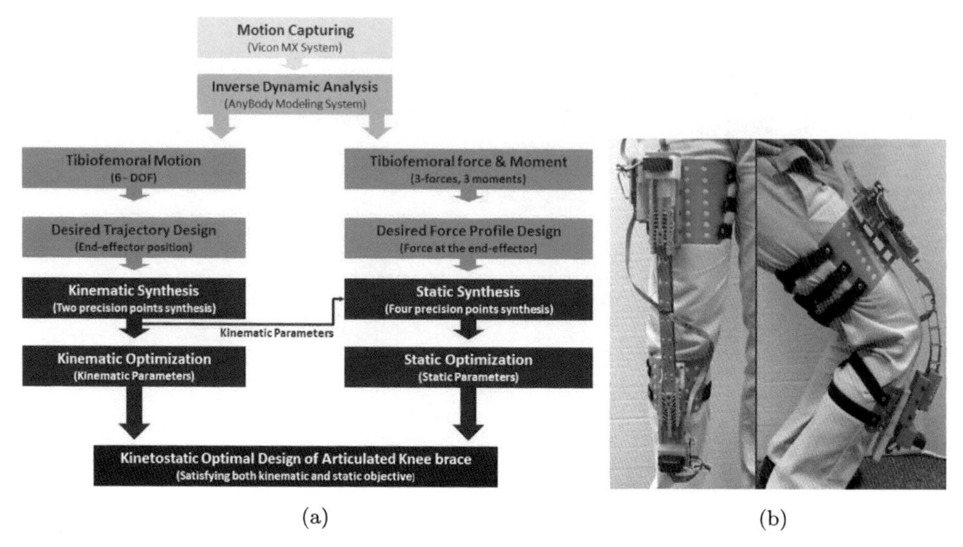

Figure 13. (a) The process of Kinetostatic optimization for articulated (4-bar linkage) knee brace and (b) semi-active PCCP/PEB knee brace.[58]

with concomitant speedup and cost reductions that facilitates the delivery of rehabilitation services is one of the goals of this work.

Most knee braces and exoskeleton designs depend on the intuition and experience of a therapist. Knee braces require customization to ensure proper fit to the thigh and shank circumferences. Therefore, we introduced a quantitative customization method, such as kinetostatic optimization and screw theoretic analysis, for knee brace design customization (see Fig. 13).[58]

4. Quantitative Progressive Exercise Rehabilitation Regimen

Most rehabilitation protocols are individualized and progressive in nature to some extent with appropriate, valid and reliable quantitative techniques. One such broad-based rehabilitative paradigm is Quantitative Progressive Exercise Rehabilitation (QPER), which is based on the quantitative measure of physiological and functional deficits of the individual[75,76] while addressing some of the limitations of standard rehabilitation strategies.

Specifically, (i) the physiological changes that occur with development and/or aging, (ii) the pathophysiologic changes that occur as a result of dystonia or disability together with the appropriate quantitative physiologic and functional deficits measurements are considered. The most suitable treatments for the individual in terms of the individual's indications and contraindications for exercise (including appropriate mode, intensity, frequency and duration of exercise) are then prescribed based on exercise physiology principles. Additional factors include immersion designed to encourage high rates of compliance and adherence; ease of program implementation; and overall cost-effectiveness.

Such QPER strategy has been successfully employed in the quantitative evaluation and treatment of several disability groups, including the frail[77] and the elderly,[78] and persons with OA[75,77] and juvenile arthritis. Our intent is to adapt QPER to allow remote prescription of individualized and progressive exercise rehabilitation programs.

There is considerable evidence that directly links functional recovery to the duration, frequency, regularity, and intensity of structured repetitive rehabilitation therapy.[75,79] Quantitative Progressive Exercise Rehabilitation addresses the limitations of standard rehabilitation strategies by measuring the appropriate physiological and functional deficits so that the progress of the underlying disease can be assessed and monitored, and appropriate therapies prescribed. However, success is dependent upon the availability of quantitative data, either acquired or simulated. In lieu of *ad hoc* behavioral conditioning cues, the quantitative models developed above will be used to provide a formal method for composing rehabilitation regimes that are customized to the individual and readily adjustable to accommodate progress of the disease and/or recovery.

A staged iterative process for inclusion of the QPER paradigm into the proposed rehabilitation framework is proposed. (1) Initially, parameterized exercise tasks will be broken down into important physiological and functional aspects, i.e. range of motion/position of different joints or links; strength, endurance and speed needed to perform tasks; muscle groups and actions involved. The emphasis will be on the selection and use of minimal numbers of orthogonal sets of measurements to facilitate maximal leveraging of the QPER approach; (2) Quantitative measurement of these variables will then be conducted using the initial prototype client interface to determine the parametric ranges on all of these variables to complete the task correctly; and (3) Each candidate exercise path will be broken down into its component parts in terms of the effects on the measured parameters. In effect, the minimal function required by the patient to correctly complete the task will be determined and then used in the determination of the QPER therapy program. The iterative nature is due to the fact that as the library of exercises is developed, step (2) needs to be repeated for each additional entry.

5. Example Implementation

A home-based rehabilitation prototype will integrate a measuring system, smart knee brace and host system. The measuring system comprises both the Kinect and Wii Balance Board to record both kinematic and force measures of respective participants. The Smart knee brace is considered a compliant mechanism, which

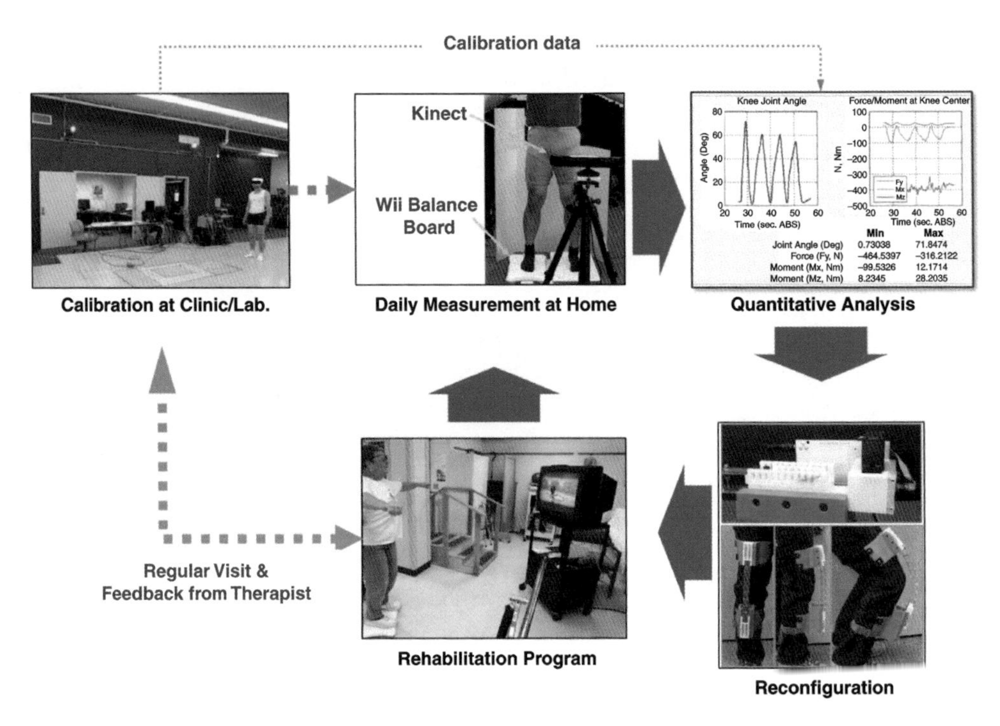

Figure 14. Home-based rehabilitation system scenario.

will consist of a servo motor, IMU sensor and a microcontroller which will communicate with the host system. The host system to be operated using a GUI will record subject's motion data transmitted from the measuring system and analyze it to modify parameters of the smart knee brace. By changing parameters, the smart knee brace provides a customized force/torque profile to the users which is based on current measurement and prescription by the therapist, as shown in Fig. 14.

During the calibration process either in the laboratory or clinic, all kinematic information (including marker and sensor position) is collected and saved into a calibration file and later transferred to the host PC in the patient's house, as shown in Fig. 14.

After calibration (in laboratory and/or clinic), patients recorded their motions using the low-cost sensor (Kinect) and PC-based application. Kinematic and quasi-static data captured by Kinect sensor and Wii balance board were transmitted to the host system, which then calculated knee load profiles during quasi-static/dynamic trails, then the desired force/torque profile based on pre-programmed prescription or by therapist can be accessed remotely.

The semi-active smart knee brace has the capability of customizing force/torque profiles in a similar level of fully-actuated exoskeletons with less power consumption, and simpler, lighter configuration. The host system that transfers the desired loading profile to the smart knee braces minimizes the error between the actual and desired knee force/torque.[58]

6. Conclusion

As previously described, home-based rehabilitation not only reduces patients' stay at the clinic, and improves access to rehabilitation, but also reduces cost, saves time, and enhances compliance of monitoring. However, development in technology accelerates the transition to a new paradigm, computer-enhanced rehabilitation at home. The new features in this paradigm are: (i) convergence of computerization, communication and miniaturization, (ii) creation of a new class of COTS, and (iii) empowering the home-based paradigm.

This paradigm has opened up immense possibilities for designing a system with integrated sensing and analysis for data-driven healthcare decision-making. This system involves integration of sensing, data acquisition, and implementing data-, information- and knowledge-driven examination of healthcare decision making processes.

References

1. C. Warlow, J. Van Gijn, M. S. Dennis, J. M. Wardlaw, J. M. Bamford, G. J. Hankey, P. A. Sandercock, G. Rinkel, P. Langhorne, C. Sudlow, *et al.* (2008). *Stroke: Practical Management.*
2. J. Patton, S. L. Small and W. Zev Rymer. (2008). Functional restoration for the stroke survivor: informing the efforts of engineers, *Topics in Stroke Rehabilitation* 15(6):521–541.
3. S. E. Fasoli, H. I. Krebs, J. Stein, W. R. Frontera, R. Hughes and N. Hogan. (2004). Robotic therapy for chronic motor impairments after stroke: Follow-up results, *Archives of Physical Medicine and Rehabilitation* 85(7):1106–1111.
4. L. Murphy, T. A. Schwartz, C. G. Helmick, J. B. Renner, G. Tudor, G. Koch, A. Dragomir, W. D. Kalsbeek, G. Luta and J. M. Jordan. (2008). Lifetime risk of symptomatic knee osteoarthritis, *Arthritis Care and Research* 59(9):1207–1213.
5. S. L. Murphy, D. M. Smith and N. B. Alexander. (2008). Measuring activity pacing in women with lower-extremity osteoarthritis: a pilot study, *The American Journal of Occupational Therapy: Official Publication of the American Occupational Therapy Association* 62(3):329.
6. K. D. Gross and H. J. Hillstrom. (2008). Noninvasive devices targeting the mechanics of osteoarthritis, *Rheumatic Disease Clinics of North America* 34(3):755–776.
7. J. M. Hootman and C. G. Helmick. (2006). Projections of us prevalence of arthritis and associated activity limitations, *Arthritis and Rheumatism* 54(1):226–229.
8. R. Amara. (2010). *Health and Health Care: The Forecast the Challenge* (2nd Edition). Jossey-Bass (A Wiley Company), CA, USA.
9. T. N. Lindenfeld, T. E. Hewett and T. P. Andriacchi. (1997). Joint loading with valgus bracing in patients with varus gonarthrosis, *Clinical Orthopaedics and Related Research* 344:290–297.
10. S. L. Wolf, D. E. Lecraw, L. A. Barton and B. B. Jann. (1989). Forced use of hemiplegic upper extremities to reverse the effect of learned nonuse among chronic stroke and head-injured patients, *Experimental Neurology* 104(2):125–132.

11. E. Taub, N. Miller, T. Novack, E. Cook 3rd, W. Fleming, C. Nepomuceno, J. Connell and J. Crago. (1993). Technique to improve chronic motor deficit after stroke, *Archives of Physical Medicine and Rehabilitation* 74(4):347–354.
12. L. Kahn, M. Zygman, W. Rymer and D. Reinkensmeyer. (2001). Effect of robot-assisted and unassisted exercise on functional reaching in chronic hemiparesis, in *Engineering in Medicine and Biology Society, 2001. Proceedings of the 23rd Annual International Conference of the IEEE* 2:1344–1347.
13. D. J. Reinkensmeyer, N. Hogan, H. I. Krebs, S. L. Lehman, P. S. Lum and D. J. Newman. (2000). Rehabilitators, robots, and guides: New tools for neurological rehabilitation, in *Biomechanics and Neural Control of Posture and Movement*. Springer, New York, NY, pp. 516–534.
14. D. Reinkensmeyer, C. Painter, S. Yang, E. Abbey and B. Kaino. (2000). An internet-based, force-feedback rehabilitation system for arm movement after brain injury, in *California State University–Northridge 15th Annual International Conference: Technology and Persons With Disabilities*, Los Angeles. Retrieved February 21, 2009.
15. D. J. Reinkensmeyer, B. D. Schmit and W. Z. Rymer. (1999). Assessment of active and passive restraint during guided reaching after chronic brain injury, *Annals of Biomedical Engineering* 27(6):805–814.
16. C. Bütefisch, H. Hummelsheim, P. Denzler and K.-H. Mauritz. (1995). Repetitive training of isolated movements improves the outcome of motor rehabilitation of the centrally paretic hand, *Journal of the Neurological Sciences* 130(1):59–68.
17. R. Dickstein, Y. Heffes, A. N. Laufer, Yocheved and E. L. Shabtai. (1997). Repetitive practice of a single joint movement for enhancing elbow function in hemiparetic patients, *Perceptual and Motor Skills* 85(3):771–785
18. H. M. Feys, W. J. De Weerdt, B. E. Selz, G. A. C. Steck, R. Spichiger, L. E. Vereeck, K. D. Putman and G. A. Van Hoydonck. (1998). Effect of a therapeutic intervention for the hemiplegic upper limb in the acute phase after stroke a single-blind, randomized, controlled multicenter trial, *Stroke* 29(4):785–792.
19. M. Paci, Physiotherapy based on the bobath concept for adults with post-stroke hemiplegia: a review of effectiveness studies, *Journal of Rehabilitation Medicine* 35(1):2–7.
20. J. H. Carr and R. B. Shepherd. (2003). *Stroke Rehabilitation: Guidelines for Exercise and Training to Optimize Motor Skill*. Butterworth-Heinemann Medical.
21. Y. Salem, E. Pappas, *et al.* (2009). Overground gait training for individuals with chronic stroke: A cochrane systematic review, *Journal of Neurologic Physical Therapy* 33(4): 179–186.
22. M. E. Dohring and J. J. Daly. (2008). Automatic synchronization of functional electrical stimulation and robotic assisted treadmill training, *IEEE Transactions on Neural Systems and Rehabilitation Engineering* 16(3):310–313.
23. P. Gregory, L. Edwards, K. Faurot, S. W. Williams and A. C. Felix. (2010). Patient preferences for stroke rehabilitation, *Topics in Stroke Rehabilitation* 17(5):394–400.
24. R. Bogey and T. George Hornby. (2007). Gait training strategies utilized in poststroke rehabilitation: are we really making a difference? *Topics in Stroke Rehabilitation* 14(6):1–8.
25. H. Barbeau and M. Visintin. (2003). Optimal outcomes obtained with body-weight support combined with treadmill training in stroke subjects, *Archives of Physical Medicine and Rehabilitation* 84(10):1458–1465.
26. E. B. Larson, M. Feigon, P. Gagliardo and A. Y. Dvorkin. (2013). Virtual reality and cognitive rehabilitation: a review of current outcome research, *NeuroRehabilitation* 34(4):759–772,.
27. S. Jezernik, G. Colombo and M. Morari. (2004). Automatic gait-pattern adaptation algorithms for rehabilitation with a 4-DOF robotic orthosis, *IEEE Transactions on Robotics and Automation* 20(3):574–582.

28. V. Fung, A. Ho, J. Shaffer, E. Chung and M. Gomez. (2012). Use of nintendo wii fit in the rehabilitation of outpatients following total knee replacement: a preliminary randomised controlled trial, *Physiotherapy* 98(3):183–188.
29. N. Hogan, H. I. Krebs, A. Sharon and J. Charnnarong. (1995). Interactive robotic therapist. US Patent 5,466,213.
30. R. J. Sanchez, J. Liu, S. Rao, P. Shah, R. Smith, T. Rahman, S. C. Cramer, J. E. Bobrow and D. J. Reinkensmeyer. (2006). Automating arm movement training following severe stroke: functional exercises with quantitative feedback in a gravity-reduced environment, *Neural Systems and Rehabilitation Engineering, IEEE Transactions on Neural Systems and Rehabilitation Engineering* 14(3):378–389.
31. A. Bardorfer, M. Munih, A. Zupan and A. Primožič. (2001). Upper limb motion analysis using haptic interface, *Mechatronics, IEEE/ASME Transactions on Mechatronics* 6(3):253–260.
32. J. Broeren, K. S. Sunnerhagen and M. Rydmark. (2007). A kinematic analysis of a haptic handheld stylus in a virtual environment: a study in healthy subjects, *Journal of NeuroEngineering and Rehabilitation* 4(1):13.
33. R. Q. Van der Linde, P. Lammertse, E. Frederiksen and B. Ruiter. (2002). The hapticmaster, a new high-performance haptic interface, in *Proceedings of Eurohaptics* 1–5.
34. D. J. Reinkensmeyer, L. E. Kahn, M. Averbuch, A. McKenna-Cole, B. D. Schmit and W. Z. Rymer. (2000). Understanding and treating arm movement impairment after chronic brain injury: progress with the arm guide, *Journal of Rehabilitation Research and Development* 37(6):653–662.
35. M. Bouzit, G. Burdea, G. Popescu and R. Boian. (2002). The rutgers master ii-new design force-feedback glove, *Mechatronics, IEEE/ASME Transactions on Mechatronics* 7(2):256–263.
36. G. Rosati, P. Gallina and S. Masiero. (2007). Design, implementation and clinical tests of a wire-based robot for neurorehabilitation, *Neural Systems and Rehabilitation Engineering, IEEE Transactions on Neural Systems and Rehabilitation Engineering* 15(4):560–569.
37. L. Legg and P. Langhorne (2004). Therapy-based rehabilitation for stroke patients living at home, *Stroke* 35(4):1022–1022.
38. C. Anderson, S. Rubenach, C. N. Mhurchu, M. Clark, C. Spencer and A. Winsor. (2000). Home or hospital for stroke rehabilitation? results of a randomized controlled trial i: Health outcomes at 6 months, *Stroke* 31(5):1024–1031.
39. C. Anderson, C. N. Mhurchu, P. M. Brown and K. Carter. (2002). Stroke rehabilitation services to accelerate hospital discharge and provide home-based care, *Pharmacoeconomics* 20(8): 537–552.
40. S. Byford, J. Geddes, M. Bonsall, *et al.* (1995). Stroke rehabilitation: a cost-effectiveness analysis of a placement scheme. Technical report.
41. J. Gladman, D. Whynes and N. Lincoln. (1994). Cost comparison of domiciliary and hospital-based stroke rehabilitation, *Age and Ageing* 23(3):241–245.
42. E. Hui, J. Woo, K. Or, L. Chu and K. Wong. (1995). A geriatric day hospital in hong kong: an analysis of activities and costs, *Disability and Rehabilitation* 17(8):418–423.
43. J. Young and A. Forster. (1991). Cost-analysis of geriatric day hospital-care, *Journal of Clinical and Experimental Gerontology* 13(4):247–262.
44. K. Diserens, N. Perret, S. Chatelain, S. Bashir, D. Ruegg, P. Vuadens and F. Vingerhoets. (2007). The effect of repetitive arm cycling on post stroke spasticity and motor control: repetitive arm cycling and spasticity, *Journal of the Neurological Sciences* 253(1):18–24.
45. K. B. Reed, I. Handžić and S. McAmis. (2014). Home-based rehabilitation: enabling frequent and effective training. In P. Artemiadis (Ed.), *Neuro-Robotics: From Brain Machine Interfaces to Rehabilitation Robotics*, Springer, pp. 379–403.

46. C. G. Burgar, P. S. Lum, P. C. Shor and H. M. Van der Loos. (2000). Development of robots for rehabilitation therapy: the palo alto va/stanford experience, *Journal of Rehabilitation Research and Development* 37(6):663–674.
47. J. Whitall, S. M. Waller, K. H. Silver and R. F. Macko. (2000). Repetitive bilateral arm training with rhythmic auditory cueing improves motor function in chronic hemiparetic stroke, *Stroke* 31(10):2390–2395.
48. S. Hesse, C. Werner, M. Pohl, J. Mehrholz, U. Puzich and H. I. Krebs. (2008). Mechanical arm trainer for the treatment of the severely affected arm after a stroke: a single-blinded randomized trial in two centers, *American Journal of Physical Medicine and Rehabilitation* 87(10): 779–788.
49. M. Sivan, J. Gallagher, S. Makower, D. Keeling, B. Bhakta, R. J. O'Connor and M. Levesley. (2014). Home-based computer assisted arm rehabilitation (hcaar) robotic device for upper limb exercise after stroke: results of a feasibility study in home setting, *Journal of Neuroengineering and Rehabilitation* 11(1):163.
50. S. Dhurjaty. (2001). Challenges of telerehabilitation in the home environment. In *Proceedings of the State of the Science Conference on Telerehabilitation* 89–93.
51. S. J. Housman, V. Le, T. Rahman, R. J. Sanchez and D. J. Reinkensmeyer. (2007). Arm-training with t-wrex after chronic stroke: preliminary results of a randomized controlled trial. In *Rehabilitation Robotics, IEEE 10th International Conference on ICORR* 562–568.
52. M. Tousignant, H. Moffet, S. Nadeau, C. Mérette, P. Boissy, H. Corriveau, F. Marquis, F. Cabana, P. Ranger, É. L. Belzile, *et al.* (2015). Cost analysis of in-home telerehabilitation for post-knee arthroplasty, *Journal of Medical Internet Research* 17(3):e83.
53. M. Huber, B. Rabin, C. Docan, G. C. Burdea, M. AbdelBaky and M. R. Golomb. (2010). Feasibility of modified remotely monitored in-home gaming technology for improving hand function in adolescents with cerebral palsy, *Information Technology in Biomedicine, IEEE Transactions on Information Technology in Biomedicine* 14(2):526–534.
54. M. Huber, B. Rabin, C. Docan, G. Burdea, M. E. Nwosu, M. Abdelbaky and M. R. Golomb. (2008). Playstation 3-based tele-rehabilitation for children with hemiplegia, in *Virtual Rehabilitation*, IEEE, 105–112.
55. M. R. Golomb, B. C. McDonald, S. J. Warden, J. Yonkman, A. J. Saykin, B. Shirley, M. Huber, B. Rabin, M. AbdelBaky, M. E. Nwosu, *et al.* (2010). In-home virtual reality videogame telerehabilitation in adolescents with hemiplegic cerebral palsy, *Archives of physical medicine and rehabilitation* 91(1):1–8.
56. C. Jadhav, P. Nair and V. Krovi. (2006). Individualized interactive home-based haptic telerehabilitation, *MultiMedia, IEEE* 13(3):32–39.
57. A. Cole and Q. Binh. (2002). Home care technologies for an aging population, in *Proceedings of the State of the Science Conference on Telerehabilitation.*
58. S. Jun. (2015). *A Home-based Rehabilitation System for Deficient Knee Patients.* PhD thesis, The State University of New York at Buffalo.
59. H. Bartlett, J. Bingham and L. H. Ting. (2012). Validation and calibration of the wii balance board as an inexpensive force plate, *American Society of Biomechanics* 1(2):3–4.
60. F. E. Zajac and M. E. Gordon. (1989). Determining muscle's force and action in multi-articular movement, *Exercise and Sport Sciences Reviews* 17(1):187–230.
61. M. Damsgaard, J. Rasmussen, S. T. Christensen, E. Surma and M. de Zee. (2006). Analysis of musculoskeletal systems in the anybody modeling system. *Simulation Modelling Practice and Theory* 14(8):1100–1111.
62. S. L. Delp, F. C. Anderson, A. S. Arnold, P. Loan, A. Habib, C. T. John, E. Guendelman and D. G. Thelen. (2007). Opensim: open-source software to create and analyze dynamic simulations of movement, *IEEE Transactions on Biomedical Engineering* 54(11):1940–1950.

63. A. M. Dollar and H. Herr. (2008). Lower extremity exoskeletons and active orthoses: challenges and state-of-the-art, *IEEE Transactions on Robotics* 24(1):144–158.
64. A. Alamdari and V. N. Krovi. (2015). Design and analysis of a cable-driven articulated rehabilitation system for gait training, *Journal of Mechanisms and Robotics*. doi: 10.1115/1.4032274. (In press).
65. A. Alamdari and V. Krovi. (2015). Parallel articulated-cable exercise robot (pacer): novel home-based cable-driven parallel platform robot for upper limb neuro-rehabilitation, in *Proceedings of the ASME 2015 International Design Engineering Technical Conferences and Computers in Engineering Conference, August 2–5*. American Society of Mechanical Engineers.
66. A. Alamdari and V. Krovi. (2015). Modeling and control of a novel home-based cable-driven parallel platform robot: Pacer, in *2015 IEEE/RSJ International Conference on Intelligent Robots and Systems (IROS)* 6330–6335.
67. A. Alamdari and V. Krovi. (2015). Robotic physical exercise and system (ropes): A cable-driven robotic rehabilitation system for lower-extremity motor therapy, in *Proceedings of the ASME 2015 International Design Engineering Technical Conferences and Computers in Engineering Conference, August 2–5*. American Society of Mechanical Engineers.
68. A. Alamdari. (2016). *Cable-Driven Articulated Rehabilitation System for Gait Training*. PhD thesis, The State University of New York at Buffalo.
69. A. M. Dollar and H. Herr. (2008). Design of a quasi-passive knee exoskeleton to assist running, in *Intelligent Robots and Systems, International Conference on IEEE/RSJ*, 747–754.
70. S. K. Banala, S. H. Kim, S. K. Agrawal and J. P. Scholz. (2009). Robot assisted gait training with active leg exoskeleton (alex), in *IEEE Transactions on Neural Systems and Rehabilitation Engineering* 17(1):2–8.
71. H. Kawamoto, S. Lee, S. Kanbe and Y. Sankai. (2003). Power assist method for hal-3 using emg-based feedback controller, in *IEEE International Conference on Systems, Man and Cybernetics* 2:1648–1653.
72. H. Kazerooni and R. Steger. (2006). The berkeley lower extremity exoskeleton, *Journal of Dynamic Systems, Measurement, and Control* 128(1):14–25.
73. R. D. Orpwood. (1990). Design methodology for aids for the disabled, *Journal of Medical Engineering and Technology* 14(1):2–10.
74. V. Krovi, V. Kumar, G. Ananthasuresh and J.-M. Vezien. (1999). Design and virtual prototyping of rehabilitation aids, *Journal of Mechanical Design* 121(3):456–458.
75. N. M. Fisher and D. R. Pendergast. (1995). Application of quantitative and progressive exercise rehabilitation to patients with osteoarthritis of the knee, *Journal of Back and Musculoskeletal Rehabilitation* 5(1):33–53.
76. N. Fisher, S. White, H. Yack, R. Smolinski and D. Pendergast. (1997). Muscle function and gait in patients with knee osteoarthritis before and after muscle rehabilitation, *Disability and Rehabilitation* 19(2):47–55.
77. N. M. Fisher, D. R. Pendergast, E. Calkins, *et al.* (1991). Muscle rehabilitation in impaired elderly nursing home residents, *Archives of Physical Medicine and Rehabilitation* 72(3): 181–185.
78. N. Fisher and D. Pendergast. (1994). 1213 muscular and cardiovascular training in well elderly subjects: A six month follow-up, *Medicine and Science in Sports and Exercise* 26(5):S215.
79. R. Perini, N. Fisher, A. Veicsteinas and D. R. Pendergast. (2002). Aerobic training and cardiovascular responses at rest and during exercise in older men and women, *Medicine and Science in Sports and Exercise* 34(4):700–708.

Chapter 9

ROBOT-ENHANCED WALKERS FOR TRAINING OF CHILDREN WITH CEREBRAL PALSY: PILOT STUDIES

Jiyeon Kang and Sunil Kumar Agrawal

Robotics and Rehabilitation (ROAR) Laboratory
Department of Mechanical Engineering
Columbia University, NY, USA

Children with cerebral palsy (CP) often suffer from movement disorders. They show poor balance and motor coordination. These children typically use passive walkers in their early years. However, there are no prior studies that document the effects of robot-enhanced walkers on functional improvements of these children. This paper reports the results of two pilot studies where children were trained to walk with a robot to perform a series of tasks with increasing levels of difficulty over a number of training sessions. The outcome measures are based on both data collected by the robot such as travel distance, average speed, and success ratio of given task and clinical variables to characterize their levels of disability and motor function. This pilot study documents the training outcomes for children with CP and compares results (i) between small and large number of training sessions and (ii) between toddlers and older children.

1. Introduction

Mobility is a key factor in a child's early development. In typically developing young children, the emergence of independent mobility is associated with advances in motor, social, emotional, perceptual, cognitive, and language skills.[1,2] However, impaired children with motor disabilities are at risk for further developmental delays due to lack of self-generated mobility.

For example, children born with cerebral palsy (CP), a prevalent cause of movement disorder, can have physical impairments on one side of the body, their lower extremities, or all four extremities.[3] The incidence of CP is 2 to 3 per 1000 live births and about 40–100 per 1000 live births among babies born very early or with very low birth weight.[4,5] Although the underlying neuropathology is not progressive, children with CP may decline in motor function as they grow older.[6] As the children with CP continue to have longer life expectancy, it is important to treat them sooner to prevent deterioration and improve their quality of life.

The cause of CP is injury to the immature brain and it is now thought that the most common time for such an injury is prenatal.[7] Problems during labor, delivery and injuries at postnatal period can also be causes of CP.[8] Premature birth is a well-known risk factor for CP and is seen in almost half of CP patients.[9,10]

Our previous studies of CP children (Sec. 2.2) were mainly focused on automated driving devices to train mobility of these children. This intervention with mobile robots adopted "top-down" approach to physical therapy.[11] Instead of acting on the physical deficit directly, driving the mobile robot has potentially an indirect influence on the neural system that is needed for coordination during ambulation.[12] Even though studies showed that driving can enhance the children's gross motor functions and social skills,[13] there are limitations due to lack of training during ambulation. If children with CP are not trained for overground walking, muscles in the lower limbs may weaken further and the distal neuromuscular activations will decline over time.

In this study, a robotic device is presented that facilitates both driving and self-ambulation during the training program. This robotic walker was designed using a conventional walker and a steering wheel to practice simultaneously overground walking and directional driving. To assess clinically the CP children who participated in this training, Pediatric Evaluation of Disability Inventory (PEDI), Quality of Upper Extremity Skills Test (QUEST), and Gross Motor Function Measure 88 (GMFM-88) were used. PEDI is a comprehensive tool to assess the development and capability of functional skills in children, with or without caregiver assistance, in three domains: self-care, mobility, and social function.[14] QUEST evaluates the quality of upper extremity function in four domains: dissociated movement, grasp, protective extension, and weight bearing. It was developed for evaluation of children who have neuromuscular dysfunction with spasticity.[15] GMFM-88 scores evaluate the change in gross motor function of children with CP as they grow older.[16]

The study reports the driving performance and clinical evaluation results when children with CP are trained to walk with a robot-enhanced walker over multiple training sessions.

2. Our Previous Work on Pediatric Rehabilitation

Various robotic interventions have being developed to enhance the mobility of children with special needs. Different robotic devices and software have been designed to show the feasibility of these as a helpful tool for impaired children to enhance their motor control. Collaborating with clinicians, conventional clinical evaluations were conducted to verify the training effects of these robotic interventions.

2.1. *Mobility interface for infants on a mobile robot by kicking*

Children with mobility impairments often do not use powered chairs until the age of five, as per current medical practice. To provide an automated mobility system at an earlier age, a robotic device was proposed, which uses a single camera-marker system to track the kicking leg motion and this information to control the translational velocity of the robot. Besides translation, the rotational velocity is controlled by a joystick, installed in front of the child (Fig. 1).

For evaluation of the feasibility of this system, two typically developing infants were recruited, 11 months and 17 months old. Experiments were performed for 2 days a week and for 4 days altogether. During each day, the infants used the interface to drive as long as possible, until they showed signs of fatigue or tried to get out of the safety straps. A caregiver stood in front of the infant and encouraged the infant to move their limbs in order to move the robot.

Two toddlers were able to move around in the environment by using the novel driving interface of the mobile robot which is activated by leg motion. It is believed that the integration of the camera-marker system, as opposed to joysticks found in conventional powered wheelchairs, can be more accessible to infants as movement of the legs requires less fine motor skills. The proposed drive interface simultaneously provides an opportunity for exercise while exploring the

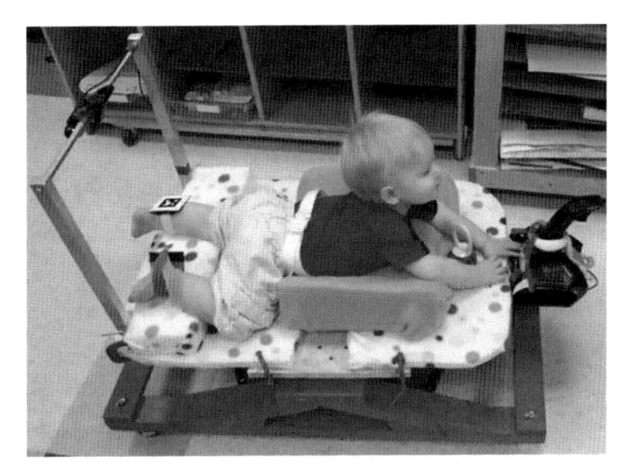

Figure 1. Overview of the infant base with the foam wedge for supporting an infant, a camera for capturing leg motion, and joystick for turning.[17]

environment. The use of two markers can imitate crawling in the robot, encouraging infants to perform rhythmic patterns with their legs.

2.2. *Studies with conventional joystick-driven power mobility*

Over the past years, our laboratory has conducted various pilot/case studies with joystick-driven power mobility devices.[18–23] Extending these studies, a controlled trial with the power mobility device was conducted for fifteen CP children.[13] The experimental group drove a mobile robot and performed different levels of driving tasks. In the experiment area, sub-regions were identified which served as the start, intermediate, or goal points. Children were asked to move between different sub-regions and practice driving straight or while making turns (Fig. 2).

The experimental group, which practiced with the robot, advanced in gross motor control, upper extremity functions, and social function, evaluated by GMFM, PEDI, and QUEST scores. In line with the findings of Refs. [13, 24], we believe that these interventions can be optimally effective for children with special needs if applied within the principles of early intervention, i.e. the interventions should (i) begin as soon as possible, (ii) be built on the current abilities of the child, and (iii) be primarily provided in the typical environment of the child such as the home, school, and community as opposed to a clinic.

However, some issues need to be overcome in the application of power mobility devices. Even among adult patients, many with mobility impairments find it uncomfortable to use the currently available power wheelchair for activities of

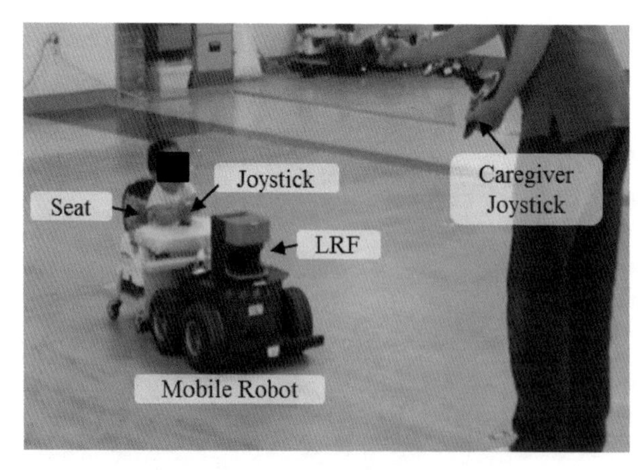

Figure 2. A CP child driving a mobile robot using a joystick. A lidar range finder was installed on the mobile robot for accurate localization of the robot. Travel distance, speed, and success ratio of the task were recorded by an on-board computer. A separate joystick were provided to the caregiver to override the inputs of the child's joystick for safety.[13]

daily living (ALD). Around 40% of the patients have reported that they find the steering and maneuvering tasks difficult or even impossible.[25] From our studies, we also observed that despite up to 6 months of training three times a week, infants displayed difficulties in learning to turn left or right.[20]

2.3. *Intelligent power mobility device with force feedback joystick*

Another effort to lower the barriers for the use of wheel chairs is to develop a system that is capable of providing force feedback to teach how to drive these. A force feedback joystick was installed on a mobile robot to guide the child's hand toward a specific targeted direction. The software for this force feedback was programmed based on "assist-as-needed" method to determine the direction and amount of the guided force. As the child's hand deviated further from the target direction, larger force was applied to gently guide the child's hand toward the desired direction (Fig. 3).

The force applied on the child's hand depended on three different regions, divided around instantaneous desired direction (Fig. 4(b)). The first region is the damping only region which is denoted as Region 1 in Fig. 4(b). This region is defined by a cone with a constant angle α, where only small damping force is applied to stabilize the joystick. Regions 2a/2b are the force field regions where restoring force is applied to bring the handle of the joystick toward the desired direction. This force is normal to the virtual wall described in Fig. 4(b) and proportional to the distance from the wall. In Region 3, with directions opposite to the desired direction, a centering force is applied on the child's hand to bring the joystick back to the center.

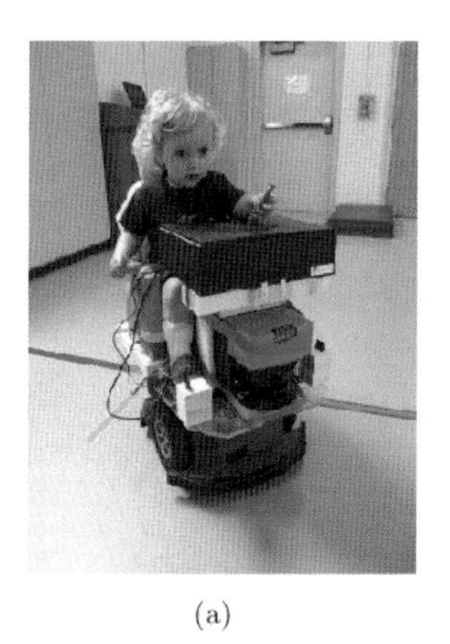

(a)

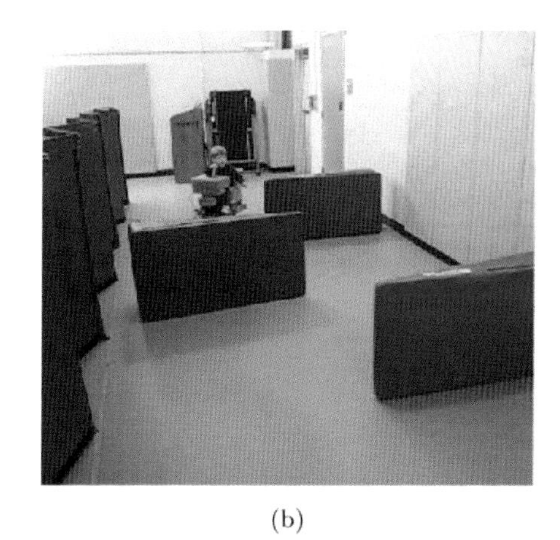

(b)

Figure 3. (a) A child driving a mobile robot with a force feedback joystick and (b) Training environment for potential field-based controller to avoid obstacles.[26,27]

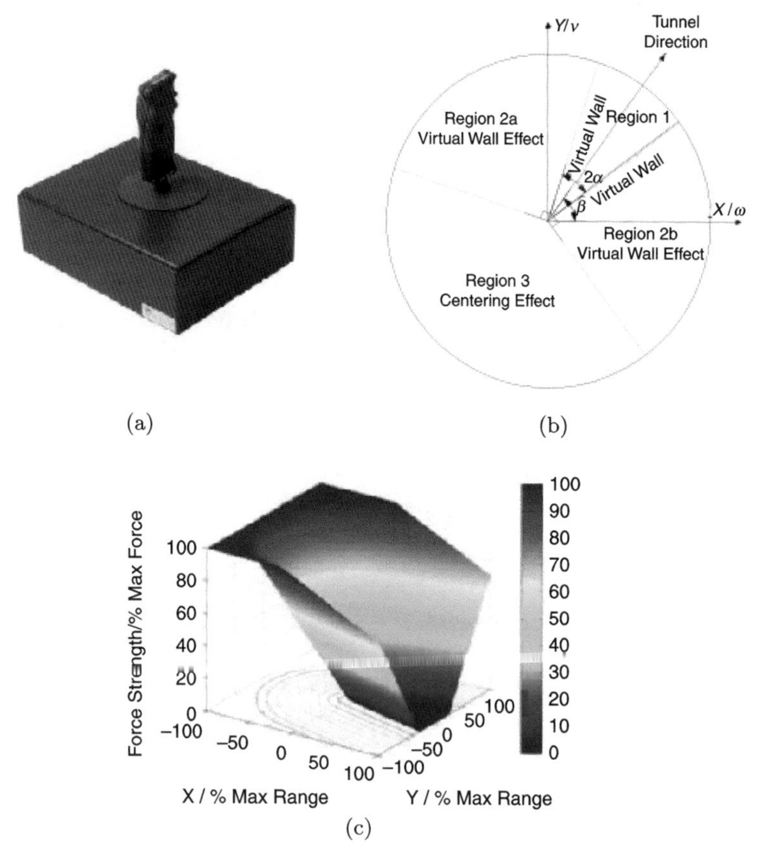

Figure 4. (a) Force feedback joystick. (Impulse Stick, Immersion Co.) (b) Force tunnel shown by a virtual wall around nominal joystick motion direction. (c) The joystick tip force outside the cone for the tunnel direction $\beta = 0$ and half tunnel width $\alpha = 15°$. Tip force within the cone is zero. The damping effect is not shown in this plot.[27]

In addition to the force feedback, a lidar scanner was installed on the mobile robot to avoid stationary or dynamic obstacles and plan the target trajectory. The sensor information is used to localize the robot in the space and detect obstacles to prevent collision. A potential field-based controller[28] is used to implement the path planning and obstacle avoidance. The algorithm allows quick calculation of the desired driving direction from any point within the maze to the goal.

A study with five experimental and control children was conducted to evaluate the training effect. The training group included five healthy toddlers with an average age 31.0 ± 2.5 months and was trained to drive with the force field. The control group also included five healthy toddlers with an average age 30.6 ± 3.9 months. They drove without the force field. Toddlers that young do not understand instructions such as "drive the robot to follow the lines on the ground". To accommodate their behavior, a trainer stood at each turning point on the path to encourage the child to come to that point. The trainer always stood one robot radius ahead of the turning point, and notified and moved on to the next turning point or the goal once the child reached the next region in the training area.

The results of the group study show that the force field algorithm helped very young children learn to navigate and avoid obstacles faster, more accurately, and with greater safety. Besides typically developing children, children with spina bifida and CP showed successfully the use of a force-feedback joystick during practice.

One natural question to ask is whether the toddlers simply learned the specifics of the path or if they really learned the behavior of steering. Also, would they be able to retain this acquired skill later after the training is complete. In order to answer these questions, subjects were retested at least 1 week after the training was complete, but in a different configuration and at a different location. The results suggest that the toddlers were in fact able to learn to steer and retained this behavior at least 1 week after the training.

2.4. *A novel mobile robot to enhance socialization of impaired children*

The lack of mobility in special needs children results in other delays in their development milestones. The walking and crawling in children affect the development of cognition, perception, and socialization.[1,2] Studies show that there is smaller social interaction between children with special needs and their typically developing peers in class rooms, gymnasium, or a playground.[31,32] This lack of social experience is known to cause emotional depression, maladjustment in classrooms, and behavioral disorders.[33] Toddler and preschool age are crucial period to acquire social skills.[34] Difficulties in social interaction in preschool remain and continue over to elementary school.[35–37] Repeated rejection from the peers in their early childhood may lead to early interaction difficulties[38] and difficulty in learning social behaviors at a later time. Early development or intervention of social skills is expected to reduce the risk of rejection from future peers.

To develop a training paradigm to enhance socialization, two different sets of studies were designed.[29,30] From previous designs,[26,27] Indoor Positioning System (IPS) from Ubisense was additionally installed in the gym where the experiment was conducted (Fig. 5). For global localization, one Ubisense was attached on the robot and the other Ubisense tag was attached on another child, a toy, or a caregiver. Inside the robot, a trajectory was planned for the robot to track the second tag. The joystick provides a force feedback to the child's hand such that the child is encouraged to move toward another child who has the ball with the tag.

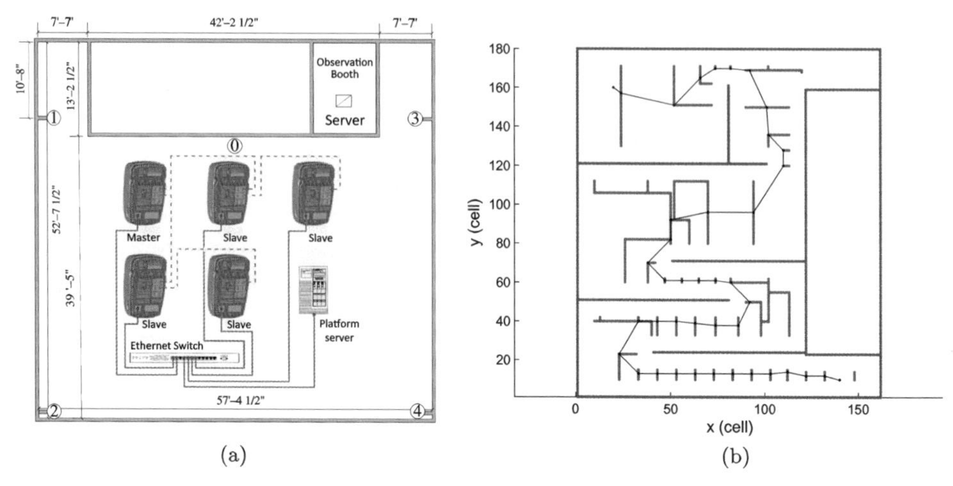

Figure 5. (a) Floor plan of the gymnasium and the Ubisense IPS: receivers and tags. The play area is of rectangular shape. Five receivers are mounted at positions 0–4 and are connected to a computer server by data cables (solid) and timing cables (dotted). (b) Simulated relaxed A* and square generation algorithm to create a target trajectory between the mobile robot and the targeted toy.[29]

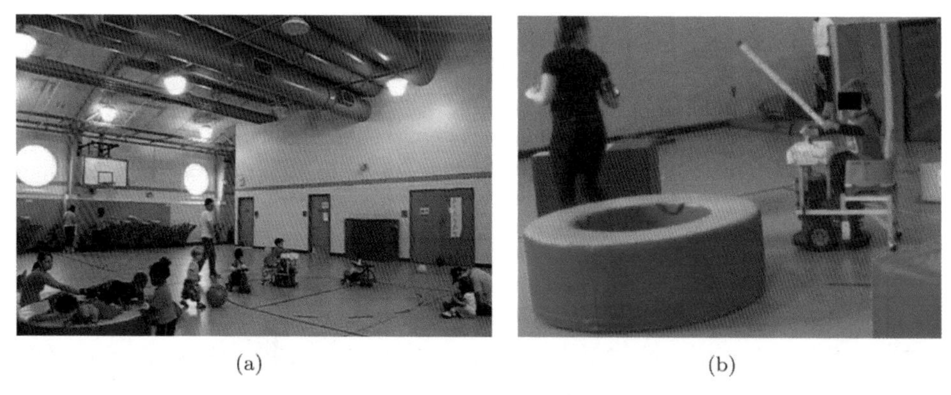

(a) (b)

Figure 6. Two experiments were conducted to show the feasibility of the new robotic training paradigms to enhance socialization (a) A child driver is driving toward the ball. (b) Chasing game to catch the tagged caregiver.[29,30]

The first study was designed to implement the tag inside a ball. In this game, a caregiver and some children pass the ball to each other on one side of the gymnasium and attract a child driver from the other side to the ball (Fig. 6(a)). If the driver successfully reaches the group, the ball is passed to him/her. The driver and the ball were separated by at least 5 m at the beginning of each trial. Note that the driver and the caregiver can start anywhere behind the start lines so that the driver does not simply learn a trajectory. Figure 6(b) shows a chase game designed to increase interactions with other children. A chaser who drives the mobile robot should tag the other child to win the game. The force feedback guidance is used within the game to promote directional movements toward the tagged peer. This role in the chase game can result in the children to interact with others unconsciously. For evaluation, a caregiver is tagged instead of other peers for consistent movement in the experiment.

The experimental results of both experiments show that all children were able to move closer to other peers or the caregiver with haptic feedback. We feel that this experiment involving an intelligent mobility device with haptic feedback can be an effective test bed for social skills training of children with mobility impairments.

2.5. *Novel assistive interface where toddlers walk with a mobile robot supported at the waist*

There have been several examples of powered assist devices, such as smart wheelchairs, robotic canes, robotic crutches, powered exoskeletons, and robotic walkers. Among these, smart wheelchairs are the most widely used devices.[40] However, due to lack of self-ambulation, muscles may further weaken and deteriorate over time.[41] Powered exoskeletons provide the external forces to facilitate limb movement, but are not ideal for very young children.[42] Robotic walkers have been developed to provide both safety and stability through external support.[43,44] These robotic walkers are designed to provide body weight support through harness and encourage users to correct upright posture. However, these assist devices tend to be heavy and bulky to train children with mobility issues. To make robotic walkers accessible to children, a novel walker is proposed to provide partial weight support and guidance forces with more compact and lighter design.

To provide proper assistance with this active walker, detection of children's intention is crucial to make the device functional and ensure safety (Fig. 7). Various methods have been suggested and tested by researchers on how to sense the intention of young subjects. Most powered mobility devices are driven by direct interfaces such as joysticks[45] or touch screens.[46] Also, hand gesture,[47] leg motion,[17] voice control,[48] EEG,[49] and EMG[50] were used to detect child's movement. In line with these studies, the proposed robotic walker is equipped with a smart harness that is designed to sense the position and orientation of the child in the device. The posture of the child is utilized in two different controllers for the robotic walker to provide effective assistance depending on child's movement.

Two different controllers were implemented in the mobile robot to follow the child, as shown in Fig. 8. Feedback linearization controller computed the control input to minimize the distance d between the child and the robot. The other controller in Fig. 8(b), which is the line following controller, defined a target direction from the potentiometers and reduced the distance/angle between the robot and the

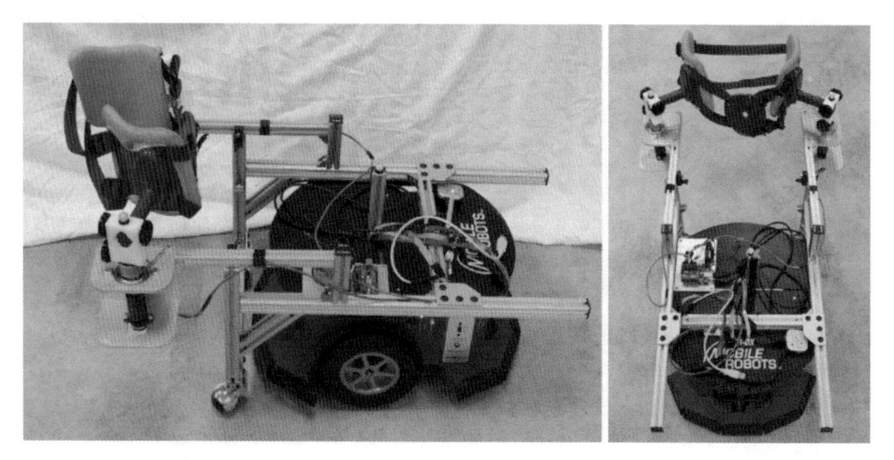

Figure 7. P3-DX robot and aluminum extension frame. Two arm structures with spring loaded hinge joints are attached on the mobile robot. Safety straps were used to secure the child's trunk and keep upright posture.[39]

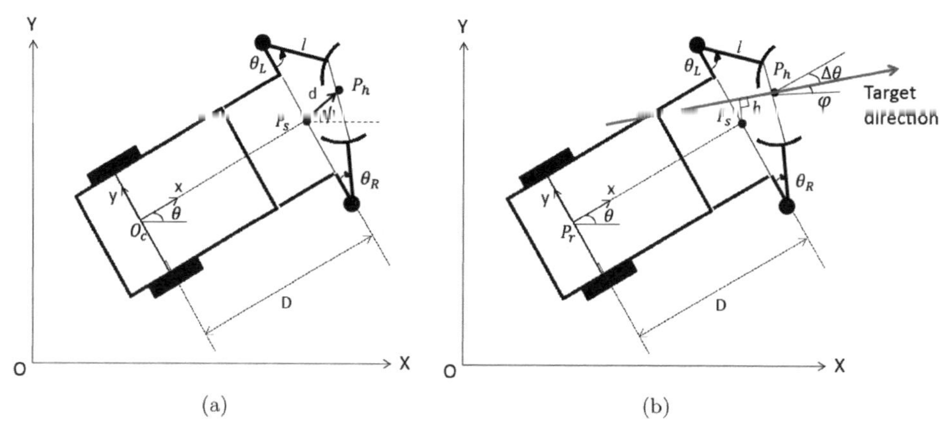

Figure 8. Schematic of two different controllers (a) Feedback linearization controller computes linear speed and angular speed of the mobile robot to reduce the distance between the robot and the child. (b) Line following controller tracks a specified path, denoted as a red arrow.[39]

target direction. Five toddlers walked in the novel assistive interface through three different levels of tasks to compare these two control algorithms. Tasks include walking straight (Task 1), turning to the right/left (Task 2), or making U-turns (Task 3). The results of five toddlers demonstrated that feedback linearization controller responded faster than the line following controller when reacting to sudden or fast movements of the toddlers. It used less time to achieve almost the same success ratio and even smaller deviation area in the first two tasks. On the other hand, the line following controller performed better in the most difficult task. It handled sharp turns in the difficult task more smoothly and could correct error faster once deviated.

3. Experiment Description

3.1. *Participating subjects*

This study was approved by the Institutional Review Board of Hanyang University Medical Center (HYUMC) in Seoul, South Korea. Participation of all children with CP in this study required parental informed consent. The children with CP were recruited from the outpatient clinic of rehabilitation medicine in HYUMC and Seongdong Community Rehabilitation Center.

The inclusion conditions in this study were: (1) diagnosis of CP, (2) the ability of children to walk independently for at least 2–3 steps, and (3) the ability of the child to hold on to the walker for at least 20 minutes. The exclusion conditions were: (1) diagnosis of additional neurologic diseases besides CP, (2) too short a height to use the robot walker, and (3) severe cognitive decline that could affect the robot-enhanced walker training.

Before training, functional scores of all participants were taken on 3 domains of PEDI (self-care, mobility, and social function), QUEST, and GMFM-88. These scores were evaluated again after every 15 sessions of training. The scores were evaluated around the same time of the day and the evaluations were carried out by a single therapist who was blinded to the study. The age of children is reported in Table 1 at the time of the first assessment of the clinical score.

3.2. *Robot hardware and interface*

The pediatric walker system was assembled using a PowerBot from Adept, a gaming steering wheel (G27 Racing Wheel, Logitech Inc.), and an off-the-shelf

Table 1. Average and standard deviation of age of children who participated in Pilot studies A and B. Pilot study A had four experimental children and one control child. Pilot study B consisted of five experimental children and five control children.

Age (months)	Study A experimental		Study A control
Subject	A1–A4		AC1
Average	40		29
Standard deviation	7.16		0
	Study B experimental young group	Study B experimental old group	Study B control
Subject	B1–B3	B4–B5	BC1–BC5
Average	44	102	31.2
Standard deviation	3.61	25.46	6.57

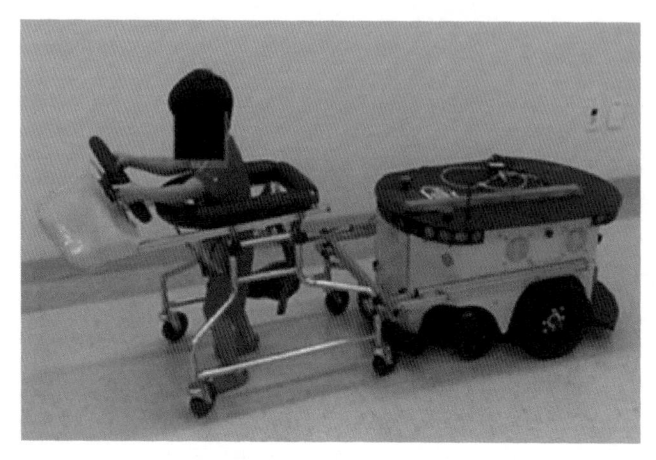

Figure 9. A child with the pediatric robotic walker. The system consists of a steering wheel, a mobile robot, a laser range finder, and the off-the-shelf walker frame. The child steers the robot with the steering wheel while the robot moves along with the child who walks at self-selected speed.

walker. As shown in Fig. 9, the off-the-shelf walker was attached to the front of the mobile robot. The child stayed roughly a meter in front of the center of the robot. A wireless joystick (FREEDOM 2.4, Logitech Inc.) enabled a caregiver to control the forward velocity of the PowerBot. The child used a steering wheel to control the direction of motion, where the rotational speed of the vehicle was selected to be proportional to the angle of rotation of the steering wheel. The user input commands from the steering wheel and the joystick were interfaced using C++ with the library of Direct X. The rotational speed ω of the robot is given below

$$\omega = \frac{IP}{IP_{\max}}\omega_{\max}, \tag{1}$$

where IP is the input command of the steering wheel, $IP_{\max}$ is the maximum value of the input command, and $\omega_{\max}$ is the maximum rotational speed. In this experiment, $IP_{\max} = 10{,}000$ and $\omega_{\max} = 26^{\circ}/\text{s}$ were applied.

Since the driving wheels of the PowerBot do not satisfy the no-slip condition, position errors accumulate over the duration of the experiments. Therefore, a particle filter localization algorithm, provided by Adept software, was applied by using the laser range finder (LMS 200, SICK Inc.). The LRF has a 180° range with three levels of angular resolution and 1° of resolution was used in the current study. As a result, an accuracy of 5 cm was obtained by repeated calibrations and measurements. During the experiment, the position of the robot was recorded in log files. An overview of the robotic pediatric walker system is shown in Figs. 9 and 10.

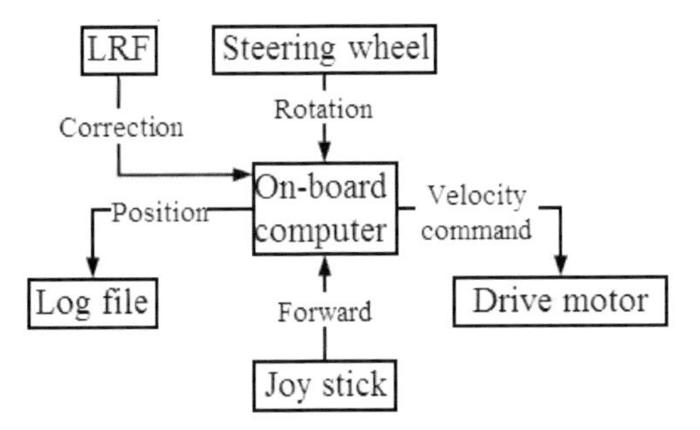

Figure 10. A schematic of the robot-enhanced walker: A steering wheel provides the direction of movement and the caregiver's joystick controls the speed of the walker. The data from encoders on the wheels and a laser range finder were used to determine the current position of the robot.

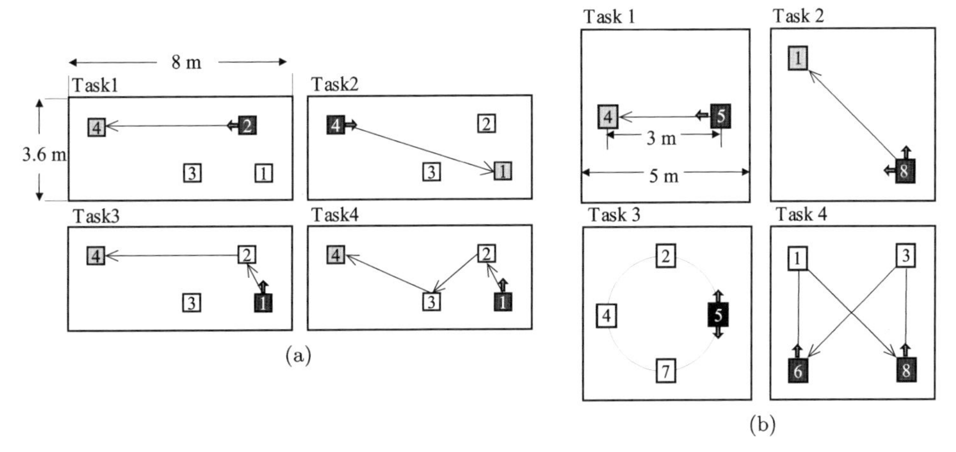

Figure 11. Four tasks with different task levels for (a) Pilot study A and (b) Pilot study B. A child with the robotic walker was asked to move across sub-regions, labeled by numbers and connected by arrows. Bold arrows indicate the start direction of a child in the robotic walker, black color shows the starting point, and grey color denotes the final end point of the task.

3.3. *Task description*

Pilot study A was conducted in a space of 8 m × 3.6 m and Pilot study B was performed in a 5 m × 5 m task area. Within the task area, numbered sub-regions were defined, as shown in Fig. 11, as the starting direction (black squares), intermediate goals (white squares), or the final goal (grey squares) of the tasks. These numbered sub-regions are connected with arrows to demonstrate the path of each task that the child needs to follow. The initial configurations of the child and the robot are expressed as bold arrows in Fig. 11. In Pilot study B, Tasks 2 and 3 are described by two bold arrows, denoting that two different starting directions are possible. For these tasks, it was randomly chosen to start with right or left turn

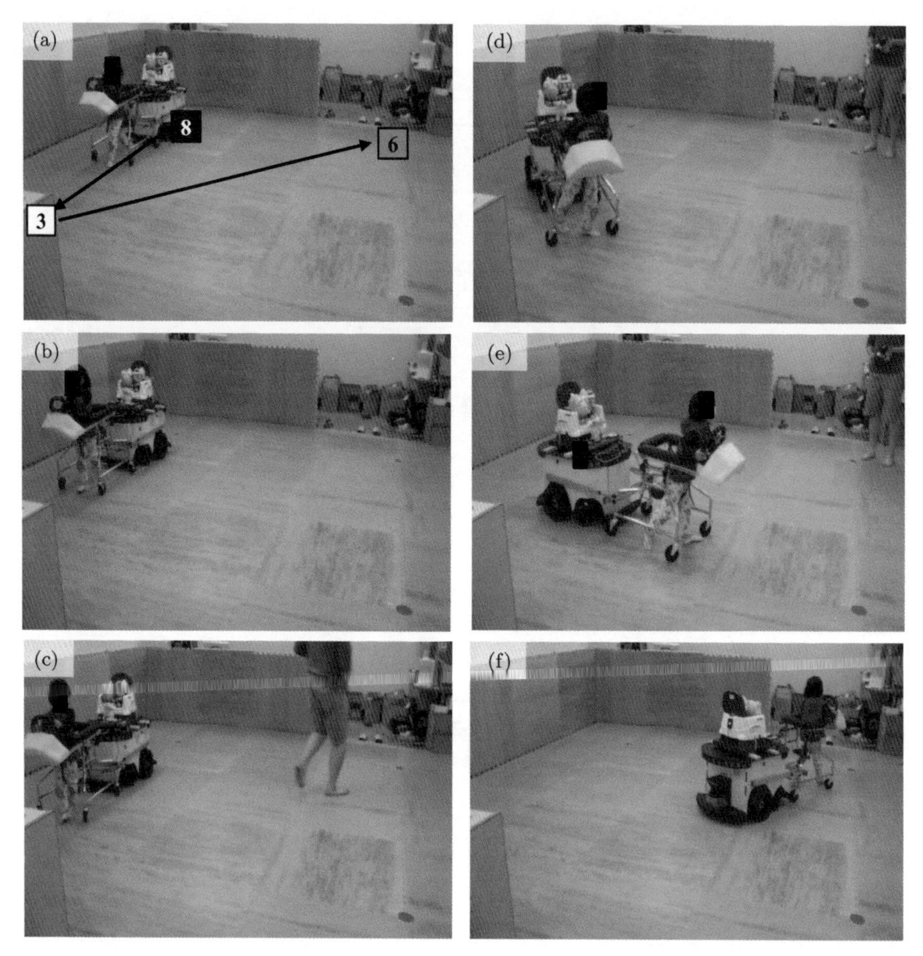

Figure 12. The motion in Task 4 of the Pilot study B. The colored squares and arrows in (a) demonstrate the path of Task 4. The child needs to move from sub-region 8 (black square) to 3 (white square), then to sub-region 6 (grey square). A caregiver encouraged the child to move towards the intermediate goals with verbal reinforcement.

toward the target. As an example, Fig. 12(a) shows Task 4 of the Pilot study B which starts in the sub-region 8, follows the arrows until the end of the task at sub-region 6 (see Figs. 12(b)–12(f)). Each pilot study consisted of four tasks which progressively became more difficult. Higher difficulty tasks required the child to make sharper turns and demonstrate better steering skills.

The forward speed of the robot was applied by a caregiver using a wireless joystick and the rotational motion was controlled using the steering wheel by the child. In Pilot study A, in order to challenge the children, the target forward speed of the robot was chosen as follows: sessions 1–5 at 0.15 m/s, sessions 6–10 at 0.17 m/s, and sessions 11–15 at 0.19 m/s. If the child walked slower than the target speed, the robot was slowed down to keep the child safe. In pilot study B where sharper turns are required, for higher safety of the children, the initial velocity of the robot was determined based on the distance between the bumper of the mobile robot and the heel of the child during experiments in the first session. Once a child got used to the velocity of the robotic walker, a caregiver gradually increased the velocity until the distance between the bumper of the mobile robot and the heel of the child roughly became 10 cm. Each child was encouraged to manipulate the steering wheel to complete the given tasks while the speed was held constant during each trial. Other specifics of the protocol were as follows:

(1) Each session started from Task 1 and moved progressively to the next task until the highest task was achieved.
(2) If the child moved too close to a wall or deviated significantly from the desired path, the caregiver reduced the speed to avoid collision using the wireless joystick. The task was declared as a failure and the child restarted the failed task.
(3) The child manipulated the rotational speed by using the steering wheel. If the child walked slower than the target speed, the robot was slowed down to keep the child safe.
(4) If a child rested or leaned on the walker or got tired, the experiment was stopped temporarily. The task was considered a failure and the child restarted the failed task.
(5) Children's songs, videos, toys, and hand gestures were used to encourage the child to continue during the experiment.
(6) Once the child and robotic walker got closer than 10 cm from an intermediate sub-region, the caregiver moved to the next designated sub-region to prompt the child to change the direction toward the next targeted sub-region.

4. Results From Pilot Study A (15 Training Sessions)

Four children participated in this study to evaluate the effect of the robotic walker training. Three outcome measures were computed from the trajectory of the walker to evaluate the performance of the child walking with the robot. Also, clinical scores were measured by the therapist before and after 15 sessions of training to assess changes due to training with the walker.

4.1. *Robot measures*

These measures show the performance of children walking during the training sessions. Using the position data of the robot, we determined how fast the children walked in the device, how well they accomplished the given task, and how far they moved within the training sessions. Below are the details of the three metrics.

- **Average velocity:** Walking speed (v_i) was recorded by the mobile robot to determine how fast a child moved with the robot over all four tasks. It was averaged with task time ($t_{f,i}$) for each ith task.

$$\text{Average velocity} = \sum \frac{\int_0^{t_{f,i}} v_i \, dt}{t_{f,i}}. \tag{2}$$

- **Success ratio:** If the child completed all assigned sub-areas for a given task, the task was considered as a success. It is computed as the number of successes (NS_i) divided by the number of trials (NT_i) for each ith task.

$$\text{Success ratio} = \sum \frac{NS_i}{NT_i}. \tag{3}$$

- **Path length:** This refers to the total driving distance during Tasks 1, 2, 3 and 4 in one session (20 min). As children spent different time periods to complete each task, we used the overall path length for consistency and have presented here accumulated path length in one session.

Figure 13 shows that the graphs increase linearly with increasing number of sessions for average velocity, success ratio, and path length. Children could walk faster with the robot (average velocity), and improved steering skills to accomplish their tasks (success ratio). Increasing average velocity signifies not only increase in the speed of movement, but also continuity of walking. If subjects pause during walking, the average velocity decreases depending on frequency and duration of pause. Comparing data among subjects, subject A1 shows higher values for all metrics compared to other subjects. It is also noticeable that subject A3 has a higher rate of improvement during 15 sessions of training as seen from the slopes of fitted lines.

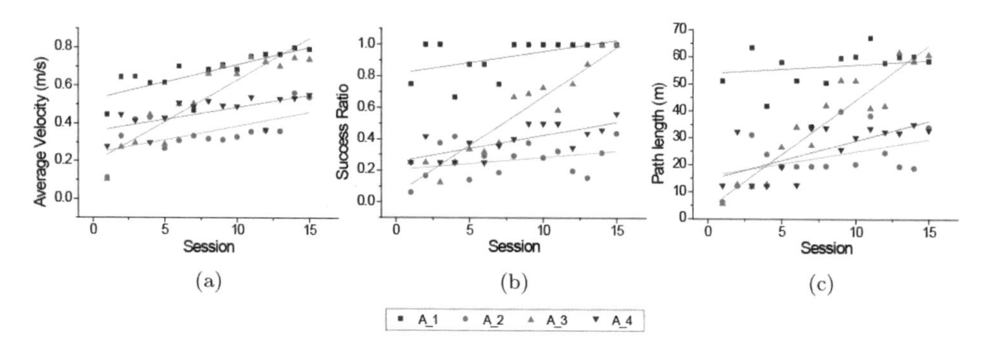

Figure 13. Average velocity, success ratio, and path length of four children in pilot study A with 15 sessions. Robotic measures showed increasing trend for all children who participated in this robotic training.

4.2. *Clinical measures*

Clinical measures were taken to assess how this robotic intervention affects measures outside the robot. Standard score sheets were used for evaluation. Assessments of children were conducted both before the first training and after the last training. Higher scores indicate more favorable changes. The list below shows the focus areas for each measure.

- GMFM: hip/knee flexion, roll, sit, kick, walk
- QUEST: shoulder/elbow/wrist flexion, grasp, weight bearing
- PEDI_C: self-care
- PEDI_M: mobility
- PEDI_F: social function

Most children showed improvements in PEDI_M and GMFM scores after the robotic training as shown in Table 2. PEDI_M and GMFM scores represent mobility in the children. Also, social function (PEDI_F) of children is enhanced as the caregiver continuously encourages the child to move toward the goal. Additionally, QUEST scores, which denote function in upper extremity, show improvements in subjects A1, A2, and A3. This may be attributed to hand movements to control the robot using the steering wheel on the robot. Comparing among subjects, A1 and A3 increased scores in all measures except PEDI_C, which is not highly correlated in this study. Subject A1 showed striking changes in PEDI_M and GMFM, followed by subject A3. As mentioned in the previous section, subjects A1 and A3 also showed substantial changes in robot measurements. A1 had the highest values and A3 had the highest slope in the fitted curves in all robotic measurements. Based on these data, we can conclude that there is a correlation between children's participation in robotic training and increased mobility scores.

Table 2. PEDI, GMFM, and QUEST scores of four subjects in pilot study A. Robot-enhanced training helped children to improve their mobility development (PEDI_M). Shaded areas represent substantial improvements before and after training. Children showed progress in lower and upper extremity movements after the robotic training.

Measure	PEDI_M		PEDI_F		PEDI_C		GMFM		QUESTS	
subject	Pre	Post	Pre	Post	Pre	Post	Pre	Post	Pre	Post
A1	43.3	54.8	59.9	70.8	50.3	51.7	82.31	89.77	76.88	86.08
A2	51.4	56.5	56.6	58.5	46	51	79.04	81.98	42.24	62.28
A3	59.1	65	65.1	70.8	59.3	60.5	80.23	84.21	73.81	82.23
A4	46.1	47	53.7	53.7	52.4	53	73.66	78.73	80.34	80.34

5. Result for Pilot Study B (30 Training Sessions)

From the results of the first study, we observed that children with average age of 40 months benefitted from 15 sessions of the robotic training. Following this first study, we extended the number of training sessions to 30 in order to observe if longer training improves the development of children. Additionally, we recruited two older children of age 7 and 10 years (subjects B4 and B5), to investigate if older children can also benefit from this robotic intervention. All detailed procedures of this experiment were identical to pilot study A.

5.1. *Robot measures*

The same metrics were used to evaluate performance of children with the robotic walker. Children sustained interest in walking until the end of 30 training sessions. Figure 14 shows the average velocity, success ratio, and path lengths of children in 30 sessions of training. For most subjects, a different trend was observed when compared to Pilot study A. First 15 sessions showed increment in all metrics similar to pilot study A, but the values plateaued after 15 sessions. The average velocity shows increasing trend during the first half of training sessions. Additionally, the success ratio in Fig. 14(b) shows that a majority of children reached the value of one toward the latter half of the training sessions. This means that they were able to accomplish all given tasks without fail. Unlike other subjects, B2 showed an increasing trend until the end of the training. Average velocity of B2 continuously increased also for the latter half of the training sessions. For this subject, the success ratio was kept below one until the end of the last training. This indicates that the given tasks were still challenging for this child until the end of the training. Two older children B4 and B5 did not show any specific trends compared to younger ones.

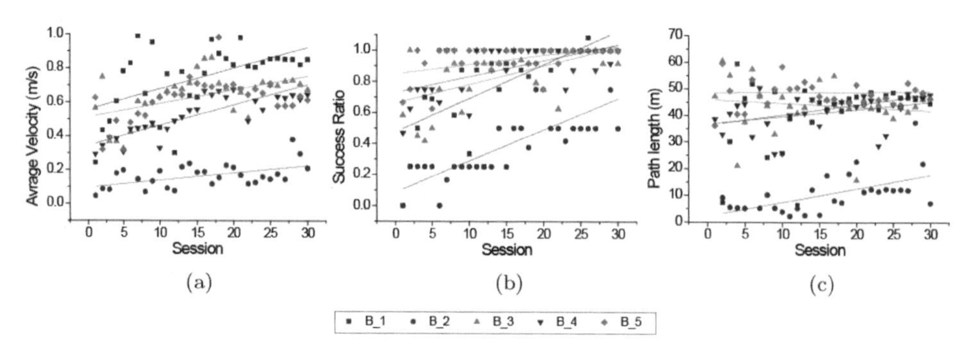

Figure 14. Average velocity, success ratio, and path length of five children in study B with 30 sessions. Robotic measurements of most children initially show increasing trend, but plateau after 15 session. Only Subject B2 showed continuous increment in these measurements.

5.2. *Clinical measures*

Clinical assessments were made to observe if the robotic training can foster improvements in other functional scores. In this experiment, we measured the scores three times, before, after 15th session, and after 30th session of training. Measurements after 15th session were performed to compare scores with the first experiment which had only 15 sessions. Same measures as in the first study were used to assess functional development of children.

In Table 3, children with higher age (subjects B4 and B5) did not show any visible increment in the clinical scores. Even though subjects B4 and B5 showed similar trends in robotic measurement as younger children, the robotic training was ineffective to enhance their clinical scores. In the younger group (B1 ~ B3), the effect of extending beyond 15 training sessions is reported below. Subjects B1 and B3 had increased PEDI_M score between first and second measurements (before training and after 15th session), but they stopped to improve mobility related scores after the second measurement. However, subject B2 improved GMFM score consistently for both former and latter halves of the training sessions. This result correlates well with robotic measurements. Subjects B1 and B3 showed plateauing in average velocity after 15 sessions of training. Additionally, subjects B1 and B3 approached the success ratio of 1 after 15th session which denotes that they succeeded in all the tasks. Children could benefit initially from the robotic training when it was challenging for them, but as the children got used to the tasks, robotic training could not promote children to enhance their functional development any more.

Table 3. PEDI, GMFM, and QUEST scores of five children who participated in robotic training for 30 sessions in study B. Shaded areas indicate substantial changes in clinical assessment. Children with higher age (B4: 7 years, B5: 10 years) showed no noticeable change in scores after robotic training.

Measure	PEDI_M			PEDI_F			PEDI_C		
Subject	Pre	Mid	Post	Pre	Mid	Post	Pre	Mid	Post
B1	73.3	89.2	89.2	55.4	62.3	62.3	64.6	66.8	66.8
B2	47.9	49.7	49.7	63.2	67.4	67.4	56.8	56.2	56.2
B3	67.4	73.3	73.3	66.2	66.2	66.2	56.8	58.6	58.6
B4	44.3	44.3	44.3	77.3	77.3	77.3	51	51.7	51.7
B5	51.4	51.4	51.4	96.3	96.3	96.3	65.3	65.3	65.3

Measure	GMFM			QUEST		
Subject	Pre	Mid	Post	Pre	Mid	Post
B1	95.64	97.31	97.31	81.26	84.78	84.78
B2	71.67	75.99	80.22	30.35	32.31	39.48
B3	95.02	96.8	97.07	40.46	40.46	40.46
B4	71.8	73.19	74.88	17.08	17.08	17.08
B5	67.35	67.35	68.81	62.39	62.39	62.39

For the case of subject B2, robotic training was challenging until the 30th training session, which caused continuous improvements in GMFM scores for all training sessions. From this observation, we found that children benefitted from robotic training, but the task levels should remain challenging for effective functional development.

6. Comparison of Results Between Experimental and Control Groups

As each experimental group had a corresponding control group, comparisons of changes in scores for all clinical measures are presented. Control group children were evaluated at the same time as their corresponding experimental group to maintain consistency. Figure 15(a) shows the score changes between pre- and post-training in pilot study A (15 sessions of training). Four experimental children and one control child are included in this graph. Even though we had one subject in the control group, all score changes in the experimental group were higher than those of the child in the control group. Figure 15(b) shows score changes between, before training, after 15th session, and after 30th training in pilot study B. Three experimental children and five control children are included in the second graph. Experimental group for study B only includes subjects B1, B2, and B3, since children with much higher age (B4: 7 years old and B5: 10 years old) did not show changes with this robotic intervention, as mentioned in the previous section of this chapter. In Fig. 15(b), dominant changes were observed in PEDI_M and GMFM

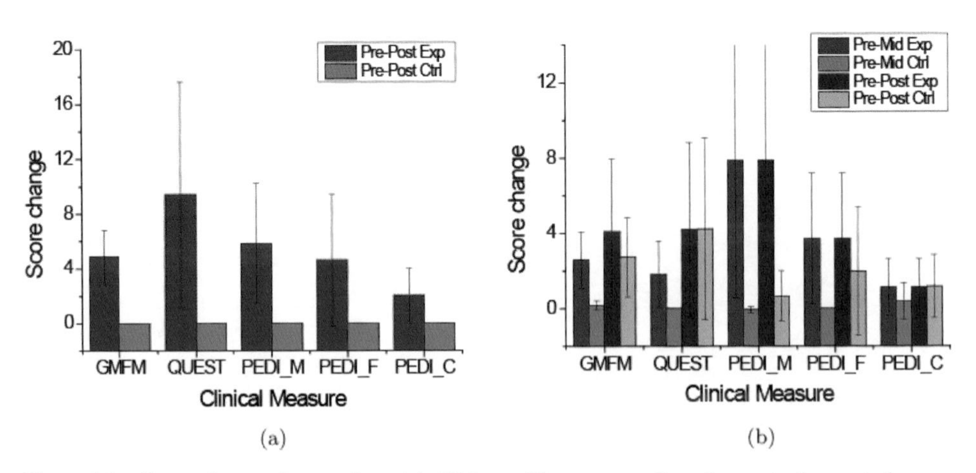

Figure 15. Score changes in experimental children with corresponding change in the control group in Pilot studies A and B. (a) Study A (15 sessions) measured clinical scores before and after training. (b) Study B (30 sessions) measured clinical scores before training, after 15th session, and after training. Pre-mid is score change between the pre-training and 15th session. Pre-post is score change between the pre-training and the post-training.

scores for experimental children compared to the control group. Other scores also show increasing trend for experimental children. From these two comparisons, we found that there is a substantial change in the various developmental measures of children who underwent this robotic intervention.

7. Conclusion

This novel study, where children were trained to walk with a robot to perform a series of tasks with increasing levels of difficulty over a number of training sessions, shows the following results: (i) Children with CP sustained interest in driving over multiple training sessions across many days. They were able to walk at a faster speed, completed their tasks, and covered larger distances. (ii) Younger children tended to benefit more in terms of driving abilities compared to older children and this was well correlated with increases in clinical measures such as PEDI-M, GMFM, and QUEST. (iii) Children trained with the robot benefited more in their clinical measures compared to the control group who did not drive the robot. (iv) With increase in the number of training sessions from 15 to 30, the children did not improve their driving measures or the clinical measures of PEDI-M, GMFM, and QUEST. A possible explanation may be that after 15 training sessions, the children were able to learn different tasks and were not significantly challenged any further.

In summary, training with robot walkers promotes young children to enhance their driving skills and improve the clinical scores such as GMFM, QUEST and specific domains of PEDI. However, this study must be interpreted with caution and performed with a larger number of subjects to assess the effects clinically.

Acknowledgments

We would like to thank M. J. Kim, Y. M. Lee, S. W. Kong, H. P. Cho, G. J. Park with Hanyang University and Hanyang Medical Center for recurring subjects and conducting the experiment. This research was supported by WCU (World Class University) program through the Korea Science and Engineering Foundation funded by the Ministry of Education, Science and Technology (No. R32-2009-000-10022-0). Partial support to the authors was provided by the NSF Behavioral and Cognitive Systems program number 1252876.

References

1. D. I. Anderson, J. J. Campos, D. E. Anderson, T. D. Thomas, D. C. Witherington, I. Uchiyama and M. A. Barbru-Roth. (2001). The flip side of perception-action coupling: locomotor experience and the ontogeny of visual-postural coupling, *Human Movement Science* 20(4–5): 461–487.

2. J. J. Campos, D. I. Anderson, M. A. Barbu-Roth, E. M. Hubbard, M. J. Hertenstein and D. Witherington. (2000). Travel broadens the mind, *Infancy* 1(2):149–219.
3. A. Eliasson, L. Krumlinde-Sundholm, B. Rosblad, E. Beckung, M. Ohrvall and P. Rosenbaum. (2006). The manual ability classification system (MACS) for children with cerebral palsy: scale development and evidence of validity and reliability, *Developmental Medicine and Child Neurology* 48(7):549–554.
4. M. Yeargin-Allsopp, K. V. N. Braun, N. S. Doernberg, R. E. Benedict, R. S. Kirby and M. S. Durkin. (2008). Prevalence of cerebral palsy in 8-year-old children in three areas of the United States in 2002: a multisite collaboration, *Pediatrics* 121(3):547–554.
5. C. M. Robertson, M. J. Watt and Y. Yasui. (2007). Changes in the prevalence of cerebral palsy for children born very prematurely within a population-based program over 30 years, *Journal of American Medical Association* 297(24):2733–2740.
6. M. Bax, M. Goldstein, P. Rosenbaum, A. Leviton and N. Paneth. (2005). Proposed definition and classification of cerebral palsy, *Developmental Medicine and Child Neurology* 47(8): 571–576.
7. C. P. Torfs, B. J. van den Berg, F. Oechsli and S. Cummins. (1990). Prenatal and perinatal factors in the etiology of cerebral palsy, *Journal of Pediatrics* 116(4):615–619.
8. T. M. O'Shea. (2002). Cerebral palsy in very preterm infants: new epidemiological insights, *Mental Retardation and Developmental Disabilities* 8(3):135–145.
9. A. F. Colver, M. Gibson, E. N. Hey, S. N. Jarvis, P. C. Mackie and S. Richmond. (2000). Increasing rates of cerebral palsy across the severity spectrum in north-east England 1964–1993, *Archives of Diseases in Childhood — Fetal and Neonatal Edition* 83(1):F7–F12.
10. B. Hagberg, G. Hagberg and R. Zetterstrom. (1989). Decreasing perinatal mortality-increase in cerebral palsy morbidity, *Acta Paediatrica* 78(5):664–670.
11. H.-F. Chen, L. Tickle-Degnen and S. A. Cermak. (2003). The treatment effectiveness of top-down approaches for children with developmental coordination disorder: a meta-analysis, *Journal of Occupational Therapy Association* 21:16–28.
12. J.-M. Belda-Lois, S. Mena-del Horno, I. Bermejo-Bosch, J. C. Moreno, J. L. Pons, D. Farina, M. Iosa, M. Molinari, F. Tamburella, A. Ramos, A. Caria, T. Solis-Escalante, C. Brunner and M. Rea. (2011). Rehabilitation of gait after stroke: a review towards a top-down approach, *Journal of Neuro Engineering and Rehabilitation* 8:1–19.
13. S. K. Agrawal, J. Kang, X. Chen, M. J. Kim, Y. Lee, S. W. Kong, H. Cho and G.-J. Park. (2016). Robot-enhanced mobility training of children with cerebral palsy: short-term and long-term pilot studies, *IEEE Systems Journal* 10(3):1098–1106.
14. S. M. Haley, W. J. Coster and R. M. Faas. (1991). A content validity study of the pediatric evaluation if disability inventory, *Pediatrics Physical Therapy* 3(3):177–184.
15. C. DeMatteo, M. Law, D. Russell, N. Pollock, P. Rosenbaum and S. Walter. (1993). The reliability and validity of the quality of upper extremity skills test, *Physical and Occupational Therapy Pediatrics* 13(2):1–18.
16. D. J. Russell, P. L. Rosenbaum, D. T. Cadman, C. Gowland, S. Hardy and S. Jarvis. (1989). The gross motor function measure: a means to evaluate the effects of physical therapy, *Developmental Medicine and Child Neurology* 31(3):341–352.
17. X. Chen, S. Liang, S. Dolph, C. B. Ragonesi, J. C. Galloway and S. K. Agrawal. (2010). Design of a novel mobility interface for infants on a mobile robot by kicking, *Journal of Medical Devices* 4(3):031006.
18. S. K. Agrawal, X. Chen, M. J. Kim, Y. M. Lee, H. P. Cho and G.-J. Park. (2012). Feasibility study of robot-enhanced mobility in children with cerebral palsy, in *Proceedings IEEE RAS and EMBS International Conference Biomedical Robotics and Biomechatronics (BioRob)*, Rome, Italy, pp. 1541–1548.

19. J. C. Galloway, J. C. Ryu and S. K. Agrawal. (2008). Babies driving robots: Self-generated mobility in very young infants, *Intelligent Service Robotics* 1(2):123–134.
20. A. Lynch, J. C. Ryu, S. K. Agrawal and J. C. Galloway. (2009). Power mobility training for a 7-month-old infant with spina bifida, *Pediatrics Physical Therapy* 21(4):123–134.
21. A. Lynch. (2009). *Robot Assisted Mobility for Very Young Infants.* PhD Thesis, University of Delaware, DE, USA (Spr.).
22. C. Ragonesi, X. Chen, S. K. Agrawal and J. C. Galloway. (2010). Power mobility and socialization in preschool: a case report on a child with cerebral palsy, *Pediatrics Physical Therapy* 22(3):322–329.
23. C. B. Ragonesi, X. Chen, S. K. Agrawal and J. C. Galloway. (2011). Power mobility and socialization in preschool: follow-up case study of a child with cerebral palsy, *Pediatrics Physical Therapy* 23(4):399–406.
24. C. T. Ramey and S. L. Ramey. (1998). Early intervention and early experience, *American Psychology* 53(2):109–120.
25. L. Fehr, W. E. Langbein and S. B. Skaar. (2000). Adequacy of power wheelchair control interfaces for persons with severe disabilities: a clinical survey, *Journal of Rehabilitation Research and Development* 37(3):353–360.
26. X. Chen, C. Ragonesi, J. C. Galloway and S. K. Agrawal. (2011). Training toddlers seated on mobile robots to drive indoors amidst obstacles, *IEEE Transaction on Neural Systems and Rehabilitation Engineering* 19(3):271–279.
27. S. K. Agrawal, X. Chen, C. Ragonesi and J. C. Galloway. (2011). Training toddlers seated on mobile robots to steer using force-feedback joystick, *IEEE Transaction on Haptics* 5(4):376–383.
28. J.-C. Latombe. (1991). *Robot Motion Planning.* Kluwer Academic Publishers.
29. X. Chen, C. Ragonesi, J. C. Galloway and S. K. Agrawal. (2014). Design of a robotic mobility system with a modular haptic feedback approach to promote socialization in children, *IEEE Transaction on Haptics* 7(2):131–139.
30. J. Kang, S. Logan, J. C. Galloway and S. K. Agrawal. (2014). A chase-game to teach children on a robot to follow moving objects, in *Proceedings IEEE International Conference on Robotics and Automation (ICRA),* Hong Kong, China, pp. 234–239.
31. F. M. Gresham. (1981). Social skills training with handicapped children: a review, *Review of Educational Research* 51(1):139—176.
32. D. Feitelson, S. Weintraub and O. Michaeli. (1972). Social interactions in heterogeneous preschools in Israel, *Child Development* 43:1249–1259.
33. G. Ladd and S. Asher. (1985). *Social Skill Training and Children's Peer Relations.* Handbook of social skills training and research, Wiley.
34. J. Mize and G. W. Ladd. (1990). A cognitive-social learning approach to social skill training with low-status preschool children, *Developmental Psychology* 26(3): 388–397.
35. G. W. Ladd and J. M. Price. (1987). Predicting children's social and school adjustment following the transition from preschool to kindergarten, *Child Development* 58(5):1168–1189.
36. D. Van Alstyne and L. A. Hattwick. (1939). A follow-up study of the behavior of nursery school children, *Child Development* 10(1):43–72.
37. M. F. Waldrop and C. F. Halverson Jr. (1975). Intensive and extensive peer behavior: longitudinal and cross-sectional analyses, *Child Development* 46(1):19–26.
38. N. Eisenberg-Berg, E. Cameron, K. Tryon and R. Dodez. (1981). Socialization of prosocial behavior in the preschool classroom, *Developmental Psychology* 17(6):773–782.
39. N. Jin, J. Kang and S. K. Agrawal. (2015). Design of a novel assist interface where toddlers walk with a mobile robot supported at the waist, in *Proceedings IEEE International Conference on Rehabilitation Robotics (ICORR)*, Singapore, pp. 577–582.

40. R. C. Simpson. (2005). Smart wheelchairs: a literature review, *Journal of Rehabilitation Research and Development* 42(4):423–436.
41. G. Lee, T. Ohnuma and N. Y. Chong. (2010). Design and control of JAIST active robotic walker, *Intelligent Service Robotics* 3(3):125–135.
42. D. Teft, P. Guerette and J. Furumasu. (1999). Cognitive predictors of young children's readiness for powered mobility, *Developmental Medicine and Child Neurology* 41(10): 665–760.
43. M. Peshkin, D. A. Brown, J. J. Santos-Munné, A. Makhlin, E. Lewis, J. E. Colgate, J. Patton and D. Schwandt. (2005). KineAssist: a robotic overground gait and balance training device, in *Proceedings IEEE International Conference on Rehabilitation Robotics (ICoRR)*, Chicago, USA, pp. 241–246.
44. K.-H. Seo and J.-J. Lee. (2009). The development of two mobile gait rehabilitation systems, *IEEE Transactions on Neural Systems and Rehabilitation Engineering* 17(2):156–166.
45. G. Bourhis and Y. Agostini. (1998). Man-machine cooperation for the control of an intelligent powered wheelchair, *Journal of Intelligent and Robotic Systems* 22:269–287.
46. L. Montesano, M. Diaz, S. Bhaskar and J. Minguez. (2010). Towards an intelligent wheelchair system for users with cerebral palsy, *IEEE Transactions on Neural Systems and Rehabilitation Engineering* 18(2):193–202.
47. R. S. Rao, K. Conn, S. H. Jung, J. Katupitiya, T. Kientz, V. Kumar, J. Ostrowski, S. Patel and C. J. Taylor. (2002). Human robot interaction: application to smart wheelchairs, in *Proceedings IEEE International Conference on Robotics and Automation (ICRA),* Washington, USA, pp. 3583–3588.
48. N. I. Katevas, N. M. Sgouros, S. G. Tzafestas, G. Papakonstantinou, P. Beattie, J. M. Bishop, P. Tsanakas and D. Koutsouris. (1997). The autonomous mobile robot SENARIO: a Sensor Aided Intelligent Navigation System for Powered Wheelchairs, *IEEE Robotics and Automation Magazine* 4(4):60–70.
49. K. Tanaka, K. Matsunaga and H. O. Wang. (2005). Electroencephalogram-based control of an electric wheelchair. *IEEE Transaction on Robotics* 21(4):762–766.
50. K. Choi, M. Sato and Y. Koike. (2006). A new, human-centered wheelchair system controlled by the EMG signal. *In Proceedings IEEE International Joint Conference on Neural Networks (IJCNN)*, Vancouver, Canada, pp. 4664–4671.

Chapter 10

FROM AUTISM SPECTRUM DISORDER TO CEREBRAL PALSY: STATE OF THE ART IN PEDIATRIC THERAPY ROBOTS

Ayanna Howard*, Yu-Ping Chen†, and Chung Hyuk Park‡

**School of Electrical and Computer Engineering*
Georgia Institute of Technology, Atlanta, GA, USA
†Department of Physical Therapy
Georgia State University, Atlanta, GA, USA
‡Department of Biomedical Engineering
The George Washington University, Washington, DC, USA

From autism spectrum disorder (ASD) to cerebral palsy (CP), there are many compelling reasons for utilizing robots in therapy and rehabilitation scenarios for children. These capabilities range from engaging children with pervasive development disorders to robot-assisted gait training for improving functional capabilities of children with motor impairments. Although there are some promising results found in the field, there are still a number of open-ended difficulties to resolve, especially in providing sufficient evidence of the long-term benefits of pediatric robots. In this chapter, we discuss the various robotic platforms that have been developed, challenges associated with their adoption, and outlooks for the future.

1. Introduction

There are an estimated 150 million children worldwide living with disabilities.[1] In the US, therapy interventions are provided for many of these children as an intervention mechanism to support the child's academic, developmental, and functional goals from birth and beyond. Many therapeutic interventions for children with disabilities focus on improving functional skills, behavioral skills, and cognitive abilities.[2,3] Physical, occupational, and speech-language therapies are typically classified as a rehabilitation service, whereas behavioral therapy

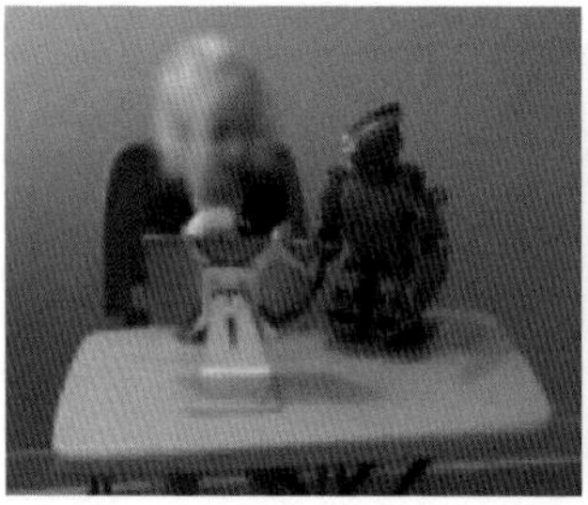
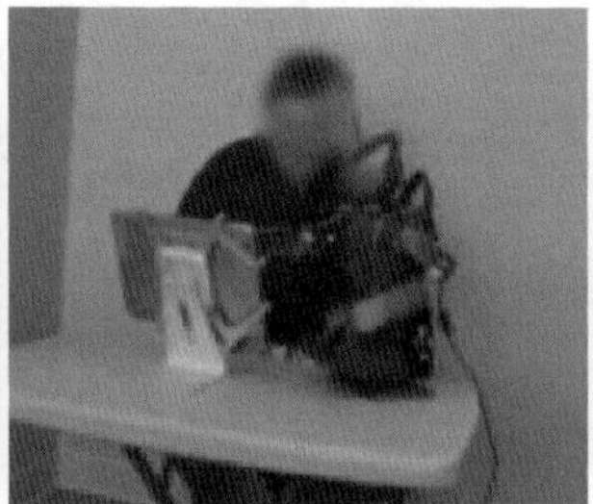
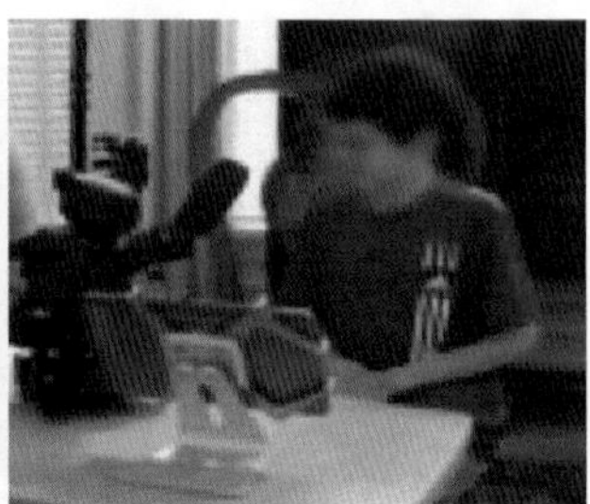

Figure 1. Various children with autism spectrum disorder interacting with a socially interactive robot used as an intervention tool for eliciting turn-taking behaviors.

or cognitive-behavior therapy is classified as a type of psychotherapy service. Although there is overlap between pediatric physical therapy and occupational therapy depending on the setting, pediatric physical therapy typically focuses on facilitating improvements in motor development and function, and improving strength and endurance. Occupational therapy, which is concerned with a child's ability to participate in activities of daily living (ADL), is used to help improve a child's motor, cognitive, sensory processing, communication, and play skills with the goal of enhancing their development and minimizing the potential for developmental delay.[4] For the purposes of this chapter, we will use these terms and roles interchangeably.

Due to a number of factors, such as costs and limits on time available for therapists to provide quality one-on-one therapy sessions, there has been interest in finding alternative ways to augment therapy sessions in between clinical visits. In recent years, the promotion of robotic platforms as an assistive therapeutic device has been gaining momentum. These pediatric robots for therapy and rehabilitation range from robotic exoskeletons for improving upper and/or lower extremity functions to socially interactive robots for behavioral therapy (Fig. 1). In this chapter, we discuss the various robotic platforms that have been developed, challenges associated with their adoption, and outlooks for the future.

2. Robots for Children with Physical Disabilities

There are many different types of physical disabilities that can affect a child, ranging from cerebral palsy (CP), spina bifida, to acquired brain and spinal injuries. A physical disability is any condition that prevents normal body movement and/or control, resulting in conditions such as delayed walking, impaired mobility and/or limitations in upper extremity function. CP is the most common motor disability in childhood and has a profound effect upon physical function.[5] The Centers for Disease Control and Prevention estimates that an average of 1 in 323 children in the US are diagnosed with CP. For such children, the goal of therapy, or rehabilitation, is to improve the child's functional skills in order to enhance their independence in ADL and quality of life. Irrespective of the type of therapy, repetitive, intensive, and task-specific movement, training is key to enhancing motor skill development. The success of this training though is strongly correlated with the ability to personalize the intervention to the specific needs of the child. As such, in recent years, alternative technologies, such as robotic rehabilitation platforms, have been developed and introduced into the clinical setting. In fact, recently, there has been a number of clinical assessments provided on the use of robots for interventions with children with CP.[6–8] In this chapter, we expand on these prior reviews, on their common findings and discuss the challenges and outlooks for the future.

2.1. *Robots for upper-extremity therapy for children with motor impairments*

About 50% of children diagnosed with CP have impaired upper extremity (UE) function (e.g. slow and jerky reaching patterns or inability to grasp and manipulate objects). Effective interventions to improve UE motor function in children with CP include repetitive practice of goal-directed tasks with sufficient visual and auditory feedback.[9,10] Recently, robotic therapy has been explored as a method for improving motor performance in children with CP.[8,11] Rehabilitation robots can provide "controlled, intensive task-specific training that is goal directed and cognitively engaging", a concept consistent with the current emphasis on therapeutic interventions for UE function in children with CP.[8,11] Robotic therapy is a relatively new method of treating children with CP. Only a few studies have examined the effects of different robotic systems on improving UE function, and those studies have a relatively small sample size. Although studies using these systems are still few, they are emerging and engineering research focused on rehabilitation robots for children with disabilities continues to grow.[12] In this section, we discuss the various robotic therapy platforms as applied to UE pediatric therapy interventions.

Cosmobot[13] is a commercially available telerehabilitation robot that was designed as an interaction tool to promote educational and therapeutic activities for children. The current configuration has been used in movement therapy in which a child's wrist and forearm gestures, identified by attached sensors, are correlated to CosmoBot movements in order to engage the child in the intervention protocol. A pilot study was conducted with three children with cerebral palsy, of ages 4–11, with UE limitations in Ref. [14]. Two of the three children showed improved functional task performance such as consistently maintaining wrist extension during a block-manipulation task and having sufficient forearm supination to open doorknobs. The therapists also noticed the longer engagement in using the robot platform than the conventional therapy session and were complimentary about the flexibility of ease of use. In a later study using randomized crossover design,[15] the CosmoBot system served as a therapist to provide instant automatic visual and/or auditory feedback to children with CP who do not reach pre-set task goals (e.g. a wrist extension angle of 45 degrees or forearm supination angle). Robotic therapy showed a trend toward improving supination angle and wrist extension angle more than conventional therapy.[15] One explanation is that the robot can be very persistent and accurate in detecting the level of resolution required to provide feedback, which a therapist would have difficulty naturally detecting through visual observation alone.

PlayROB[16] is a tele-operated 3-DOF robot with Cartesian configuration that was designed to allow children with physical disabilities the ability to manipulate LEGO bricks. The robot is controllable using a variety of access methods in order to engage the wide demographics of children with disabilities, including a 5-key input device, a joystick, and a head switch. The system was evaluated in a 2-year study involving five to ten children at three Austrian institutions beginning in 2004.[17] The authors state that the resulting data provide preliminary evidence that, through robot usage, there is a corresponding increase in children's endurance and concentration as well as spatial perception.

The Handy Robot[18] is a tele-operated 5-DOF arm and gripper designed to assist individuals with disabilities in the accomplishment of a variety of ADL, such as eating and drinking. Control of the robot is accomplished by a single-switch input device in which a sequential scan of an array of LEDs activates different robot behaviors. Although its primary use has been on assisted manipulation, it was deployed in a single subject study (Handy Artbox) to encourage independent thinking, practice and learn creativity, and help improve motor skills and spatial awareness. The Handy Artbox Robot was used over a 1-month period with a single child subject at a special school in Newcastle, Staffordshire in art and drawing play activities. Based on this preliminary case study, the authors concluded that the system could have the potential of being a useful aid for children with severe disabilities.

In Ref. [19], a 6-DOF arm for use in play-related tasks was presented, in which individual joints of a robot arm could be controlled by children through various control interfaces including large push buttons, keyboards, laser pointers, and head-controlled switches. A pilot study[20] was conducted that included 12 children with severe physical disabilities from 6 to 14 years of age for 12–15 sessions over a period of 4 weeks. Preliminary results indicated improvement in all children in operational control of the robot, which translated to varying levels of increase in functional skill development that carried over to tasks performed in the classroom environment.

Another prototype of a robotic arm was deployed by Howell and Hay (1989)[21] during an 18-month pilot project in the Columbus Public School with the intent of fostering cognitive, affective, and psychomotor development in students with severe orthopedic disabilities.[22] Based on results derived from seven children with severe orthopedic disabilities, issues involving accessibility, software design, and curriculum integration were identified.

Finally, the studies,[23–30] focused primarily on evaluating the clinical effectiveness of various contact robotic therapy systems for children with CP. The robotic devices used in these studies were mainly from two systems: InMotion2,[24,25,27,28] and NJIT-RAVR.[26,29,30] The InMotion2 and NJIT-RAVR systems are placed to be in contact with the user, i.e. the child's arm is physically in contact with the robotic arm, typically using an orthosis or brace to fix the participant's arm onto the robotic arm. The force of InMotion2 can be adjusted to either assist or resist the participant's arm while practicing reaching movements and can provide visual and auditory feedback. The NJIT-RAVR combines a robotic arm with virtual reality games to train children. Similar to InMotion2, the NJIT-RAVR system can provide either assistance or resistance to a child's upper arm movements. Generally, most of these studies involved 60-minute sessions but varied in weekly frequency and total intervention weeks. Clinical outcome measures used in these studies included kinematic variables, range of motion, muscle tone, muscle strength, and clinical assessment tools. Among the studies using InMotion2 system, after 6 or 8 weeks of robotic therapy, muscle tone decreased, kinematic variables (e.g. increased speed, decreased duration, improved smoothness) improved as did the outcome measures using clinical assessment tools.[24,25,27,28] Children in the three studies using NJIT-RAVR improved their reaching kinematics after a 3-week intervention; however, their improvements using clinical assessment tools such as the Melbourne were inconsistent.[26,29,30]

Robotic therapy to improve UE function in children with CP is still a novel approach, as such, evidence of its effectiveness is still minimal. The current research shows that robotic therapy has a potential benefit in improving UE function in children with CP, but it requires more robust research as the majority of the evidence comes from case series. One possible mechanism by which robotic therapy might work in the long term is the inherent capabilities robotic therapy has in providing an environment to encourage children to repeatedly practice their arm movements. Evidence shows that intensively repetitive task practice advances functional abilities for children with CP, especially when repeated practice occurs in near-natural contexts.[31] Thus, robotic therapy might be able to provide an intensive practice environment, which can subsequently provide a better transfer and generalization of function to daily life.

2.2. *Robots for lower-extremity therapy for children with motor impairments*

Many children who have neurological disorders, such as cerebral palsy, may not only have difficulties in UE movements but may have limitations in lower extremity movements as well. Such children may have difficulties in sitting, standing, and walking. Balance problems and/or stiffness in their gait can range from barely noticeable to the need for a wheelchair. As such, using lower-extremity (LE) robots provides another means of therapy for such children. The most widely used LE robots found in the pediatric domain are focused on imposing whole-body movements, e.g. robot-assisted locomotor trainers such as the Lokomat, which provides partial body-weight support during treadmill walking.[32] Another popular locomotor trainer system used in the pediatric domain is the Gait Trainer, which moves the legs via footplates to simulate a stance- and swing-phase.[33] Although robots for lower limb therapy endure the same fate as robots for UE therapy in terms of the lack of a sufficient evidence base, there is a growing body of clinical literature that shows robot-assisted gait training is a feasible and safe treatment method for children with neurological disorders, including children with CP.[34,35] In fact, a systematic review that included studies assessing the effectiveness of robot-assisted gait training for children was provided.[7,8,36] To counter some concerns with respect to findings that state task-specificity and goal-orientedness are crucial aspects in the treatment of children versus passive training for motor learning,[37] researchers have also begun to investigate the coupling of robotic lower-extremity systems with scenarios involving play. For example, in Ref. [38], a pilot study with 10 patients with different neurological gait disorders showed that virtual reality robot-assisted therapy approaches induced an immediate effect on motor output equivalent to conventional approaches with a human therapist. Another case study showed that using custom rehabilitation games with a robotic ankle orthosis for a child with cerebral palsy was clinically more beneficial than robotic rehabilitation in the absence of the video games.[39] Through these studies, the common theme found in this domain is that majority of children are highly motivated when using robot-assisted locomotor trainers, especially if used in conjunction with virtual-reality (VR) games for feedback and motivation (Fig. 2).[6,40,41] In fact, interactive games, irrespective of their delivery mechanism, have been shown to be a viable means of engaging children with CP in various therapy protocols (Fig. 3).[42,43]

Going beyond locomotor trainers, there has been some research efforts that have targeted training of individual joints, such as the ankle. In Ref. [44],

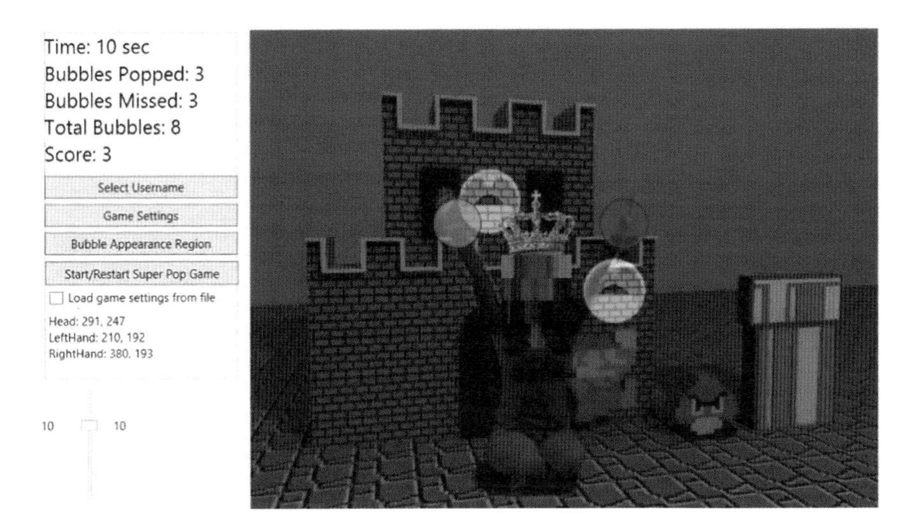

Figure 2. SuperPop VR game for interactive therapy.

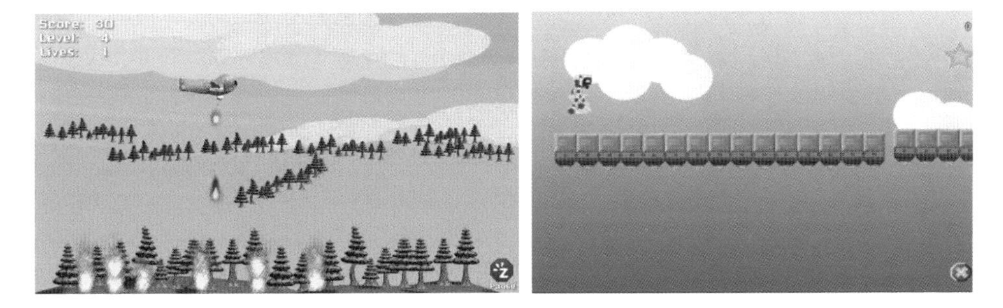

Figure 3. Interactive games used for therapy with children with disabilities.

the validity of an ankle robot for ankle rehabilitation, the pediAnklebot, was evaluated for adapting the difficulty of the therapy exercise with three children with disabilities over a 3-week period. Two of the children were diagnosed with CP and the other was diagnosed with a lesion of the common peroneal nerve. Although no direct conclusions were made with respect to therapeutic efficacy, the study implies that implicit motor learning is possible with the pediAnklebot. The Rutgers Ankle Rehabilitation System has also been adopted in a number of studies with children with CP. Systems such as the Rutgers Ankle provide assistance to the injured ankle during the exercise protocol. In Ref. [39], a study with a youth with CP using an augmented Rutgers Ankle showed that patient's motor functions and quality of life improved based on increased ankle strength and motor control after 36 rehabilitation sessions. Burdea *et al.*[45] provided further evidence by designing a similar study that included three children with CP. Also, another study[46] using a similar device with children with CP demonstrated improvements in joint biomechanical properties, motor control performance, and functional capability in balance and mobility.

Although this research area is still pushing to provide a sufficient evidence base for using robots for lower-extremity rehabilitation, this domain is the closest to validating its efficacy through clinical studies. General challenges identified by researchers in this area primarily discuss the need for creating new game designs in order to maintain participant's motivations, as well as the need for further research with a larger number of participants both in the clinical as well as in the home environment.

2.3. *Summary*

The state of the art in robotic systems for children with motor impairments show the potential of increasing function for children with CP. Robotic systems for enhancing motor skills has the potential of not only providing enhanced motivation through visual and auditory feedback, but can also be tailored to appropriate levels of task difficulty that correlates with the ability of the child. Based on motor learning theories, all of these components are essential when learning and improving a motor skill.[10,47] Thus, these components may be part of the underlying explanation for why robotic therapy works. Future research could explore the effect of each component (e.g. feedback, level of task difficulty) on the improvement of function to understand the mechanism behind use of robotic therapy. In addition, as shown in the work of Brown *et al.*,[48] using non-contact robots in intervention protocols with children with CP to provide corrective feedback for improving function might be another avenue of investigation for this domain (Fig. 4).

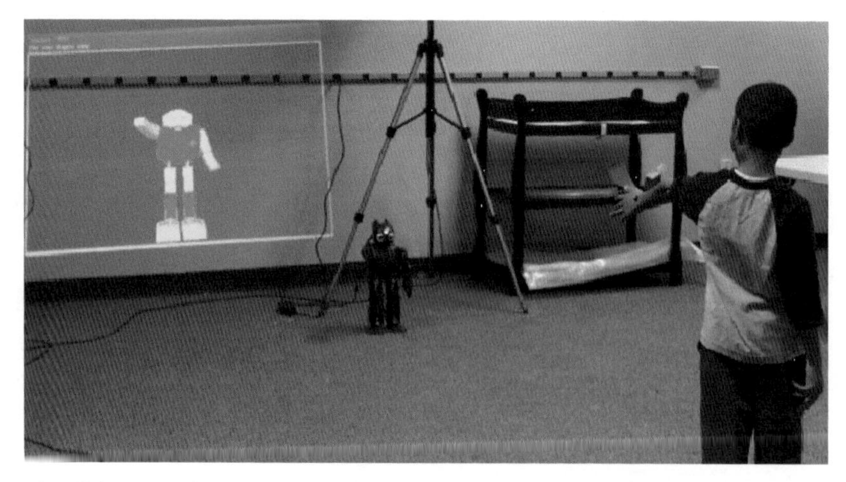

Figure 4. Using a social therapy robot to provide corrective feedback during an intervention protocol.

3. Robots for Children with Autism Spectrum Disorder

Recent estimates in the United States show that about one in six, or about 15%, of children aged 3–17 years have one or more developmental disabilities.[49] One of the largest demographics of children with developmental disabilities are children diagnosed with autism spectrum disorder (ASD). The Center for Disease Control and Prevention estimates that about 1 in 68 children in the US are diagnosed with ASD. ASD refers to a group of developmental disabilities that can cause significant social, communication and behavioral challenges.[50] Children with ASD often exhibit a diverse and multifaceted range of symptoms. The corresponding symptoms range from having difficulties in basic social skills and interaction, problems with speech and language comprehension, to exhibiting restrictedness, rigidity, and/or obsessiveness in their behaviors, activities, and interests. One of the most efficient ways of reducing the symptoms of children with ASD is through early cognitive-behavioral intervention programs. Since the most common symptoms in children with ASD largely manifests themselves as social deficits,[51] including lack of empathy, poor eye contact, and lack of awareness of others, various therapeutic interventions focus on improving a child's social interaction and communication skills. As such, behavioral therapy using robots has been of particular interest for several reasons. First, based on a clinical evidence base, it has been shown that children with ASD are capable of learning and altering their behaviors when teaching is provided using clear instructions, repetition and practice, and immediate reinforcement of correct responses. This use of repetition and feedback in teaching has been well established in a variety of prior and recent clinical studies.[52,53] Robots in their basic incarnation are well suited to provide consistent actions in a repetitive fashion.[48] It has also been shown that children with and without disabilities naturally find robots to be engaging and respond favorably to social interactions with them, even when the child typically does not respond socially with humans. Finally, it has been proposed that passive sensing used in conjunction with robots could help provide metrics of assessment for children with disabilities (Fig. 5).[54,55] Metrics associated with the child's movement parameters, gaze direction, and dialogue during interaction with the robot can provide outcome measures useful to the clinician for diagnosing and determining suitable intervention protocols for children with developmental disabilities. In fact, based on this interest in recent years, a number of critical reviews providing an in-depth assessment of the field have been conducted.[51,56–58] Using various inclusion criteria, these assessments discussed the different robot–child studies conducted, provided an overview of the robot platforms used, and reflected on the challenges for robot-assisted therapy for ASD. In this chapter, we summarize their common findings, challenges, and provide outlooks for the future.

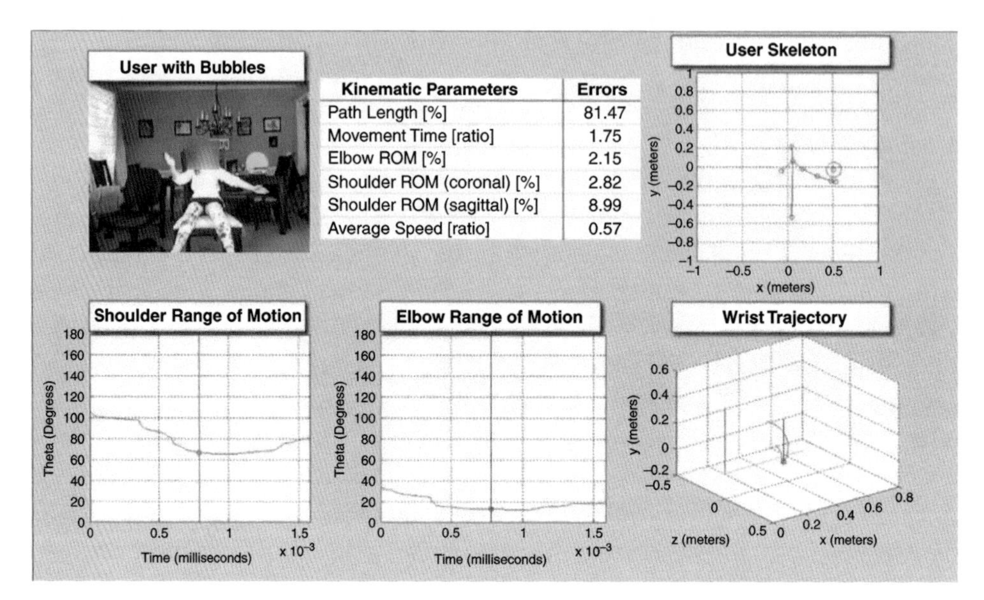

Figure 5. Kinematic metrics for assessment of a child's motor skill using passive vision-sensing methods.

3.1. *Robots for social-interactive therapy for children with ASD*

Pediatric therapy differs from adult therapy in that many times clinicians will incorporate therapy in play to provide an engaging and motivational intervention that may enhance the child's participation in the therapy session. No one will argue about how important play is during childhood. The role of play in the development of children has been extensively studied, and a large body of work exists to discuss the importance and nature of play in children. Piaget's book "Play, dreams, and imitation in childhood" is one of the earlier references showing the importance of play in the learning of cognitive, social, and physical skills.[59] With respect to robotics, most robots for behavioral therapy incorporate aspects of play, or engagement, into the protocol.

If we examine the common themes found in therapy robots for children with ASD, they can be classified into two primary roles: (1) the robot is designed to model, teach, and then have the child practice/repeat a behavioral skill or (2) the robot is designed to provide a prompt in order to elicit a response, followed by reinforcement (attention or praise) to commend the child on a positive response. The research associated with these various roles tend to result in five primary types of studies — exploring the response of children with ASD to a robotics platform; using a therapy robot for diagnosis, using a therapy robot to elicit specific behaviors in a child with ASD; using a therapy robot to model or teach a skill; using a robot to provide feedback and encouragement to a child with ASD.

If we examine the capabilities required to enable these studies, there are four primary technology capabilities (or challenges) that are required for a robot to be effective in behavioral therapy applications:

- Robot has the ability to imitate (or has the ability to learn to imitate) body movements, imitate tasks through interaction with the environment, and/or imitate facial expressions.
- Robot has the ability to exhibit or develop joint attention capabilities. Joint attention (also known as shared attention) is realized when one individual notifies another about an object by means of eye-gazing, pointing or other verbal or non-verbal indications.
- Robot has the ability to assess the child's behavioral state and engagement level in order to provide effective, and timely, responses during the intervention.
- Robot has the ability to be socially interactive, which involves incorporating aspects of emotional expressions, user engagement, and physical appearance.

While the following studies discussed in the subsequent section show preliminary evidence of the benefits of robots in behavioral therapy, current approaches typically restrict themselves to a Wizard-of-Oz (WOZ) setup.[51,60] WOZ setups involve a scenario in which the robot is remotely controlled by a human operator unbeknown to the child. In these types of scenarios, the human operator enables the required "technology" capabilities (such as commanding the robot such that it exhibits joint attention capabilities). The benefits of using a WOZ setup is that it allows for the evaluation of the behavioral intervention protocol in a repeatable manner without having to address the technological challenges associated with implementation. Unfortunately, the true benefit of therapy robots is in their potential of providing long-term, persistent, therapeutic interventions, which a WOZ setup cannot provide without the consistent presence of a therapist.

In the following section, we will provide an overview of the studies that focus specifically on behavior therapy, i.e. teaching or reinforcing specific behavioral skills. Other areas that might interest the reader are studies that explore the response of children with ASD to different robot platforms, using robots to provide feedback and encouragement to a child with ASD, or using robots to elicit, measure, and classify behavior for diagnostic purposes. The authors encourage the reader to refer other works[51,56–58] for examination of similar such studies.

3.2. *Robots that teach and/or reinforce specific behavioral skills*

One method for teaching and/or reinforcing positive behavioral skills in children with ASD is through the use of a method called prompting.[61] Prompting is defined as instructions, gestures, demonstrations, and/or touches that are instituted by a

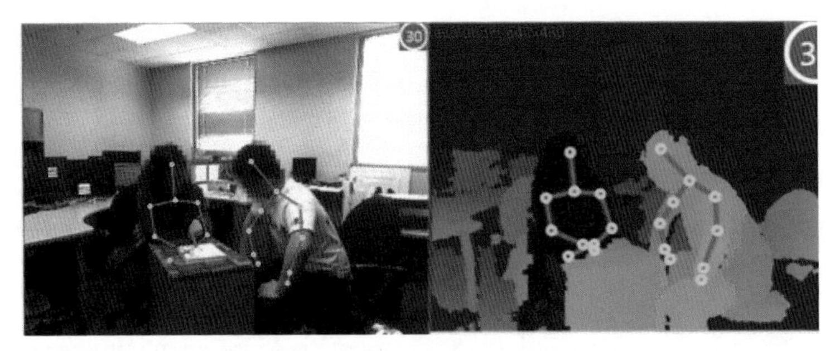

Figure 6. Prompting action (pointing and tapping) and object (a book) affordances modeled using an RGB-D video.

therapist (or parent) in order to increase the likelihood that a child will learn and respond over time with a correct response to a given task. For a therapist, prompting requires, first, determining what type of prompt to administer and then deciding on what type of information should be shared in order to emphasize the correct behavioral skill (Fig. 6).[62] There are various types of prompts that can be used, including verbal, textual, gestural, and physical prompts. Effective prompting involves systematically reducing the number of prompts as the child learns to complete the skill independently. Robots in the context of a therapeutic intervention can also provide prompts to teach and encourage positive behavioral skills. In this section, we review a few of the studies that examine the use of robots in this context of teaching and encouraging behavioral skills.

The Aurora project[63] is a research effort to aid in the therapy and education of children with ASD. The overall goal is to encourage the development of basic communication and social interaction skills. In one associated project, scientists utilized a humanoid robotic doll, named Robota,[64] in behavioral studies using imitation-based games to engage low-functioning children with ASD. Quantitative results from these longitudinal study show that Robota can successfully elicit imitative behaviors in children with ASD and qualitative results through video analysis reveal changes in various aspects of social interaction skills. In Ref. [65], a child-sized robot named KASPAR (Kinesics and Synchronisation in Personal Assistant Robotics) was designed as a social mediator and combined facial expressions and gestures to encourage children with ASD to interact with other people. The goal was to provide a mechanism for teaching social interaction skills through the use of joint attention and imitation. Published trials, which have included three children with ASD, have shown that these children could transfer imitation skills learned with the robot to other people.

Roball[66] is a spherical-shaped robot with intentional self-propelled movement designed to facilitate interaction with young children. Initial trials were performed to determine how effective Roball was for interacting with young children, with the goal of understanding the potential of such a robot to encourage skill acquisition (motor, language, intellectual, social, etc.) during the child-development process. Eight children between the ages of 12 and 18 months participated in this study. Although the quantitative results were somewhat inconclusive, anecdotal results describing successful interactions between children with ASD and other robot toys having the same underlying objective can be found in Ref. [67]. In general, it was found that, although many different robot designs had been evaluated over a number of years, children with ASD enjoy playing with mobile robotic toys and respond differently to them than to other people or non-interactive toys.

Another robotic platform that has been developed for therapy is Keepon, a robot designed to engage children with developmental disorders in playful interaction that was generally initiated and directed by the child (i.e. without any experimental setting or instruction). Several studies have been performed using the Keepon robot including a 2-year study involving 25 children with ASD and other developmental disorders from three age groups: 6–12 months, 12–24 months, and over 2 years old.[68] Longitudinal observations provided by the study discussed the emergence of various types of actions that arose in relation to the robot interaction.

De Silva *et al.*[69] performed a study in which it was shown that five individuals with ASD were able to follow social referencing behaviors made by a robot. Another study, which examined whether a robot can be used to elicit social behaviors that is transferrable between a child with ASD and another individual,[70] showed that two individuals with ASD continued to play a ball game with each other after learning from the robot. In Ref. [71], a humanoid robot was used to help four young children with ASD practice imitation behaviors in a series of intervention sessions using positive reinforcement.

Finally, in Scassellati *et al.*,[51] a review of robotics for use in autism research is presented, in which an overview is provided of the common design characteristics found in the field as well as the observations made on the types of evaluation studies performed in therapy-like settings using these robot platforms. An interesting observation is made that, despite productive collaborations between several robotics and clinical groups, the differences found between robotics research and clinical psychology often hinder the development of a common acceptable experimental standard. This is not only a common theme found in robotics-based autism research, but in most research involving robotics and pediatric therapy.

Since the publication of different reviews in Refs. [51, 56–58], there have been a few more recent studies published in the literature, but they still suffer from the same limitations as earlier studies. In a study with 11 children with

ASD,[72] researchers showed that children interacting with the humanoid robot Probo, who provided positive/negative feedback during task learning, elicited less stereotypical social behaviors than when compared with children interacting with adults alone. The study was inconclusive in showing increase in eliciting specific social behaviors. Another study in Ref. [73] used joint attention prompts in a protocol with six preschool children with ASD. Although they were examining the feasibility of using an adaptive algorithm for generating the prompts, their preliminary assessment showed that children with ASD required a higher level of prompting with the robot than with the human. Finally, researchers,[74] who presented a study for imitation skill training with robots and children with ASD and Ref. [75], which focused on training social skills in children with ASD using two different robot platforms, provided promising results associated with the integration of algorithms that help increase the autonomy of the robot interventions.

3.3. *Summary*

The preliminary results with respect to the use of therapy robots and children with ASD seem to indicate that an intervention designed using robots has some potential in eliciting specific behavioral skills in children. Most of the published studies on this topic though have small sample sizes and are constrained to a single therapeutic session. Thus, evaluation of the actual robot effectiveness is still limited. There is thus still a need for conducting studies that engage a larger sample size of children, over a longer period of time. In addition, few of the existing approaches in this domain involve robots that function autonomously. Most still use the Wizard-of-OZ technique and thus have no or little autonomy and, more importantly, are therefore not yet reducing the workload of the therapist. Recent work though has started to incorporate more autonomy into the robot, and examine its use in studies with children with ASD. For example, Park and Howard,[76] collected data during the robot–child interaction scenarios and used them to autonomously refine and adapt the intervention in a study with two children with ASD. Ge *et al.*[62] showed how spatio-temporal features could be identified during robot interventions to enable real-time prompting by the robot to engage the child in the intervention. In Refs. [77–79], the researchers discuss processes for integrating music in interactive therapy interventions using robots for children with ASD. This study provides therapy for emotional and social behaviors through multi-sensory interactions and aims to design individualized autonomy for increasing social and emotional interactions (Fig. 7). Although this work has not provided results from interaction with children as of yet, it provides a framework for enhancing the autonomy of therapy robots.

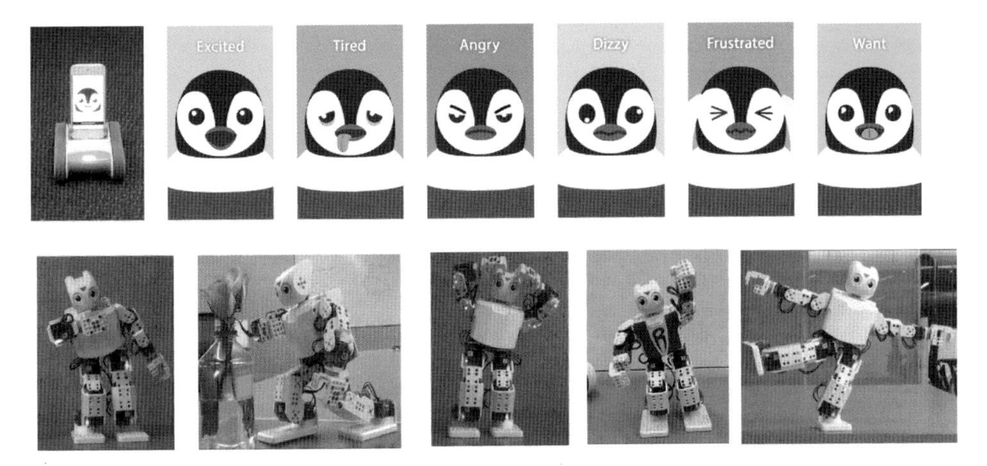

Figure 7. Interactive robots for emotional and social interaction for children with ASD.[79]

4. Discussion and Conclusion

From ASD to CP, there are many compelling reasons for utilizing robots in therapy and rehabilitation scenarios for children. These capabilities range from engaging children with pervasive development disorders to robot-assisted gait training for improving functional capabilities of children with motor impairments. Although much of the presented studies are encouraging, one of the primary shortcomings in this domain is the limited amount of quantitative results validating the long-term efficiency of utilizing robots in pediatric therapy settings. Many papers highlight case studies to show that children with disabilities will interact with the robots and, in many cases, achieve a therapeutic benefit. However, very few papers present quantitative results showing clear benefits to children derived from interaction with robots in long-term interventions across the different outcome measures. Additional substantial quantitative evidence as well as longitudinal studies that demonstrate the effectiveness of robots for therapeutic play are still necessary for validating the efficacy of these systems for pediatric therapy settings. Another shortcoming in this domain is the limited commercial availability and the high cost of the robots, which restrict the utilization for children in a home environment. An affordable, low-cost robotic platform that is commercially available outside of the research setting may enhance more clinical trials to further quantify the evidence.

The overall research presented herein brings up several interesting observations regarding the use of robotics in pediatric therapy. Many of the papers discussed the difficulty of performing studies involving children. Common reasons included distraction from outside stimuli, engaging with the robot outside of the designed protocol, and the wide variances found in children's abilities. Another observation is the stress that many of the researchers placed on robustness and iteration in design. For example, in many of the studies, especially in studies with children with ASD, children interacted with the robots in unexpected ways — ways that could potentially damage the robot if not designed in a robust fashion.

It is interesting to note that most of the above-discussed robots that could have manipulation capability (i.e. have a humanoid form with arms) did not physically manipulate objects. It appears that one area that has been largely unexplored in this domain is the utilization of autonomous robotic playmates capable of engaging children in shared manipulation-based play. Perhaps, this area as a research thread, along with an increased emphasis on providing quantitative results from child–robot interaction studies, emerges as the next step in the domain of robots for pediatric therapy. Despite these current limitations, as technology continues to advance and supporting components such as voice recognition, adaptive learning, improved sensor technology and actuation mechanisms, continue to evolve, robots will continue to have a role in providing therapy interventions for children.

Acknowledgments

This research was partially supported by the National Science Foundation under Grant No. 1208287.

References

1. UNESCO, Education for all 2000–2015: achievements and challenges (EFA Global Monitoring Report 2015), Paris, 2015, http://unesdoc.unesco.org/images/0023/002322/232205e.pdf
2. H.-W. Park and A. Howard. (2010). Case-based reasoning for planning turn-taking strategy with a therapeutic robot playmate, *IEEE International Conference on Biomedical Robotics and Biomechatronics 2010* (*BioRob'10*) 40–45.
3. L. Roberts, H.-W. Park and A. M. Howard. (2012). Robots and therapeutic play: evaluation of a wireless interface device for interaction with a robot playmate, *34th Annual International Conference of the Engineering in Medicine and Biology Society 2012* (*EMBC'12*) 6475–6478.
4. A. J. Punwar. (2000). Developmental disabilities practice, *Occupational Therapy: Principles and Practice* (Eds.: A. J. Punwar, S. M Peloquin). pp. 159–174.
5. M. W. Jones, E. Morgan, J. E. Shelton and C. Thorogood. (2007). Cerebral palsy: introduction and diagnosis (Part I), *Journal of Pediatric Health Care* 21(3):146–152.
6. Y. P. Chen, S. Lee and A. Howard. (2014). Effect of virtual reality on improving upper-extremity function in children with cerebral palsy: a meta-analysis, *Pediatric Physical Therapy* 26(3):289–300.
7. A. Meyer-Heim and H. J. van Hedel. (2013). Robot-assisted and computer-enhanced therapies for children with cerebral palsy: current state and clinical implementation, *Seminars in Pediatric Neurology* 20(2):139–145.
8. S. E. Fasoli, B. Ladenheim, J. Mast and H. I. Krebs. (2012). New horizons for robot-assisted therapy in pediatrics, *American Journal of Physical Medicine and Rehabilitation* 91(11 Suppl 3):S280–S289.

9. R. N. Boyd, M. E. Morris and H. K. Graham. (2001). Management of upper limb dysfunction in children with cerebral palsy: a systematic review, *European Journal of Neurology* 8(5): 150–166.
10. L. Sakzewski, J. Ziviani and R. Boyd. (2009). Systematic review and meta-analysis of therapeutic management of upper-limb dysfunction in children with congenital hemiplegia, *Pediatrics* 123(6):e1111–e1122.
11. H. I. Krebs, B. Ladenheim, C. Hippolyte, L. Monterroso and J. Mast. (2009). Robot-assisted task-specific training in cerebral palsy, *Developmental Medicine and Child Neurology* 51(4):140–145.
12. Y. P. Chen and A. Howard. (2014). Effects of robotic therapy on upper-extremity function in children with cerebral palsy: a systematic review, Developmental Neurorehabilitation, doi:10.3109/17518423.2014.899648.
13. C. Lathan, A. Brisben and C. Safos. (2005). CosmoBot levels the playing field for disabled children. *Interactions* 12(2):14–16.
14. K. C. Wood, C. E. Lathan and K. R. Kaufman. (2009). Development of an Interactive Upper Extremity Gestural Robotic Feedback System: From Bench to Reality, in *Annual International Conference of the IEEE in Engineering Medicine and Biology Society* 5973–5976.
15. K. C. Wood, C. E. Lathan and K. R. Kaufman. (2013). Feasibility of gestural feedback treatment for upper extremity movement in children with cerebral palsy. *IEEE Transactions on Neural Systems and Rehabilitation Engineering* 21(2):300–305.
16. G. Kronreif, B. Prazak, S. Mina, M. Kornfeld, M. Meindl and M. Fürst. (2005). Playrob-robot-assisted playing for children with severe physical disabilities. 9th *IEEE International Conference on Rehabilitation Robotics (ICORR 05)* 193–196.
17. G. Kronreif, B. Prazak, M. Kornfeld, A. Hochgatterer and M. Fuirst. (2007). Robot Assistant "PlayROB" — User Trials and Results. *16th IEEE International Conference on Robot & Human Interactive Communication 2007* (RO-MAN'07) 113–117.
18. M. Topping. (2002). An overview of the development of handy 1, a rehabilitation robot to assist the severely disabled. *Journal of Intelligent and Robotic Systems* 34(3):253–263.
19. A. M. Cook, M. Q. Meng, J. J. Gu and K. Howery. (2002). Development of a robotic device for facilitating learning by children who have severe disabilities. *Neural Systems and Rehabilitation Engineering* 10(3):178–187.
20. A. M. Cook, B. Bentz, N. Harbottle, C. Lynch and B. Miller. (2005). School-based use of a robotic arm system by children with disabilities. *Neural Systems and Rehabilitation Engineering* 13(4):452–460.
21. R. Howell and K. Hay. (1989). Software-based access and control of robotic manipulators for severely physically disabled students. *Journal of Artificial Intelligence in Education* 1(1): 53–72.
22. R. Howell. (1989). A Prototype Robotic Arm for Use by Severely Orthopedically Handicapped Students. Final Report. Ohio: 102.
23. K. Coleman Wood, C. E. Lathan and K. R. Kaufman. (2013). Feasibility of gestural feedback treatment for upper extremity movement in children with cerebral palsy. *IEEE Transactions on Neural Systems and Rehabilitation Engineering* 21(2):300–305.
24. L. Masia, F. Frascarelli, P. Morasso, G. Di Rosa, M. Petrarca, E. Castelli and P. Cappa. (2011). Reduced short term adaptation to robot generated dynamic environment in children affected by Cerebral Palsy. *Journal of NeuroEngineering and Rehabilitation* 8:28.
25. S. E. Fasoli, M. Fragala-Pinkham, R. Hughes, N. Hogan, H. I. Krebs and J. Stein. (2008). Upper limb robotic therapy for children with hemiplegia. *American Journal of Physical Medicine and Rehabilitation* 87(11):929–936.
26. G. G. Fluet, Q. Qiu, D. Kelly, H. D. Parikh, D. Ramirez, S. Saleh, *et al.* (2010). Interfacing a haptic robotic system with complex virtual environments to treat impaired upper extremity motor function in children with cerebral palsy. *Developmental Neurorehabilitation* 13(5):335–345.

27. F. Frascarelli, L. Masia, G. Di Rosa, P. Cappa, M. Petrarca, E. Castelli, *et al.* (2009). The impact of robotic rehabilitation in children with acquired or congenital movement disorders. *European Journal of Physical Rehabilitation and Medicine* 45(1):135–141.
28. H. I. Krebs, S. E. Fasoli, L. Dipietro, M. Fragala-Pinkham, R. Hughes, J. Stein, *et al.* (2012). Motor learning characterizes habilitation of children with hemiplegic cerebral palsy. *Neurorehabilitation and Neural Repair* 26(7):855–860.
29. Q. Qiu, S. Adamovich, S. Saleh, I. Lafond, A. S. Merians, G. G. Fluet. (2011). A comparison of motor adaptations to robotically facilitated upper extremity task practice demonstrated by children with cerebral palsy and adults with stroke. *IEEE International Conference of Rehabilitation Robotics* 5975431.
30. Q. Qiu, D. A. Ramirez, S. Saleh, G. G. Fluet, H. D. Parikh, D. Kelly, *et al.* (2009). The New Jersey Institute of Technology Robot-Assisted Virtual Rehabilitation (NJIT-RAVR) system for children with cerebral palsy: a feasibility study. *Journal of Neuroengineering and Rehabilitation* 6:40.
31. H. H. Huang, L. Fetters, J. Hale, A. McBride. (2009). Bound for success: a systematic review of constraint-induced movement therapy in children with cerebral palsy supports improved arm and hand use. *Physical Therapy* 89(11):1126–1141.
32. G. Colombo, M. Joerg, R. Schreier and V. Dietz. (2000). Treadmill training of paraplegic patients using a robotic orthosis, *Journal of Rehabilitation Research and Development* 37:693–700.
33. S. D. Hesse and D. Uhlenbrock. (2000). A mechanized gait trainer for restoration of gait, *Journal of Rehabilitation Research and Development* 37:701–708.
34. I. Borggraefe, J. Klaiber, T. Schuler, D. Warken, S. Schroeder, F. Heinen, *et al.* (2010). Safety of robotic-assisted treadmill therapy in children and adolescents with gait impairment: a bi-center survey. *Developmental Neurorehabilitation* 13(2):114–119.
35. A. Meyer-Heim, C. Ammann-Reiffer, A. Schmartz, J. Schaefer, F. H. Sennhauser, F. Heinen and I. Borggraefe. (2009). Improvement of walking abilities after robotic-assisted locomotion training in children with cerebral palsy. *Archives of Disease in Childhood* 94(8):615–620.
36. D. L. Damiano and S. L. DeJong. (2009). A systematic review of the effectiveness of treadmill training and body weight support in pediatric rehabilitation. *Journal of Neurologic Physical Therapy: JNPT* 33(1):27.
37. A. S. Papavasiliou. (2009). Management of motor problems in cerebral palsy: a critical update for the clinician. *European Journal of Paediatric Neurology* 13(5):387–396.
38. K. Brütsch, T. Schuler, A. Koenig, L. Zimmerli, S. Mérillat, L. Lünenburger and A. Meyer-Heim. (2010). Influence of virtual reality soccer game on walking performance in robotic assisted gait training for children. *Journal of Neuroengineering and Rehabilitation* 7(1):15.
39. D. Cioi, A. Kale, G. Burdea, J. Engsberg, S. Janes and S. Ross. (2011, June). Ankle control and strength training for children with cerebral palsy using the Rutgers Ankle CP, in *IEEE International Conference on Rehabilitation Robotics (ICORR)* 1–6.
40. T. Schuler, K. Brütsch, R. Müller, H. J. van Hedel and A. Meyer-Heim. (2011). Virtual realities as motivational tools for robotic assisted gait training in children: a surface electromyography study, *NeuroRehabilitation* 28:401–411.
41. K. Brütsch, A. Koenig, L. Zimmerli, S. Mérillat-Koeneke, R. Riener, L. Jäncke, H. J. van Hedel and A. Meyer-Heim. (2011). Virtual reality for enhancement of robot-assisted gait training in children with central gait disorders, *Journal of Rehabilitation Medicine* 43:493–499.
42. Y. P. Chen, S. García-Vergara and A. Howard. (2015). Effect of a home-based virtual reality intervention for children with cerebral palsy using SuperPop VR™ evaluation metrics — a feasibility study, *Rehabilitation Research and Practice* 2015:9 pages.

43. A. Howard and J. MacCalla. (2014). Pilot study to evaluate the effectiveness of a mobile-based therapy and educational app for children, *ACM Sensys Workshop on Mobile Medical Applications — Design and Development*. Memphis, TN.
44. K. P. Michmizos, S. Rossi, E. Castelli, P. Cappa and H. I. Krebs. (2015). Robot-aided neurorehabilitation: a pediatric robot for ankle rehabilitation. *IEEE Transactions on Neural Systems and Rehabilitation Engineering* 23(6):1056–1067.
45. G. C. Burdea, D. Cioi, A. Kale, W. E. Janes, S. A. Ross and J. R. Engsberg. (2013). Robotics and gaming to improve ankle strength, motor control, and function in children with cerebral palsy — a case study series. *IEEE Transactions on Neural Systems and Rehabilitation Engineering* 21(2):165–173.
46. Y. N. Wu, M. Hwang, Y. P. Ren, D. Gaebler-Spira and L. Q. Zhang. (2011). Combined passive stretching and active movement rehabilitation of lower-limb impairments in children with cerebral palsy using a portable robot, *Neurorehabil Neural Repair* 25(4): 378–85.
47. I. Novak, S. McIntyre, C. Morgan, L. Campbell, L. Dark, N. Morton, *et al.* (2013). A systematic review of interventions for children with cerebral palsy: state of the evidence, *Developmental Medicine and Child Neurology* 55(10):885–910.
48. L. Brown, S. Garcia-Vergas and A. Howard. (2015). Evaluating the effect of robot feedback on motor skill performance in therapy games. *IEEE International Conference on Systems, Man, and Cybernetics*, Hong Kong.
49. C. A. Boyle, S. Boulet, L. Schieve, R. A. Cohen, S. J. Blumberg, M Yeargin-Allsopp, S. Visser and M. D. Kogan. (2011). Trends in the prevalence of developmental disabilities in US children, 1997–2008. *Pediatrics* 127(6):1034–1042.
50. Autism Society of America, Retrieved Jan 1, 2016, from http://autism-society.org
51. B. Scassellati, H. Admoni and M. Matarić. (2012). Robots for use in autism research, *Annual Review of Biomedical Engineering*, 14:275–294.
52. O. I. Lovaas. (1981). *Teaching Developmentally Disabled Children: the ME Book*. Baltimore, MD: University Park Press.
53. J. L. Crockett, R. K. Fleming, K. J. Doepke and J. S. Stevens. (2005). Parent training: acquisition and generalization of discrete trials teaching skills with parents of children with autism, *Research in Developmental Disabilities* 28(1):23–36.
54. D. Brooks and A. Howard. (2012). Quantifying upper-arm rehabilitation metrics for children through interaction with a humanoid robot, *Applied Bionics and Biomechanics* 9(2): 157–172.
55. S. Garcia-Vergas, M. Serrano, Y. P. Chen and A. Howard. (2014). Developing a baseline for upper-body motor skill assessment using a robotic kinematic model, *IEEE International Symposium on Robot and Human Interactive Communication* (*RO-MAN*), Edinburgh, Scotland, August.
56. S. Boucenna, A. Narzisi, E. Tilmont, F. Muratori, G. Pioggia, D. Cohen and M. Chetouani. (2014). Interactive technologies for autistic children: a review, *Cognitive Computation* 6(4):722–740.
57. S. Thill, C. Pop, T. Belpaeme, T. Ziemke and B. Vanderborght. (2012). Robot-assisted therapy for autism spectrum disorders with (partially) autonomous control: challenges and outlook, *Paladyn Journal of Behavioral Robotics* 3(4):209–217.
58. J. Diehl, L. Schmitt, M. Villano and C. Crowell. (2012). The clinical use of robots for individuals with autism spectrum disorders: a critical review, *Research in Autism Spectrum Disorders* 6(1): 249–262.
59. J. Piaget. (1951). *Play, Dreams and Imitation in Childhood*. London: Routledge and Kegan Paul Ltd.

60. L. D. Riek. (2012). Wizard of Oz studies in HRI: a systematic review and new reporting guidelines, *Journal of Human Robot Interaction* 1(1):119–136.
61. A. Fitzer and P. Sturmey. (2007). Autism spectrum disorders: applied behavior analysis, evidence, and practice, in *Behavior Analytic Teaching Procedures: Basic Principles, Empirically Derived Practices*, W. H. Ahearn, W. V. Dube, R. MacDonald and R. B. Graff (Eds.), Austin, TX, pp. 31–72.
62. B. Ge, H. W. Park and A. Howard. (2015). Learning spatio-temporal features of prompting during robot intervention for children with autism, *IEEE International Conference on Robotics and Automation* (*ICRA*). Seattle, WA.
63. K. Dautenhahn and I. Werry. (2004). Towards interactive robots in autism therapy, *Pragmatics and Cognition* 12(1):1–35.
64. A. Billard, B. Robins, K. Dautenhahn and J. Nadel. (2007). Building robota, a mini-humanoid robot for the rehabilitation of children with autism, *RESNA Assistive Technology Journal* 19(1):37–49.
65. J. B. Robins, K. Dautenhahn and P. Dickerson. (2009). From isolation to communication: a case study evaluation of robot assisted play for children with autism with a minimally expressive humanoid robot. *Proceedings Second International Conference Advances in CHI* (ACHI'09), 205–211.
66. F. Michaud, J. Laplante, H. Larouche, A. Duquette, S. Caron, D. Letourneau and P. Masson. (2005). Autonomous spherical mobile robot to study child development, *IEEE Transactions on Systems, Man, and Cybernetics* 35(4):471–480.
67. F. Michaud and C. Théberge-Turmel. (2002). Mobile robotic toys and autism. *Socially Intelligent Agents — Creating Relationships*, Kluwer Academic Publishers, pp. 125–132.
68. H. Kozima and C. Nakagawa. (2006). Social robots for children: practice in communication-care. 9th *IEEE International Workshop on Advanced Motion Control* 768–773.
69. P. R. S. De Silva, K. Tadano, A. Saito, S. G. Lambacher and M. Higashi. (2009). Therapeutic-assisted robot for children with autism, *IEEE/RSJ International Conference on Intelligent Robots and Systems*. New York, NY: ACM Press, pp. 3561–3567.
70. S. Costa, C. Santos, F. Soares, M. Ferreira and F. Moreira. (2010). Promoting interaction amongst autistic adolescents using robots, in *IEEE Annual International Conference of Engineering in Medicine and Biology Society (EMBC)*, 3856–3859.
71. A. Duquette, F. Michaud and H. Mercier. (2008). Exploring the use of a mobile robot as an imitation agent with children with low-functioning autism, *Autonomous Robots* 24: 147–157.
72. C. A. Pop, S. Pintea, B. Vanderborght and D. O. David. (2014). Enhancing play skills, engagement and social skills in a play task in ASD children by using robot-based interventions, *A Pilot Study. Interaction Studies* 15(2):292–320.
73. E. Bekele, J. A. Crittendon, A. Swanson, N. Sarkar and Z. E. Warren. (2013). Pilot clinical application of an adaptive robotic system for young children with autism, *Autism* 18(5): 598–608.
74. Z. Zheng, E. M. Young, A. Swanson, A. Weitlauf, W. Zachary and N. Sarkar. (2015). Robot-mediated imitation skill training for children with autism. *IEEE Transactions on Neural Systems and Rehabilitation Engineering*, 682–691.
75. S. S. Yun, H. Kim, J. Choi and S. K. Park. (2016). A robot-assisted behavioral intervention system for children with autism spectrum disorders. *Robotics and Autonomous Systems* 76:58–67.
76. H. W. Park and A. Howard. (2014). Engaging Children in Social Behavior: interaction with a robot playmate through tablet based apps. *Rehabilitation Engineering and Technology Society of North America (RESNA) Annual Conference*. Indianapolis, IN.

77. C. H. Park, N. Pai, J. Bakthavatchalam, Y. Li, M. Jeon and A. Howard. (2015). Robotic framework for music-based emotional and social engagement with children with autism, *AAAI-15 Workshop on Artificial Intelligence Applied to Assistive Technologies and Smart Environments*. Austin, TX.
78. C. H. Park, M. Jeon and A. Howard. (2015). Robotic Framework with Multi-Modal Perception for Physio-Musical Interactive Therapy for Children with Autism, *5th International Conference on Development and Learning and on Epigenetic Robotics*. Providence, RI.
79. C. H. Park, M. Jeon and A. Howard. (2016). Interactive Robotic Framework for Multi-sensory Therapy for Children with Autism Spectrum Disorder, *ACM/IEEE International Conference on Human-Robot Interaction (HRI)*. New Zealand.

INDEX

L

M

N

O

P